ACLS: Rapid Review and Case Scenarios

ACLS: Rapid Review and Case Scenarios

Ken Grauer, MD, F.A.A.F.P.
Professor
Department of Community Health and Family Medicine
Assistant Director, Family Practice Residency Program
College of Medicine, University of Florida, Gainesville
ACLS Affiliate Faculty for Florida

Dr. Grauer can be reached by:

Mail- Dr. Ken Grauer
Family Practice Residency Program
625 S.W. 4th Avenue
P.O. Box 147001
Gainesville, Florida 32614

Fax- (352) 332-9154
e-Mail- grauer@fpmg.health.ufl.edu
Home page-http://www.med.ufl.edu/chfm/people/grauer/

Daniel Cavallaro, REMT-P
Senior Medical Officer for Lifeguard Air Ambulance
President of the Center for Medical Research, Tampa Florida
Past ACLS National Affiliate Faculty

Dan Cavallaro can be reached by:

e-Mail- danlcav@aol.com

Mosby Lifeline

St. Louis Baltimore Boston Carlsbad Chicago Naples New York Philadelphia Portland
London Madrid Mexico City Singapore Sydney Tokyo Toronto Wiesbaden

Mosby Lifeline
Dedicated to Publishing Excellence

Vice-President and Publisher: David Dusthimer
Editor-in-Chief: Claire Merrick
Managing Editor: Julie Scardiglia
Senior Assistant Editor: Kay Beard
Project Manager: Chris Baumle
Production Editor: Dave Orzechowski
Book Design: E.L. Graphics
Cover Design: Nancy McDonald

Printed in the United States of America
Composition by: E.L. Graphics
Printing/binding by: Courier Kendallville, Inc.

Mosby-Year Book, Inc.
11830 Westline Industrial Drive
St. Louis, Missouri 63146

International Standard Book Number 0-8151-3623-4

98 99 00/ 9 8 7 6 5 4 3

PREFACE to ACLS: Rapid Review and Case Scenarios

Since publication of our two volume ACLS set (*ACLS: Certification Preparation*- Volume I; and *ACLS: A Comprehensive Review*- Volume II) nearly four years ago, numerous advances have been made in the field of cardiopulmonary resuscitation and emergency cardiac care. In response to these advances, and especially in response to recent revision of the ACLS course format by the American Heart Association, the need was felt to revise this book.

In the interest of facilitating preparation for the ACLS Provider Course according to the new course format, we have completely rewritten and consolidated the content contained within our previous edition. While still maintaining our thought provoking and reader-friendly style, we have enhanced our consistency with AHA recommendations by frequent reference throughout our book to page numbers in the 1994 American Heart Association ACLS Textbook on which relevant discussion of the topic can be found. In this way, the reader can rapidly access detailed information on specific AHA Guidelines for the topic at hand.

How To Use This Book

This new edition of our book contains four basic chapters. Key points of interest to be found within each chapter include the following:

Chapter 1: Overall Approach to Cardiopulmonary Arrest: *Algorithms for Treatment*. The essence of the ACLS course is contained in this first chapter. Included within is general discussion of key concepts involved with assessment of the patient in cardiopulmonary arrest, application of the *Universal Algorithm* for adult emergency cardiac care, and guidelines for use of the *Automatic External Defibrillator* (**Section 1A**). Subsequent sections in this chapter specifically address each of the major algorithms for treatment- including *V Fib/Pulseless VT* (**Section 1B**); the patient with *Tachycardia* (**Section 1C**); and *Bradyarrhythmias* including *PEA/Asystole* (**Section 1D**). Detailed discussion of each of these major rhythms stresses a practical approach to management with close correlation (and frequent page reference) to the AHA ACLS Textbook.

Chapter 2: Essential Drugs and Treatment Modalities. Extensive coverage in an easy-to-use format is provided in this chapter for the major drugs and treatment modalities that are used in cardiopulmonary resuscitation and emergency cardiac care. The chapter begins in **Section 2A** with focused discussion of general principles for drug delivery (which IV route is best; when and how to use endotracheal drug administration, etc.)- and brief review of how to apply clinically our understanding of the role of the autonomic nervous system (alpha- and beta-adrenergic receptors; selection of a pressor agent; determinants of cardiac performance). There follows specific sections detailing the dosing and clinical use of each of the major drugs. *KEY Drugs* used in ACLS are detailed in **Section 2B** (including Epinephrine, Lidocaine, Atropine, Dopamine, Adenosine, Magnesium, and others). *Additional Drugs* used in emergency cardiac care are covered in **Section 2E** (including Digoxin, Esmolol, Amiodarone, and Aminophylline). *Deemphasized Drugs* (i.e., Sodium Bicarbonate, Calcium Chloride, and Isoproterenol) are described in **Section 2F**, with focus on the remaining appropriate indications for use of these agents. An easily mastered approach for *Simplified Calculation of IV Infusions* is presented in **Section 2C**, that should readily allow even the most novice of caregivers to appropriately formulate IV infusions for the most commonly used drugs.

Although the focus of this book is clearly on management of adult-related emergency cardiac care- overview principles of *Pediatric Resuscitation* are briefly discussed in **Section 2G**, with specific recommendations (in tabular form) for drug dosing of pediatric patients of various body weights.

Finally, the major *Diagnostic/Therapeutic Modalities* involved with ACLS and emergency cardiac care are discussed in **Section 2D**- including defibrillation, synchronized cardioversion, the precordial thump and cough version, pacemaker therapy, and clinical use of the various vagal maneuvers.

Chapter 3: Key Clinical Issues in ACLS/Airway Management. This section serves as a targeted review of the *KEY* concepts needed for management of cardiopulmonary arrest (and for successfully completing the ACLS course). Key clinical issues are presented in a practical format- always with close correlation (and specific page reference) to the AHA ACLS Textbook. Examples of issues addressed in **Section 3A** include:

- *What if V Fib is refractory?*
- *When might use of high-dose Epinephrine be appropriate?*
- *How to evaluate (and treat) the patient with a wide-complex tachycardia?*
- *What if the rhythm is torsade de pointes?*
- *How to approach the patient with hypotension?*
- *What if the monitor shows a flat line rhythm?*

- and many more relevant issues in cardiopulmonary resuscitation.

Section 3B concludes this informative chapter with a detailed practical (and fully illustrated) review of *Airway Management and Ventilation-* including a user-friendly clinically oriented algorithmic approach to the patient with respiratory difficulty or arrest.

Chapter 4: Putting It All Together: *Practice for MEGA Code*. This expanded feature has traditionally been the most popular section of our book. Simulated case scenarios that closely correlate with those that are used in the new course format are presented. *The reader is then put to the test.* A brief scenario and rhythm strip is shown- after which you are asked to detail your approach to management. Fully explained answers follow each management step- with important *Teaching Points* integrated along the way for full comprehensiveness. Reference is made throughout to concepts discussed earlier in our book- as well as to specific pages in the AHA ACLS Textbook. This chapter truly *"puts it all together"* and prepares the reader for the situation at hand.

Appendix: Value Added Drug Table. This new feature facilitates ready recall of the essentials for use of the 20 most important drugs in ACLS. A separate page is devoted to each agent that details dosing and highlights key features of the drug.

Regardless of one's clinical background and training, there should be more than enough material in this book to confidently allow successful completion of the ACLS course according to the new course format- as well as providing a ready reference source for daily use in the management of emergency cardiac care situations.

For the Reader Who Wants More . . . .

In 1993 we published the second edition of our flash cards in conjunction with our two-volume ACLS book (*ACLS: Mega Code Review/Study Cards*- Mosby Lifeline, St. Louis). The aim of these cards was twofold:

i) To provide another type of *study aid* that might supplement the 1993 edition of our book.

ii) To provide an additional method of preparing for the challenging MEGA CODE station that would simulate testing conditions, but at the same time allow the student to individualize their preparation- *and proceed at their own pace.*

The first goal was easily accomplished by posing a clinical question or simply listing a drug or arrhythmia on the front of a card, and providing explanatory discussion on the back. The latter goal was attained by incorporating a portion of the cards into simulated code scenarios in which the front of a card presented the patient's rhythm and clinical status, and the back of that card indicated our suggested approach to treatment.

We have completely revised and rewritten the cards in this study aid (***ACLS: Rapid Study Card Review****- Third Edition,* Mosby Lifeline, 1996). In addition to being closely integrated to material contained in our new book, the 1996 edition of our *Study Cards* is specifically designed for the new course format. As in our new book, frequent reference is again made to page numbers in the AHA ACLS Textbook indicating where relevant discussion of each topic addressed can be found. Utilization of these ***Study Cards*** therefore provides an additional, time-effective way of reviewing the essentials of cardiopulmonary resuscitation that *complements* the content in our new book, facilitating preparation for the AHA ACLS Provider Course according to the new course format.

Still to come within the next few months- revision of the 1994 edition of our ***ACLS Pocket Reference****-* and publication of a new book, ***Arrhythmia Interpretation: ACLS Preparation & Clinical Approach.***

We are excited about these new publications. We sincerely hope you enjoy reading our ACLS material, and find it clinically useful. It was written with YOU- the reader- in mind.

AUTHOR's NOTE

Our recommendations for management in the key algorithms of cardiopulmonary resuscitation are generally *very* consistent with those put forth by the American Heart Association. However, we do not always adhere strictly to their guidelines. In cases where we differ, we clearly state the rationale for our views, and openly discuss any points of contention.

We do *not* feel such differences of opinion represent a departure from the objectives of the American Heart Association, since this agency freely acknowledges that their algorithms for treatment are not all inclusive. On the contrary, we firmly believe that acknowledging areas of controversy and presenting potential alternative approaches for selected situations is beneficial and may lead to improved emergency care. Our book is therefore aimed to *complement* the American Heart Association ACLS Textbook. We hope combined use will not only prove insightful, but also add an extra dimension to the learning experience of the reader.

To my wife,

Anita Wofford-Grauer

for her ever present love and support while I wrote this book.

About the Authors:

KEN GRAUER, M.D., F.A.A.F.P., is a professor in the Department of Community Health and Family Medicine, College of Medicine, University of Florida, and assistant director of the Family Practice Residency Program in Gainesville. He is board certified in family practice, and is ACLS Affiliate Faculty for Florida (and former National ACLS Affiliate Faculty). He is also a former contributor to the American Heart Association ACLS Textbook who served on the Task Force for ACLS Post-Testing. In addition to this book, Dr. Grauer is the principal or sole author of the following books and teaching resources: *ACLS: Mega Code Review/Study Cards* (Third edition, Mosby Lifeline- *in press*), *1996 ACLS Pocket Reference* (Third edition, Mosby Lifeline- *in press*), *A Practical Guide to ECG Interpretation* (Mosby-Year Book, 1992), *ECG Interpretation Pocket Reference* (Mosby-Year Book, 1992), *Clinical Electrocardiography: A Primary Care Approach* (Second edition-Blackwell Scientific Publications, 1992), and *ACLS Teaching Kit: An Instructor's Resource* (Mosby-Year Book, 1990). His ACLS materials are featured on the Mosby Lifeline CD-ROM products, *ACLS Infobase: The ACLS Omnibus Resource*, and *ACLS Review* (User's Manual and Instructor's Version). He has lectured widely and is primary author of numerous articles on cardiology for family physicians, including several "ECG of the Month" columns that have been published for more than a decade in various primary care journals. He also has served on the Editorial Board of the following journals: Family Practice Recertification, Procedural Skills and Office Technology, and Internal Medicine Alert, Emergency Medicine Alert, and ACLS Alert.

Dr. Grauer has become well known throughout Florida and nationally for teaching ACLS courses and ECG/arrhythmia workshops to diverse medical audiences including nurses, paramedics, medical students, physicians in training, and physicians in practice. His trademark has always been the ability to simplify otherwise complicated topics into a concise, practical, and easy-to-remember format.

DAN CAVALLARO, REMT-P, is senior medical officer for Lifeguard Air Ambulance, and President of the Center for Medical Research in Tampa, Florida. He is a former ACLS National Affiliate Faculty member, and a former contributor to the American Heart Association ACLS Textbook who served on the Task Force for ACLS Post-Testing. In addition to coauthoring this book, he has coauthored the following teaching resources: *ACLS: Mega Code Review/Study Cards* (Third edition, Mosby Lifeline- *in press*), *ACLS Pocket Reference* (Third edition, Mosby Lifeline- *in press*), *ACLS Teaching Kit: An Instructor's Resource* (Mosby-Year Book, 1990), and the Mosby Lifeline ACLS CD-ROM products. Clinically, he has worked in the critical care, emergency medical, and surgical fields for the past 20 years. During that time, he has also been extremely active developing and participating in courses on pre-hospital care and emergency medicine, and has taught in well over 200 ACLS courses.

Acknowledgments:

I am indebted to the following people whose contributions were instrumental to the preparation of this book:

Dan Cavallaro, whose expertise has continued to enrich my knowledge over the years, and whose friendship and enthusiasm kept me going during the seemingly "endless" period it took to complete the writing (and constant rewriting) of this book. His contributions to all of our ACLS materials have truly been *invaluable* to me.

John Gums, Pharm D, for his assistance in reviewing those aspects of our ACLS materials that relate to cardiovascular pharmacology. Nowhere could there possibly be another Pharm D the equal of John, whose encyclopedic, photographic memory and unfathomable clinical insight become the instant envy of all who are lucky enough to work with him. And he keeps getting better . . . .

Julie Scardiglia- formerly of Mosby Lifeline- who during her years with the company was "the force" that enabled the writing of this book. Her endless patience, ever encouraging enthusiasm, and unwavering support throughout the entire process meant more to us than words can say. May the success that Julie so richly deserves flow forever forth in her new life.

Kay Beard- for her superb assistance to Julie Scardiglia, and now for carrying the task through to its completion. We are truly indebted to Kay!

Claire Merrick- for her support and encouragement from above that helped make this project possible. Thank you Claire!

Rick Griffin, **Stephanie Ivey**, and **Paul Ivey**- for their friendship and support at the best (!) restaurant in Gainesville- ***Ivey's Grill***- which provided me with the peaceful, pleasant, and inspiring environment for writing (and forever rewriting), and reviewing much of this text (and for the tofu and fruit to keep my coronaries clean). Thanks also to my favorite waiters and waitresses at Ivey's, who truly make up the *best* and friendliest staff anywhere!

Maria Alvarez and **Ray Parris**- those best teachers (and great friends) at the ***Maria Alvarez Imperial Dance Studio***, who have forever been instrumental in helping me to maintain my sanity (and still have fun by dancing) for much of the time I was working on this book.

Judy Niverson- for her friendship and individual attention and support that helped to further improve our dancing (and maintain my sanity).

Barney Marriott, MD, and **William P. Nelson,** MD- *for teaching me more about ECGs than I can ever say.* I will always remember their teachings!

The Cardiology staff at Alachua General Hospital (Burt Silverstein, MD; Steve Roark, MD; Mike Dillon, MD; and Marshall Decker, MD)- for their tremendous support of me, and for teaching cardiology to our residents.

To *all* of the other excellent cardiologists who have inspired me, and from whom I have learned.

To *all* those who have knowingly (and unknowingly) provided me with tracings and other nuggets of information through the years.

And last but far from least- to *all* the nurses, medical students, residents, and other paramedical personnel who through the years have allowed me to learn by teaching them.

Ken Grauer, MD

Contents

Chapter 1: Overall Approach to Management of Cardiopulmonary Arrest: *Algorithms for Treatment*

Section A: *Overview of Cardiac Arrest*

Section B: *V Fib/Pulseless VT*

Section C: *Tachycardia*

Section D: *Bradyarrhythmias (including PEA/Asystole)*

Chapter 3: *Key Clinical Issues in ACLS/Airway*

Section A: *KEY Clinical Issues in ACLS*

Appendix: *Value Added Drug Table*

CHAPTER 1

Overall Approach to Management of Cardiopulmonary Arrest: Algorithms for Treatment

---

Section 1A: *Overview of Cardiac Arrest*

The goal of this introductory chapter is to provide a brief overview of the approach to the management of ***cardiopulmonary arrest***- and to introduce the ***Algorithms for Treatment***. At first glance, the thought of having to learn all the material contained herein may seem to be no less than an overwhelming task. *This need not be the case.* If one breaks down the topic of cardiac arrest into those rhythms that are usually associated with the initial event (i.e., *primary* or precipitating mechanisms of the arrest), and the rhythms that are most likely to follow conversion out of ventricular fibrillation (i.e., *secondary* mechanisms or *post-conversion* rhythms)- organization of the problem becomes much simpler (Table 1A-1).

Table 1A-1: Primary and Secondary Mechanisms of Cardiopulmonary Arrest

- ***Primary*** (i.e., *precipitating*) ***Mechanisms of Arrest***
  - Ventricular tachycardia (VT)
  - Ventricular fibrillation (V Fib)
  - Bradycardia (including PEA rhythms and asystole)
- ***Post-Conversion Rhythms*** (i.e., *secondary* mechanisms)
  - VT
  - Bradycardia (including PEA rhythms and asystole)
  - A *supraventricular* rhythm with a *rapid* heart rate (i.e., a supraventricular *tachyarrhythmia*)
  - A *supraventricular* rhythm with a *controlled* heart rate (and an adequate blood pressure).

ACLS *Algorithms* for Treatment

Although it may initially seem like innumerable therapeutic options are available, the essentials of management are contained within the basic algorithms presented in this chapter. Mastery of these algorithms will provide you with the information needed to effectively run most codes (and to do well on the *MEGA CODE* and other *Teaching Stations*).

A major reason for emphasizing the algorithms is that they provide an overall perspective for the management of cardiac arrest. *They are the **essential foundation** upon which the building blocks of treatment are laid.* While some may object to the thought of dependence on algorithms (on the grounds that they sometimes restrict thinking, and do not always apply to the particular situation at hand)- the use of algorithms for training emergency care providers to manage cardiac arrest has clearly been shown to *expedite* clinical decision making. Perhaps nowhere in medicine does the ability to rapidly decide on a rational course of therapy have as much impact on survival as it does at the scene of a cardiopulmonary arrest.

With practice and application, recall of the various algorithms becomes automatic. Such *"automaticity"* is extremely beneficial during an arrest situation- because it helps prevent the emergency care provider from forgetting basic material that was so well known under less stressful circumstances. Algorithms are *not* meant to be a substitute for judgement. On the contrary, reflexive recall of the framework of management *facilitates* organization of one's thinking, the setting of priorities, and institution of appropriate therapeutic measures.

> We emphasize that the ***ACLS Algorithms*** do *not* account for all possible permutations of management. *They are not meant to*- since doing so would entail specification of an endless number of uncommonly used treatment alternatives that would not only confuse the issue, but also defeat the original purpose of the algorithm- namely, *organization*, *simplicity*, and *practicality*.

AHA Guidelines stress the importance of viewing the algorithms as a *"summary and memory aid"*- rather than as an *'end-all answer'* to every conceivable clinical situation (AHA Text- Pg 1-11). The algorithms should *not* be used blindly. Instead- *flexibility* is not only accepted but *encouraged* in adapting one's approach to the clinical situation at hand. Above all, AHA Guidelines admonish- ***"Treat the patient- NOT the monitor"*** !!!

Primary Mechanisms of Cardiopulmonary Arrest

Most cases of adult cardiopulmonary arrest occur *outside* the hospital. As suggested in Table 1A-1, the three principal ***primary* mechanisms** for out-of-hospital cardiopulmonary arrest are:

i) Ventricular tachycardia (VT)
ii) Ventricular fibrillation (V Fib)
iii) Bradycardia (including PEA rhythms and asystole).

Of these three primary mechanisms, ***V Fib*** is by far the most common in this setting. It occurs in almost two thirds of cases. In contrast, ***VT*** is a relatively infrequent mechanism of out-of-hospital cardiac arrest. In only 5-10% of cases is ventricular tachycardia documented as the initial rhythm (i.e., as the *presumed* precipitating mechanism of the arrest) by emergency medical service (EMS) personnel at the time of their arrival on the scene. The remaining patients (a little less than one third of the total) are initially found in some type of ***bradyarrhythmia*** (including the PEA rhythms and asystole).

The literature suggests that *ventricular tachycardia* is a much more common precipitating mechanism of cardiac arrests that occur *inside* the hospital. Perhaps this is simply a result of the fact that the time from onset of the arrest until discovery by trained personnel is significantly less in a hospital setting. In other words, it is likely that many cases of out-of-hospital cardiac arrest *began* as VT- but have *already* deteriorated to V Fib (and/or to asystole) by the time they are first recognized.

Primary respiratory arrest is also an important precipitating mechanism of arrests that occur *inside* the hospital. As is the case for VT- the finding of *pure* respiratory arrest as a precipitating mechanism is probably a reflection of the *earlier* discovery that is likely to occur in a hospital setting (i.e., discovery of the victim at a point *after* breathing has stopped- but *before* there has been progression to full cardiac arrest). In contrast, identification of a victim in *pure* respiratory arrest is much less likely to be seen *outside* of the hospital setting because deterioration of the rhythm (to V Fib or a bradyarrhythmia) will have almost always occurred by the time the victim is finally discovered.

Clinical Implications of the Primary Mechanisms

Management of the three principal *primary* mechanisms of cardiac arrest is discussed in the sections that follow in this chapter. The point we stress here relates to the fact that awareness of what the *precipitating* mechanism of a cardiac arrest is may provide important insight to the likely prognosis of the patient. Such awareness may also assist with selection of the most appropriate treatment for the situation at hand. For example, patients who are found on the scene by EMS personnel in either pure *respiratory arrest* or *ventricular tachycardia* tend to have a much better chance of being successfully resuscitated than those who are found in V Fib. In fact, successful resuscitation is likely for many (if not most) patients who suffer pure respiratory arrest since the treatment approach (supportive ventilation) is easily implemented once trained personnel arrive on the scene. The principal determinant of long-term survival (and the expected extent of neurologic recovery) will depend primarily on the *duration* of time that the patient was apneic *prior* to initiation of ventilation- and on the patient's underlying medical condition. Patients initially found on the scene in sustained VT *with* a pulse also have a generally good long-term prognosis- since synchronized cardioversion tends to be very effective in converting this rhythm to a supraventricular mechanism. In contrast, patients who are found on the scene in a *bradyarrhythmia* (including PEA rhythms or asystole) as the mechanism of out-of-hospital cardiac arrest have a dismal long-term prognosis. Even if a pulse is initially restored in such patients, the chance for ultimate survival with intact neurologic function is exceedingly small. Intermediate between these two extremes is the large group of patients who present with *V Fib* as the primary mechanism of their arrest. The likelihood of meaningful long-term survival for these patients is estimated to be between 5-25% (depending on a host of *difficult-to-control-for* variables).

The goal of cardiopulmonary resuscitation and emergency cardiac care is clear- arrive on the scene at a point in the process *before* irreversibility has set in (i.e., ideally *before* deterioration of the initial rhythm to V Fib or asystole).

Selection of treatment priorities by the emergency care provider may also be a function of the mechanism of arrest. This is especially true with regard to the use of ***Epinephrine***- for which the dose of drug required to optimize coronary and cerebral perfusion during resuscitation appears to vary according to *duration* of the arrest and the *initial* (precipitating) rhythm. Specifically- higher doses of drug (i.e., ***HDE*** or *High-Dose Epinephrine*) are likely to be needed *sooner* in a patient who has been unresponsive for a longer period of time (as is usually the case for out-of-hospital cardiac arrest). In contrast, a lower dose of Epinephrine (i.e, ***SDE*** or *Standard-Dose Epinephrine*) may be adequate (at least some of the time) for treatment of cardiac arrest that is *promptly* attended to in a hospital setting. Patients with no electrical activity at all (i.e., victims who are initially found in asystole) are also likely to require higher doses of drug *sooner* than patients with evidence of partial (albeit inadequate) contractile function (as may be the case for some patients with EMD). Regardless of the precipitating mechanism, if the decision is made to *initially* try SDE but the drug *fails* to produce the desired response- consideration should be given to the potential benefits of *increasing* the dose (i.e., to HDE).

The *Chain* of Survival

As alluded to above, meaningful survival from cardiac arrest (i.e., long-term survival with *intact* neurologic status) is *critically* dependent on the interrelation between a series of interventions that are said to make up the ***"links"*** in a ***Chain of Survival*** (AHA Text- Pg 16-4). Analogy to a "chain" is made because if *any* of the links are faulty- the end result is likely to be the same (i.e., a very *poor* chance for long-term survival). The *Chain of Survival* consists of 4 links:

- Link #1 = ***Early Access***

  Prompt *recognition* of the arrest (or impending arrest)- with rapid notification of (and immediate response by) the EMS system.

- Link #2 = ***Early CPR***

  After calling for help-"***Bystander CPR*** *is the best treatment a cardiac arrest patient can receive until arrival of a defibrillator and ACLS care"* (AHA Text- Pg 16-7). Performance of ***BLS*** (*Basic Life Support*) measures on the scene is a critical step for preserving neurologic function.

- Link #3 = ***Early Defibrillation***

  This is by far the *most* important link in the *chain* (and the one with the best chance of improving ultimate survival).

- Link #4 = ***Early ACLS***

  Performance of ***ACLS*** (by paramedics on arrival at the scene- and/or by hospital providers) is the *final* critical link in the *Chain of Survival.*

> AHA Guidelines emphasize how distinction between BLS and ACLS has become "blurred" with development of AEDs, use of endotracheally administered medication, and other new developments. Practically speaking- ***ACLS*** *is just the other end (of a continuum) that begins with* ***recognition*** *of the arrest and* ***BLS*** (AHA Text- Pg 1-3).

The Brain and the Patient

Although the *initial* step in cardiopulmonary resuscitation is clearly to restart the heart- ***cerebral resuscitation*** is the *ultimate* goal. For the end result to be judged successful, the patient must therefore be restored to their *prearrest* level of neurologic functioning. Practically speaking- this is unlikely to occur unless there is *prompt* implementation of *both* BLS and ACLS measures.

AHA Guidelines emphasize that *despite* multiple simultaneous actions occurring at the scene of a cardiac arrest- one thought must remain prominent in the mindset of the emergency care provider (AHA Text- Pg 1-27):

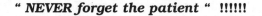

> ***" NEVER forget the patient "*** **!!!!!!**

The *KEY* to accomplishing successful cardiac (and cerebral) resuscitation will hinge on being able to *"constantly return to the overall view"* of how *each* intervention affects the patient (AHA Text- Pg 1-2). Equally important tasks for the emergency care provider to assume are continued consideration of what may have *caused* the arrest in the first place (*potentially correctable* factors?)- and *ongoing* monitoring of key clinical parameters (patency of the airway? efficacy of ventilation? adequacy of CPR? - etc.).

Secondary Mechanisms of Cardiopulmonary Arrest

If a patient in V Fib is successfully converted out of this rhythm, one of four ***secondary*** **mechanisms** of cardiac arrest is likely to be seen (Table 1A-1):

i) Ventricular tachycardia
ii) A *bradyarrhythmia* (including PEA rhythms and asystole)
iii) A *supraventricular* rhythm with a *rapid* heart rate (i.e., a supraventricular *tachyarrhythmia*)
iv) A *supraventricular* rhythm with a *controlled* heart rate (and an adequate blood pressure)

Clinically- the treatment of VT or bradycardia that arises as a *secondary* mechanism (i.e., as a *post-conversion* rhythm following defibrillation) is similar to that recommended for these rhythms when they arise as the *primary* mechanism of an arrest. This simplifies the approach of the emergency care provider- since the same evaluative process and algorithms for treatment (that we discuss in Sections 1C and 1D) can be used- *regardless* of when in the code these rhythms occur.

Alternatively- defibrillation of the patient may convert V Fib into a supraventricular mechanism *other than* bradycardia. Clinically, the treatment approach to a *non* bradycardic supraventricular rhythm will again depend on the specific mechanism of the rhythm, as well as its hemodynamic effect on the patient. If the heart rate of the post-conversion rhythm is controlled and blood pressure is adequate- *no additional treatment may be needed.* On the other hand, if defibrillation produces a supraventricular *tachyarrhythmia* (and/or a supraventricular rhythm associated with hypotension)- specific interventions aimed at converting the rhythm (or at least controlling the rate) become immediately indicated.

The Phased-Response Approach

No matter *where* an arrest occurs- and *no matter* how many personnel are involved- the principles of the ***Phased-Response Approach*** to ACLS are the *same* and should be applied (AHA Text- Pg 1-69). We summarize the 7 phases of this approach (that are described in more detail in the AHA Text):

- **Phase I**- *Anticipation* (mental/technical preparation for the code to come). Resuscitation equipment should be routinely checked in advance- and readily available for any emergency. Designation of team membership and delineation of specific duties is ideally accomplished *before* the code occurs.
- **Phase II**- *Entry* (arrival on the scene of the ***Team Leader***- with rapid initial assessment of preceding/precipitating events that led up to the code).
- **Phase III**- *Resuscitation* (working the code- application of BLS/ACLS interventions- with *ongoing* assessment of the patient's response).
- **Phase IV**- *Maintenance* (stabilization of the situation)- which must *not* dissuade the team from continued vigilence over all related aspects of management.
- **Phase V**- *Family notification* (of events that transpired)- at the *earliest* appropriate moment.
- **Phase VI**- *Transfer of the patient* (to the appropriate facility/provider team as transition is made to the *post-resuscitation* care phase).
- **Phase VII**- *Critique Process* (constructive *"soul-searching"* of events that transpired- an *invaluable* source of feedback- and an *essential* step after *every* code!). Learning from events that transpired is the best way to reinforce those actions that were optimally effective- and to improve on performance of those that were not.

Grading of AHA Recommendations

Application of scientific evidence to the *nearly-impossible-to-control-for* clinical situation of cardiopulmonary arrest poses a true dilemma. A ***Grading System*** for classifying ***Therapeutic Interventions*** in ACLS has been developed in an attempt to integrate in the most objective manner possible the relative strength of *available* supporting evidence for recommendations put forth in the AHA Guidelines. Grading according to this classification is as follows (AHA Text- Pg 1-10):

- **Class I**- a therapetuic option that is *usually indicated*, always acceptable- and considered useful and effective.

- **Class II**- a therapeutic option that is *acceptable*, is of uncertain efficacy- and may be controversial:

  - **Class IIa**- a therapeutic option for which the weight of evidence is *in favor* of its usefulness and efficacy.

  - **Class IIb**- a therapeutic option that is *not* well established by evidence, but may be helpful (and probably is *not* harmful).

- **Class III**- a therapeutic option that is inappropriate, is without scientific supporting data- and may be harmful.

The grading classification may be *summarized* as follows:

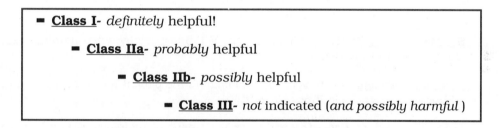

- **Class I**- *definitely* helpful!
  - **Class IIa**- *probably* helpful
    - **Class IIb**- *possibly* helpful
      - **Class III**- *not* indicated (*and possibly harmful*)

The reason for developing a grading system is simple: a need existed for more objective (and more scientific) discrimination between the various treatment options available. Clinicians were faced with sifting through an extensive literature with many difficult to interpret results. Problems encountered with many of the studies in the literature on cardiac arrest included a lack of suitably matched control groups and the absence of prospective randomization in true blinded fashion. Other problems with the studies were the differing definitions used for neurological and clinical outcome (and even for the very state of cardiac arrest), a frequent inability to prospectively witness and accurately record (and time) initial events (i.e., patient collapse) in the sequence, and the virtual impossibility of conclusively proving true treatment effect for one intevention amidst the multitude of variables (and other interventions) inherent to the management of any cardiopulmonary arrest. Selection of a panel of experts to meticulously (and scientifically) review and assess the relative merits (and drawbacks) of those studies that have been performed- and to integrate this information into a clinically useful grading system is a laudable and critically important step toward conveyance of the *relative* strength of the clinical recommendations proposed in the AHA Guidelines.

Practical Considerations of the AHA Grading System

As helpful as having graded recommendations is, the clinician is still left with a problem: ***What to do at the bedside (or on the scene)**- when the patient is **coding** and universally accepted beneficial (i.e., Class I) interventions are simply **not** working?*

Each code situation is different- just as each patient is different. Unfortunately, support in the literature is *not* always forthcoming for every nuance of each treatment intervention. Certain interventions may seem plausible (such as use of HDE for persistent asystole)- but may not have been adequately studied to receive a Class I recommendation. Alternatively- the particular situation you are suddenly faced with may not have been reproduced in a clinical study.

> **Bottom Line**- Application of Class I recommendations is clearly preferable whenever this is possible. Interventions graded as Class III are to be avoided. However, in between- ***judgement is needed*** *on the part of the emergency care provider* to determine the most suitable management approach for the particular clinical situation at hand . . . .

Examples of Grading ACLS Interventions

Insight into the ***Grading System*** for ACLS interventions is probably best provided by citing clinical examples for the more commonly used therapies in each class.

- Examples of ***Class I*** (i.e., *definitely* helpful) interventions:
  - *Standard-Dose Epinephrine* (**SDE**) = 1 mg IV every 3-5 minutes in the treatment of V Fib.
  - ***"Stacked" Defibrillations***- for persistent V Fib (especially when administration of medication is delayed).
  - ***Sodium Bicarbonate***- is Class I- *IF* (*and only if*) the patient has known *preexisting* hyperkalemia (AHA Text- Pg 1-20).
  - ***Lidocaine*** and/or ***Procainamide***- for treatment of *wide-complex* tachycardia of *uncertain* etiology.
  - ***Magenesium Sulfate***- for cardiac arrest/Acute MI when there is known (or suspected) magnesium deficiency; and/or for suppression of *Torsade de Pointes*.

- Examples of ***Class IIa*** (i.e., *probably* helpful) interventions:
  - ***Antifibrillatory Agents*** (i.e., ***Lidocaine***- ***Bretylium***)- for persistent V Fib. (In reality, the efficacy of these drugs in the latter stages of cardiopulmonary resuscitation is unknown).
  - ***Adenosine***- for treatment of a *wide-complex* tachycardia of *unknown* etiology (although this drug is unlikely to be helpful if the rhythm turns out to be VT).
  - *TransCutaneous Pacing* (***TCP***)- is a Class IIa recommendation for drug resistant bradycardia when there is an escape rhythm.

> **NOTE**- Pacing is a **Class I** recommendation for hemodynamically compromising bradycardias- *but* it is **Class IIb** for asystole (because TCP is *unlikely* to save such patients- unless started very *early* in the code).

- Examples of ***Class IIb*** (i.e., *possibly* helpful) interventions:
  - Use of *higher doses* of Epinephrine (i.e., ***HDE***) during resuscitation in cases when an initial 1 mg IV dose (i.e., SDE) does not work.

- Routine use of less well studied antifibrillatory agents (i.e., ***Magnesium-Procainamide***) for persistent V Fib.

> **NOTE**- Use of ***Magnesium*** becomes a **Class IIa** recommendation in the treatment of cardiac arrest for patients with low (or suspected low) serum magnesium levels.

- ***TransCutaneous Pacing (TCP)***- for asystole (with the *KEY* to success being to institute pacing as soon as possible).

- ***Atropine***- for asystole or severe AV block.

■ Examples of ***Class III*** (i.e., *not* indicated and *possibly* harmful) interventions:

- ***Verapamil/Diltiazem***- for treatment of a *wide-complex* tachycardia of *unknown* etiology.

- ***Sodium Bicarbonate***- has a *variable* status- depending on the clinical situation! It is designated as:

  - **Class I**- if the patient has *preexisting* hyperkalemia.

  - **Class IIa**- if the patient has known (or suspected) preexisting bicarbonate-responsive metabolic acidosis- or to alkalinize serum in severe tricyclic overdose.

  - **Class IIb**- for *intubated* patients in prolonged cardiac arrest- and/or after return of a pulse following prolonged arrest.

  - **Class III**- for patients with *hypoxic* lactic acidosis (as is likely to occur in *nonintubated* patients with prolonged cardiopulmonary arrest)- for whom *improved ventilation* (*and not Bicarb!*) is the treatment of choice!

Suggested *Initial Approach* to Cardiopulmonary Emergency

AHA Guidelines recommend a series of specific *sequential actions* in the ***Initial Approach*** to the victim with impending (or ongoing) cardiorespiratory arrest (AHA Text- Pg 1-4). The approach consists of:

i) ***Preliminary* First Actions**
ii) Performance of a ***Primary* Survey**
iii) Performance of a ***Secondary* Survey**

Sequential application of the steps and actions included in the above approach delineates the components of the ***Universal* Algorithm**. For clarity, we first discuss each of the elements in the above approach *separately*- and then *put them together* as they appear in the *Universal Algorithm* for adult emergency cardiac care.

> AHA Guidelines emphasize that the steps and actions encompassed by the Primary and Secondary Surveys are *identical* to those that comprise the Universal Algorithm. They acknowledge that some emergency care providers may find it easier to remember the steps in the *Universal Algorithm*- whereas others will prefer the memory aid afforded by the alphabetical (ABCD) acronym that highlights the elements in the *Primary* and *Secondary Surveys*. AHA Guidelines stress that whichever approach *"works best for the learner is acceptable"* (AHA Text- Pg 1-11).

The importance of total familiarity with the steps and actions encompassed by the Primary and Secondary Surveys cannot be overemphasized. Regular performance of these actions is recommended *not only* for treatment of patients in full cardiopulmonary arrest- but *also* for patients encountered in the *"pre-arrest"* state- for patients you care for in the *"post-arrest"* state (i.e., immediately *after* successful resuscitation)- and at *all* major decision points that occur *during* a difficult resuscitation effort (AHA Text- Pg 1-4).

Preliminary First Actions

Three ***Preliminary "First Actions"*** should be *immediately* performed the moment you arrive at the scene. Using 3 letters- ***" A - C - P "*** - as a memory aid helps to recall these sequential actions:

A = *Assess*

C = *Call*

P = *Position*

Specific points to keep in mind regarding performance of *Preliminary First Actions* include:

- *Assess the victim.* The first thing to do on arrival at the scene is to *assess* the victim. Determine *responsiveness* (or the *lack* thereof). Work from the assumption that *any* person found "down" is the victim of cardiorespiratory arrest- *until proven otherwise!*

  AHA Guidelines continue to recommend the traditional *"shake and shout"* to establish unresponsiveness. However, they caution that "shaking" should be *gentle*- and coordinated with asking the downed victim, *"Are you OK?"* (AHA Text- Pg 1-5). They further caution that shaking should be *avoided* if there is *any* suspicion of C-spine injury (in which case use of an even more gentle *"talk and touch"* approach is advised).

- *Call for help* ***FAST !*** Ideally- *assessing* the victim will take only seconds. As soon as this is done, a call for help should *immediately* be made. The "call" may consist of verbal shouting (if others are within hearing distance)- or momentarily *leaving* the patient to find a phone to access EMS (calling the operator or local 911 system). Realistically speaking- the principal determinant of successful resuscitation (and long-term survival) will be rapid application of advanced care measures (primarily rapid defibrillation). For this reason- AHA Guidelines give *high priority* to the ***Call for Help*** once a state of unresponsiveness has been verified (AHA Text- Pg 1-5).

> **Note**- The principal *exception* to the general rule of calling for help as soon as you verify unresponsiveness- is when an advanced care provider *strongly* suspects airway obstruction (rather than cardiac arrest) as the cause. In this situation- AHA Guidelines allow for performance of the initial A and B steps of CPR *prior* to leaving the victim to call for help (AHA Text- Pg 1-5).
>
> Clinically- situations in which *pure* respiratory arrest are more likely to be the cause of the problem include sudden loss of consciousness in a child or infant- and adult drug overdose, drowning, post-ictal state, or lightning strike. In these situations, ensuring adequate ventilation (and oxygenation) may be lifesaving measures. In almost all other cases- realistic chance for survival depends on defibrillating the patient at the earliest opportunity.

- *Position the victim- and yourself!* As soon as the *Call for Help* has been made- *return to the victim!* If the victim is unresponsive from cardiac arrest- carefully roll the victim over *as a unit* onto their back. Place one hand on the back of the victim's head and neck, and maintain the victim's cervical spine in a *straight* line as you roll the victim over (being especially careful if C-spine injury is suspected).

  After positioning the victim- *properly position yourself.* As the rescuer, you will best be able to care for the victim by *kneeling* at the level of the victim's shoulders (which should allow movement from the victim's mouth to their chest *without* having to get up to reposition your knees).

> **Note**- As will be discussed momentarily- the unresponsive victim of cardiac arrest who is breathing normally should be placed in the ***recovery position*** instead of on their back (to minimize the risk of aspiration)- provided that there is *no evidence* of C-spine trauma (*See Figure 1A-1*).

Completion of *Preliminary First Actions* is indication to *immediately* move on to the *Primary Survey . . . .*

Primary Survey

Steps in the ***Primary Survey*** are conveniently recalled by the 4-letter alphabetical (***A - B - C - D***) acronym:

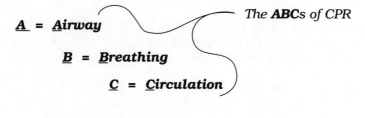

A = Airway

B = Breathing

C = Circulation

*The **ABC**s of CPR*

plus

D = Defibrillation

Performance of the *Primary Survey* entails both assessment and intervention. The Primary Survey is initiated *after* completion of *Preliminary First Actions* (i.e, *initial **A**ssessment* of the patient with establishment of unresponsiveness- ***C**alling* for help- and ***P**ositioning* yourself and the patient). Attention now turns to the ***A**irway* (which is the "**A**" component of the Primary Survey). Specific points to keep in mind regarding this first component- as well as for the remaining three ("**B** - **C** - **D**") components of the *Primary Survey* include the following:

- ***A****- Open the **A**irway.* The mouth is opened and inspected for the presence of foreign objects, vomitus, or blood. AHA Guidelines recommend removal of such material if found (AHA Text- Pg 1-6). This may either be done manually with the rescuer's fingers (covered with gauze or a piece of cloth)- and/or by turning the patient onto their side (being especially careful to *stabilize* the neck if C-spine injury is likely).

  The airway should now be opened and maintained. This may either be done with the *head tilt-chin lift* maneuver- or the *jaw-thrust* technique (with this latter technique being especially useful when the possibility of C-spine injury exists).

- ***B****- Assess for the presence and adequacy of **B**reathing.* Opening the airway facilitates determining whether the patient is spontaneously breathing- and if so, whether or not such breathing is likely to be adequate. While maintaining the victim's airway (by applying the head tilt-chin lift maneuver)- the rescuer assumes a position in which their head is lowered with one ear placed almost next to the victim's mouth. Looking straight ahead from this position- the rescuer can now ***"look- listen-** and **feel"*** for chest rise and/or air movement from the victim.

  If the victim is breathless- *begin artificial ventilation.* AHA Guidelines urge use of some type of barrier device (such as a pocket face mask). Ventilations should be delivered *slowly* (i.e., over **1** to **2 seconds**)- so as not to exceed esophageal opening pressure. Doing so greatly reduces the chance of producing gastric distention, regurgitation, and/or aspiration. Be sure to verify that ventilations are effective (i.e., that air enters the chest to produce gentle chest rise- and then passively escapes during expiration). Failure to produce air movement in this manner suggests the possibility of airway obstruction. If not easily rectified by *repositioning* the victim's head (and then *reapplying* the head tilt-chin lift maneuver)- initiate the protocol for treatment of airway obstruction (i.e., with abdominal thrusts, etc.).

- ***C****- Check for spontaneous **C**irculation.* Palpate for the presence of a carotid pulse. Be sure to carry out the pulse check for *at least* 5 (and up to 10) seconds- since the presence of a weak and/or slow pulse could easily be overlooked with less persistent palpation.

  If a pulse is present, but the victim is *not* breathing- continue rescue breathing (aiming for delivery of a breath every 5-6 seconds in the adult victim- or a rate of **10-12 rescue breaths/minute**).

  If the victim is pulseless- *begin chest compressions* (aiming for a rate of between **80-100 compressions/minute**). The absence of a pulse in a breathless, unresponsive patient defines the condition of ***full* cardiac arrest**.

- ***D***- If V Fib (or pulseless VT) is present- ***D**efibrillate the patient as soon as possible!* As emphasized earlier- the most important "link" in the *Chain of Survival* is ***early defibrillation***. The overwhelming majority of adults who do survive non-traumatic cardiac arrest are resuscitated from V Fib. Assuming there is no underlying irreversible disease process- the most important determinant of successful defibrillation will be the amount of time from the onset of arrest until delivery of electrical countershock. AHA Gudelines therefore stress the need to expedite EMS access- and then *"hunt for V Fib"* the moment a defibrillator or AED arrives on the scene (AHA Text- Pg 1-7).

If V Fib (or pulseless VT) is found- *defibrillate promptly.*

> **Summary**- When suddenly confronted with an individual who is "down":
>
> - *Think "**A** - **C** - **P** "*
>
> - *then "**A** - **B** - **C** - **D** "*
>
> Use of these lettered acronyms should facilitate recall of the *sequence* for implementation of *Preliminary First Actions*- followed closely by the *Primary Survey.*

Secondary Survey

Completion of the *Primary Survey* is indication to proceed to the ***Secondary Survey***. Like the Primary Survey just discussed, steps in the Secondary Survey may also be recalled by a 4-letter alphabetical acronym- albeit with some *modifications* in the ABCD format. Specifically, a more *advanced* level of care is implied for the "**A**" and "**B**" components of the acronym- a *second* "**C**" is added to the third component- and a *double* "**D D**" is now used to recall the final component. These changes result in the following format:

A = *Airway Assessment/Definitive Airway Control*

B = *Breathing Reassessment (at a more advanced level)*

C (& ***C***) = *Circulation/IV Access (& Cardiac Medications)*

D D = *Differential Diagnosis*

Specific points to keep in mind regarding performance of the *Secondary Survey* include:

- ***A***- *Airway Assessment/Definitive Airway Control.* Adequacy of the airway that had been secured in the Primary Survey is reassessed. At this point in the code, attention can now be given to achieving *more definitive* airway control (including endotracheal intubation- if/as appropriate).

- ***B***- *Reassessment of Breathing.* Clinically assess the efficacy of ventilation and oxygenation. This can be done by looking for appropriate chest rise with each ventilation, inspecting the patient's skin color (for cyanosis), and assessing the work of breathing (if spontaneous respiration is present). Auscultate over the lungs. If the patient is intubated, check for the presence (and equality) of bilateral breath sounds- and the *absence* of sounds over the epigastric area. Verify proper endotracheal (ET) tube placement by at least one way *in addition to* chest auscultation (i.e., proper ET tube position just above the carina on stat portable chest X-ray, increased end-tidal CO_2 reading, etc.).

> **Note**- In clinical practice, many of the steps and actions in the Secondary Survey will often be performed almost *simultaneously*- especially when a highly skilled team of emergency care providers is actively working at the bedside. AHA Guidelines emphasize that rather than strict application of therapeutic inteventions in a *specified* sequence (as suggested by the Secondary Survey)- *"common sense should prevail"* (AHA Text- Pg 1-9). Thus, despite giving higher "priority" to endotracheal intubation than to obtaining IV access- there clearly are times when IV access may be achieved first. In such cases, medication may end up being given *before* the patient has been intubated.

- *C (& C) - Circulation Assessment/Administration of Cardiac Medications.* The first " **C** " in this component relates to assessment of *Circulatory* parameters. Specifically- *Is there a pulse?* If so- *is perfusion adequate?* What is the blood pressure? Monitor leads should be attached (if they are not already on)- and determination made of the *Cardiac rhythm.*

  The second " **C** " in this component relates to *establishing* ***IV access*** (i.e., access *into* the Circulation)- so as to enable administration of *Cardiac Medications* appropriate to the clinical situation at hand.

- ***D D****- Differential Diagnosis of the cause of arrest.* AHA Guidelines stress the importance of determining (whenever possible) the *underlying* cause of arrest- and specifically devote the " **D** " component of the Secondary Survey to this consideration. Clearly, there are times when "the *only* possibility of successfully resuscitating a person lies in *searching* for- *finding*- and *treating* a reversible cause of the arrest" (AHA text- Pg 1-10). The primary reason for adding this component to the paradigm is therefore to *avoid* a narrow-minded (automatic) "rhythm-drug response" on the part of the ACLS provider- and instead to *expand* the management approach to encompass what is going on with the 'whole patient' and with the *entire* resuscitative effort (AHA Text- Pages 1-8, 9).

Differential Diagnosis of the Secondary Survey

As noted above- special attention is given to determining (whenever possible) the *cause* of the arrest in each particular case. This is because the chance for successful resuscitation will often depend on identifying the *underlying* cause and *correcting* precipitating factors. Clues to the etiology of cardiopulmonary arrest will often be forthcoming from brief review of the patient's history or medical chart. Specifically- note should be made of any medications that the patient is taking, of associated medical problems, and especially of the history *immediately* preceding and/or precipitating the acute event. Laboratory test results may suggest electrolyte or acid-base disturbance- and/or other potentially relevant abnormalities (i.e., severe anemia, hypoxemia, or renal failure). Determination of the cardiac rhythm (and evaluation of a 12-lead ECG- *if available*) may provide additional clues, such as *unsuspected* acute myocardial infarction, *Torsade de Pointes*, and/or preceding bradycardia or tachycardia.

In an attempt to facilitate recall of the most common ***potentially* reversible** (or at least *potentially* treatable) ***causes*** of cardiopulmonary arrest, we have separated potential etiologies into 3 major categories (Table 1A-2). These categories are *potentially reversible* ***respiratory*** causes- ***circulatory*** causes- and ***metabolic/miscellaneous*** causes of cardiopulmonary arrest. As an additional *memory aid*- note the prevalence of **H**'s and **T**'s among the causes that are listed in this table.

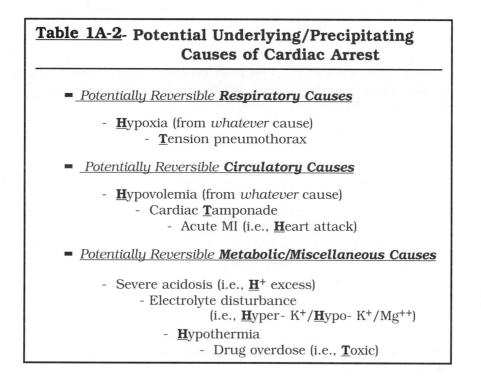

Table 1A-2- Potential Underlying/Precipitating Causes of Cardiac Arrest

- *Potentially Reversible* ***Respiratory Causes***
  - **H**ypoxia (from *whatever* cause)
  - **T**ension pneumothorax
- *Potentially Reversible* ***Circulatory Causes***
  - **H**ypovolemia (from *whatever* cause)
  - Cardiac **T**amponade
  - Acute MI (i.e., **H**eart attack)
- *Potentially Reversible* ***Metabolic/Miscellaneous Causes***
  - Severe acidosis (i.e., H^+ excess)
  - Electrolyte disturbance (i.e., **H**yper- K^+/**H**ypo- K^+/Mg^{++})
  - **H**ypothermia
  - Drug overdose (i.e., **T**oxic)

The Universal Algorithm for Adult ECC (Emergency Cardiac Care)

AHA Guidelines advise regular use of the ***Universal Algorithm*** for the *initial* approach to adult *ECC* (*Emergency Cardiac Care*). A decided advantage of this approach is that its steps are applicable to virtually any emergency situation (Figure 1A-1).

> The steps and actions encompassed in the ***Universal Algorithm*** are virtually *identical* to those that comprise the ***Primary*** and ***Secondary Surveys*** that were just discussed. As noted earlier- use of whichever approach *"works best for the learner is acceptable"* (AHA Text- Pg 1-11).

Specific points to keep in mind regarding use of the *Universal Algorithm* include the following:

- Classification of the patient (and the initial management approach) is determined by the answers to three basic questions:

  i) Is the patient ***responsive*** ?
  ii) Is the patient ***breathing*** ?
  iii) Is there a ***pulse*** ?

- Calling for help assumes *high priority* in the algorithm. Except for a few *special* situations (*see below*)- the ***Call for Help*** should be made *as soon as* the rescuer determines that the victim is unresponsive.

- If the patient is unresponsive, *NOT* breathing, and there is *NO* pulse- then by definition, the patient is in ***full* cardiac arrest**. Carefully roll the patient over (if they are not already on their back)- and *begin* ***CPR***. Specifics of subsequent management will depend on the *mechanism* of the arrest. The three major mechanisms of cardiac arrest are ***V Fib/Pulseless VT*** (the most common mechanism)- ***PEA*** *or Pulseless Electrical Activity* (when electrical activity in the form of an ECG rhythm is present but the patient is pulseless)- and ***asystole*** (when there is *no* electrical activity and *no* pulse). Management of these conditions is discussed in detail in Sections 1B, 1C, and 1D of this chapter.

- If the patient is *unresponsive*- but *IS* breathing- then the patient is *not* in full arrest (i.e., a pulse *will* be present). The patient's airway should be maintained while the rescuer assesses the efficacy of breathing. If breathing appears to be normal, and there is *no suspicion* of C-spine injury- the patient should be placed in the ***recovery position*** (*see Page 18*). On the other hand, if breathing appears to be *abnormal*- the rescuer should *reposition* the airway and reassess the situation. As will be described in detail in Section 3B (*see Figure 3B-48*)- the objectives of management at this point are to achieve optimal airway control, to rule out any component of airway obstruction- and to ensure that ventilation and oxygenation are both adequate.

Note- It is important to appreciate that if a pulse *is* present- then by definition, the patient is *not* in full arrest. In this situ-ation, one of three types of respiratory patterns may be present:

i) normal breathing
ii) abnormal breathing
iii) no breathing at all.

Figure 1A-1- *Universal Algorithm for Adult ECC*

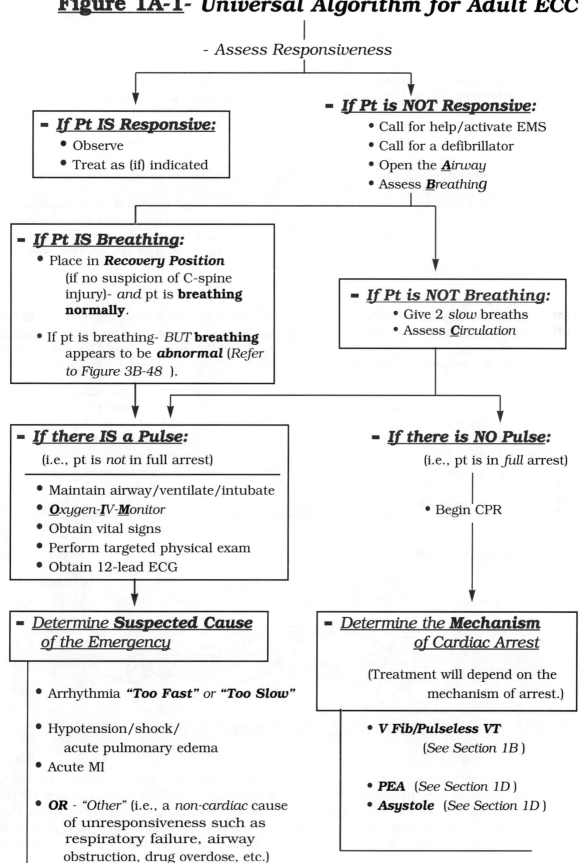

- *Assess Responsiveness*

- *If Pt IS Responsive:*
- Observe
- Treat as (if) indicated

- *If Pt is NOT Responsive:*
- Call for help/activate EMS
- Call for a defibrillator
- Open the ***A****irway*
- Assess ***B****reathing*

- *If Pt IS Breathing:*
- Place in ***Recovery Position*** (if no suspicion of C-spine injury)- *and* pt is **breathing normally**.
- If pt is breathing- *BUT* **breathing** appears to be ***abnormal*** (*Refer to Figure 3B-48*).

- *If Pt is NOT Breathing:*
- Give 2 *slow* breaths
- Assess ***C****irculation*

- *If there IS a Pulse:*
(i.e., pt is *not* in full arrest)

- Maintain airway/ventilate/intubate
- ***O****xygen*-***I****V*-***M****onitor*
- Obtain vital signs
- Perform targeted physical exam
- Obtain 12-lead ECG

- *If there is NO Pulse:*
(i.e., pt is in *full* arrest)

- Begin CPR

- *Determine **Suspected Cause** of the Emergency*
- Arrhythmia ***"Too Fast"*** *or* ***"Too Slow"***
- Hypotension/shock/ acute pulmonary edema
- Acute MI
- ***OR*** - *"Other"* (i.e., a *non-cardiac* cause of unresponsiveness such as respiratory failure, airway obstruction, drug overdose, etc.)

- *Determine the **Mechanism** of Cardiac Arrest*
(Treatment will depend on the mechanism of arrest.)

- ***V Fib/Pulseless VT*** (*See Section 1B*)
- ***PEA*** (*See Section 1D*)
- ***Asystole*** (*See Section 1D*)

- For the patient who is *not* in full arrest- initial efforts are again aimed at ensuring that ventilation and oxygenation are both adequate. After accomplishing this, attention is directed at determining the predominant/underlying *cause* of the cardiopulmonary emergency. It should be emphasized that a *combination* of factors is often responsible for the patient's condition. For example, acute myocardial infarction may precipitate cardiogenic shock if the infarct is large- *resulting in* hypotension, pulmonary edema, and ventricular tachyarrhythmias. Bradycardia might also be seen if an extensive infarction affects the conduction system. Superimposed development of severe 2° or 3° AV block would certainly aggravate the patient's already compromised hemodynamic condition. As might be imagined, treatment will depend on identifying the primary cause(s) of hemodynamic decompensation- and intervening appropriately.

- Note should be made of the point that a *non-cardiac* cause may also be responsible for the patient's condition. Important ***non-cardiac* causes** of *unresponsiveness* to consider include respiratory failure, complete airway obstruction, drug overdose, CNS catastrophe (such as a stroke or intracerebral hemorrhage), severe electrolyte abnormality, post-ictal state- and others.

- Finally- we draw attention to a series of actions that should be initiated near the beginning of most of the AHA algorithms for treatment. These actions include maintenance of the airway/ventilation/intubation; ***O**xygen-**I**V-**M**onitor*; obtaining vital signs (as appropriate); performance of a *targeted* physical exam; and obtaining a 12-lead ECG (as soon as this becomes clinically feasible).

> AHA Guidelines suggest thinking of the action "***O**xygen-**I**V-**M**onitor* " as a *single* "word"- that should be *memorized* for easy recall and rapid implementation in cardiac emergencies (AHA Text- Pg 1-27). Specifically, use of this action entails provision of *supplemental **O**xygen*- establishment of ***I**V access*- and attach-ment of ***M**onitoring leads* to the patient- all of which should be accomplished at the earliest feasible moment.

The Recovery Position

As noted in the *Universal Algorithm* shown in Figure 1A-1- if the patient is unresponsive but is breathing normally, use of the ***recovery position*** is advised (Figure 1A-2).

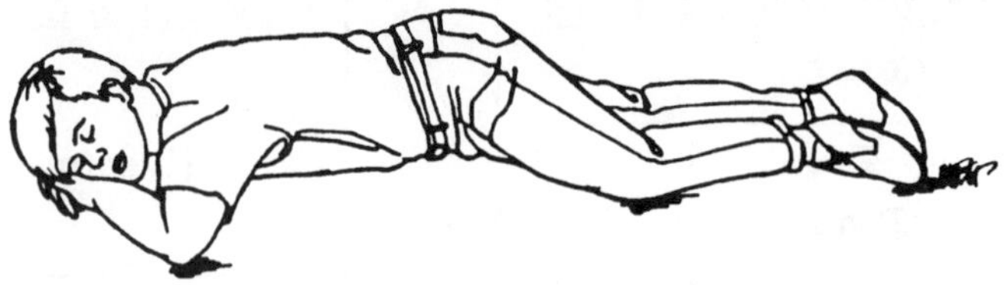

Figure 1A-2: The Recovery Position

Placement of the victim into the recovery position should *not* be attempted if there is *any* suspicion of C-spine injury. However, in the absence of this concern- moving the patient into this position minimizes the chance of developing airway obstruction that could otherwise be precipitated in the supine position (by the tongue falling back to occlude the airway). Use of the recovery position also minimizes the chance of aspiration by facilitating spontaneous drainage of the victim's secretions.

Special Situations: The *Lone* Rescuer

A dilemma arises when a trained health care provider finds himself/herself *alone* on the scene of a cardiopulmonary arrest- and *no one* is able to hear the call for help. The problem confronting the ***lone rescuer*** is what to do next:

i) *Stay with the victim* (and perform 1-rescuer CPR)?

or

ii) *Leave the victim* (to try to find help)?

In the past, AHA Guidelines called for the *single* rescuer to remain with the victim and perform 1-person CPR for an initial *one minute* prior to activating the EMS system. Despite its intuitive appeal, in practice this recommendation frequently led to significant delays in defibrillation. Awareness of time passage at the scene of an actual arrest is often imprecise- and if left to their own, trained *single* rescuers tend to perform CPR for much *longer* than the recommended "minute" before calling EMS. Practically speaking, the overwhelming majority of adults with sudden non-traumatic out-of-hospital cardiac arrest who are *potentially salvageable* will be in V Fib by the time EMS personnel arrive on the scene. For many of these patients, delay for the minute (or more) that it takes to access the EMS system could spell the difference between neurologically intact survival and a far less optimal outcome.

On the other hand, concern about recommending that the rescuer *always* leave the victim to immediately access EMS is valid. This is because *some* adults (who have either pure *respiratory* arrest or a completely *obstructed airway*) may be *inappropriately* treated by delaying full assessment of the victim and initial ventilatory support for the time that it takes to activate the EMS system. If the duration of this delay is at all prolonged (as it is likely to be if the *lone* rescuer is isolated from a phone or other access modality)- failure to *immediately* initiate ventilatory assistance could result in failure to save the patient (or in resuscitation with a less than optimal neurologic outcome). Clearly then- there *are* situations in which ensuring a patent airway and initiating rescue breathing assume *higher priority* than leaving the victim to immediately access EMS.

> **Bottom Line**- Judgement is needed (and *individualized* decision making is advised) on the part of the single *trained* rescuer for deciding what to do *FIRST* at the scene of an apparent cardiopulmonary arrest (AHA Text- Pg 1-5).

Specific points to keep in mind regarding the approach we suggest for the ***lone* rescuer** are listed below. Note that the approach recommended *differs* for the trained rescuer than for the layperson rescuer.

- For the *untrained* ***Lay* Rescuer**:

  - AHA Guidelines emphasize the need for a clear and *simple* message (in order to encourage action- yet minimize the chance of confusion). Lay individuals are easily intimidated by (and have difficulty remembering) complex decision analysis protocols- especially when called upon to render assistance in a life or death situation in which the victim may be a loved one. AHA Guidelines have therefore *simplified* the message to the single lay rescuer to- ***"Phone FIRST"*** - as soon as they encounter an unresponsive victim.

- For the *trained* ***Professional*** **Rescuer** (who is *able to appreciate* the subtleties involved):

  - If *pure* ***respiratory*** **arrest** is suspected (i.e., from airway obstruction, drowning, drug overdose, etc.)- ***STAY*** *at the scene* with the victim. *Immediately* initiate rescue breathing, since this action could be *lifesaving* in this situation.

  - Application of a Heimlich maneuver (i.e., abdominal thrusts)- *is* appropriate as an *initial* measure for the victim who is *known* (or strongly suspected) to have foreign-body airway obstruction. The most common clinical example of this situation involves the sudden collapse of a healthy adult in a restaurant setting- especially when the victim is last seen abruptly getting up from the table and rushing toward the bathroom.

  - If ***cardiac*** **arrest** is suspected as the cause of collapse, and help is "nearby" (i.e., *within* 1-2 minutes away)- ***LEAVE*** *the victim and run to get help.* Call EMS. Then *return* to the victim *as soon as you can* and initiate CPR until the EMS unit arrives on the scene.

  - Remember that the overwhelming majority of *adult* victims of sudden death die from *cardiac* arrest (and *not* from respiratory arrest). Defibrillation at the earliest possible moment holds the *KEY* for improving survival. Placing the call to activate the EMS system *immediately* after discovering the victim is the best way to expedite the process.

  - If *doubt* exists as to the cause of an arrest- always assume a *cardiac* etiology and act accordingly (i.e., *call EMS first!*). Then *return* to the victim and perform CPR until the EMS unit arrives on the scene. Take comfort in the fact that even trained rescuers often have great difficulty and may be *unable* to distinguish between primary cardiac arrest, and collapse that is secondary to airway or breathing problems.

  - Admittedly, if you are ***all alone*** at the scene when the victim collapses, and **help is *not* nearby**- *"You face some tough decisions"* (AHA Text- Pg 1-6). AHA Guidelines cite the example of sudden collapse of a jogging partner on an isolated trail *remote* from any assistance or phone contact. Sudden development of pulselessness in a jogger is almost certain indication of V Fib or pulseless VT. Realistically speaking, if help is far away (i.e., *more* than 5-10 minutes away)- the chance of accessing such help *in time* to save a collapsed victim in V Fib is practically nil. In this situation AHA Guidelines state that "common sense suggests the trained health care professional will ensure an open airway, attempt several precordial thumps, and continue CPR for at least 10 to 15 minutes" (AHA Text- Pg 1-6). Practically speaking- *not much else can be done* when you are all alone without access to a defibrillator . . . . .

  - The approach recommended for the lone rescuer is different if the victim is an infant or a child. In this situation, rapid assessment to rule out respiratory obstruction, and action to ensure adequate ventilation should be done *first* (i.e., *before* accessing EMS)- because of the much greater likelihood that an airway problem will be the primary cause of collapse or distress. AHA Guidelines advise the lone rescuer to provide an *initial* one minute of rescue support *before* seeking to access EMS personnel (AHA Text- Pg 16-7).

Use of Barrier Devices: *Practical Considerations*

Because of concern about the possibility of disease transmission, health care providers may be reluctant to initiate CPR on an unknown victim of cardiopulmonary arrest. In acknowledgement of this potential risk, we emphasize the following specific points:

- Statistically, out-of-hospital cardiac arrest is most likely to occur in the home. As a result- *layperson* CPR will most often be administered by an individual who is either related to and/or aware of the victim's health status. In such cases, there is usually little reluctance to perform CPR (including mouth-to-mouth ventilation)- provided that the rescuer is capable of doing so.

  In contrast, health care providers who encounter an *out-of-hospital* situation in which they are called on to administer CPR will usually *not* know the victim- and therefore *not* be aware of the victim's health status. Not knowing this information is a major reason why health care providers may choose not to perform mouth-to-mouth rescue breathing in this situation.

- There clearly *is* potential opportunity for saliva exchange to occur between victim and rescuer during mouth-to-mouth resuscitation. However, the *actual* risk of transmitting either hepatitis B virus or HIV infection as a *direct* result of performing CPR appears to be exceedingly small. This risk is even less if the skin around the lips and within the oral mucosa of the rescuer is intact.

- Administration of mouth-to-mouth rescue breathing may entail a somewhat greater risk of disease transmission to the rescuer if the recipient is infected with herpes simplex, Neisseria meningitidis, tuberculosis, and/or certain other types of pulmonary infections. Fortunately, even in these cases- the *overall* risk of disease transmission is probably still quite small.

- Increased availability and use of ***barrier* methods** (i.e., latex gloves, face masks or face shields, bag-valve devices, etc.) should help to *minimize* the risk of disease transmission to the rescuer. Ready availability of these devices will hopefully also reduce the reluctance of health care providers to perform rescue breathing.

- Be aware of the clinical reality that if you encounter a victim of cardiopulmonary arrest *outside* of a hospital (or other medical setting) and *YOU* do not perform CPR- *the chances are good that no one else will.* In this situation the patient will probably die. If the cause of the arrest is *purely* respiratory in nature (as it is likely to be with victims of drowning or drug overdose)- prompt adminstration of rescue breathing could be a potentially *lifesaving* intervention . . . .

- On the other hand, if a patient arrests *within* a hospital (or other medical setting) and you *know* help (and a *barrier* respiratory device) is on the way- it is probably reasonable to wait a few moments for such help to arrive. VT/V Fib is by far the most common cause of cardiopulmonary arrest in this setting- for which *defibrillation* is the treatment of choice. Putting off management of the airway for a few moments (although less than ideal) will probably *not* adversely affect outcome in most instances.

- Knowledge that nothing in the patient's history *even remotely* suggests that he/she might be HIV positive or have hepatitis B, herpes, active tuberculosis, or meningococcal meningitis- is information that *might* affect your decision of whether to administer mouth-to-mouth rescue breathing.

- If you decide *NOT* to administer rescue breathing- ***Remember*** *that performing a few cycles of external chest compressions is BETTER than doing nothing.* A primary cardiac arrest victim usually still has a certain amount of oxygenated blood in his or her system- and performance of chest compressions (at least for a *few* cycles) may help to circulate some of this blood.

- Greater ***anticipation*** (on the part of health care providers) should help to facilitate more widespread and appropriate use of respiratory barrier devices. For example, hospital staff could work to identify which acutely ill patients are at greatest risk of developing respiratory or cardiac arrest. They could then make it a point to have barrier devices routinely available at the bedside of these high risk patients.

  An even more fundamental ***anticipatory issue*** to address in hospitalized patients (*before* the arrest occurs!) is the question of whether cardiopulmonary resuscitation is even indicated or desired at all . . . . .

> Consider setting aside a moment *NOW* for ***self-reflection*** on your part- as to how ***YOU*** feel it will be most appropriate to act in the event you are one day confronted with the problematic issue of whether to administer mouth-to-mouth resuscitation to a non-breathing victim of cardiopulmonary arrest. A moment of anticipatory reflection *at THIS time* may be *invaluable* for facilitating the decision-making process (as well as *expediting* your actions) in the event that you do encounter this situation at some time in the future (*which you probably will!*). You might also consider the purchase of an inexpensive, portable barrier device (from your neighborhood pharmacy) to either keep in your car or on your person- *just in case . . . . .*

The Importance of CPR

Good technical performance of CPR *is* important. Having stated this, we feel it important to emphasize the clinical reality that by itself- performance of even perfect CPR will *not* prevent V Fib from deteriorating to asystole. What prompt initiation of CPR may do is *delay* deterioration of the rhythm- and in so doing *preserve viability* (i.e., responsiveness to defibrillation) for at least a short period of time (of perhaps 1-2 minutes). Prolonging the period of potential viability could prove to be *lifesaving* if defibrillation can then be accomplished in a timely manner.

Despite a tremendous amount of research in this area- the actual mechanism for explaining how CPR works is not yet completely clear. Theories attempting to account for how CPR works invoke the existence of a *cardiac pump* mechanism (in which the heart serves as a pump to circulate blood)- a *thoracic pump* mechanism (in which blood flow is more passive, and results from the difference in pressure that develops between intra- and extrathoracic compartments)- a *high-impulse* (i.e., force-momentum) model- and/or some combination of the above. Regardless of what the true mechanism for blood flow happens to be, however- the one conclusion that *does* seem clear is that the *efficacy* of CPR can be enhanced by attention to several key parameters. These include:

- **Ventilating *slowly* and effectively**. Ventilations should be delivered over an inspiratory time of *at least* 1.0 (and preferably closer to 2.0) seconds per breath. In addition to ventilating slowly, the rescuer should ensure that the chest actually rises with each breath delivered. The sensation of air as it enters and expands the lungs should be *felt* by the rescuer with each respiration. If this does not occur- then the airway is *not* completely patent. This may either be due to inadequate airway control (which should resolve, or at least improve with *repositioning* of the victim)- or to a mechanical cause (such as a foreign body).

As already emphasized, the importance of ventilating *slowly* is that this intervention improves the efficiency of rescue breathing by allowing adequate time for chest expansion. An additional reason for slowing the rate of ventilation in the *nonintubated* patient is that doing so reduces the risk of producing gastric distention (with resultant regurgitation/aspiration)- because it lessens the chance that esophageal opening pressure will be exceeded during any given rescue breath.

- **Compressing with *adequate* (but *not* excessive) force**. One should *not* use 'rib-breaking' force- but enough force to *adequately* depress the sternum. Failure to do so may significantly reduce the impetus for blood flow during CPR. AHA Guidelines recommend depressing the chest by 1.5-2.0 inches with each compression in the adult victim.

> We caution that performance of CPR is *not* benign. In addition to the almost universal subjective complaint of "sore chest" reported by CPR survivors- more serious complications (i.e., pneumothorax, pericardial tamponade, flail chest) occur in a significant percentage of patients. Although some of these injuries are clearly unavoidable- others (i.e., fractures of the *lateral* portion of a rib, or fractures of the *lower* ribs) could possibly have been prevented if CPR technique was more proficient (using correct hand placement over the lower half of the sternum, avoiding finger contact on the lateral chest wall when compressing, not being overzealous with application of force, etc.).

- **Compressing at the *higher end* of the rate range**. The recommended range for adults is to compress at a rate of between **80-100/minute**- and *not* at a rate of 1 per second as is still all too commonly done! Cardiac output during CPR is directly related to the *duration* of chest compression. As the rate of compression increases, the relative *percentage* of time that comprises the compression phase of CPR becomes proportionately greater (compared to the time that comprises relaxation). In addition, rescuers tend to apply greater *force* with each compression when working at a faster rate (*high-impulse CPR*). Thus the end result of increasing the recommended rate for chest compressions is improved efficiency of CPR- because the faster rate *proportionately* lengthens the period of compression duration as it increases the *force* applied with each compression. Aiming for the *upper end* of the rate range for compressions (i.e., compressing as close to a rate of 100/minute as possible- especially during the early minutes of the resuscitation effort) may be the most effective noninvasive way to optimize blood flow during CPR.

- **Considering use of *Epinephrine* at the *earliest* opportunity**. Without CPR, blood will *not* flow in the arrested heart. With properly performed two-rescuer CPR- cardiac output may approach up to 25% of normal values. However, despite this beneficial effect, the unfortunate clinical reality is that by itself- CPR is *not* an effective way to achieve adequate blood flow to the organs that count (i.e., to the heart and the brain). Practically speaking, unless vasoconstrictor medication such as Epinephrine is used, blood flow to these essential organs is virtually nil in the arrested heart (even when excellent quality CPR is being performed!). Use of Epi-nephrine is therefore recommended at an *early* point in the treatment of cardiac arrest- and the drug should be repeated *often* (i.e., at 3 to 5 minute intervals) if the patient fails to respond.

- ***Monitoring the process***. All too often, cardiopulmonary resuscitation at the bedside of a hospitalized patient becomes an overcrowded event. An important function that extra health care providers may serve at the bedside is to *monitor* the quality of CPR being performed, and constructively provide *ongoing* feedback to rescuers on parameters of CPR that they may not be aware of. For example- when left to their own, emergency care providers tend to slow down the rate of external chest compression as the code progresses. Furthermore, many health care providers are completely *unaware* of the actual rate at which they are compressing.

  We ask you to prove this to yourself. The next time you are an "extra" person at the scene of a cardiopulmonary arrest- *stand back* for a moment, and *monitor* the overall process. *Count the compression rate.* Observe other aspects of CPR performance (i.e., whether a bed board is used, compression technique, efficacy of ventilation, etc.). Given the importance of optimizing blood flow during CPR- your ***ongoing* feedback** could make a difference in the ultimate cutcome of the code.

> Consideration might be given to the use of some *objective* method for timing (and pacing the rate of) cardiac compressions. This may be done with a ***metronome*** (as is used to keep time in music) or an *audiorecording.* Use of an audio-prompted, rate-directing signal in this manner is a simple, practical way to ensure *awareness* of the correct rate of compressions. This not only facilitates the ability of rescuers to *maintain* the rate of compressions within the correct range *throughout* the resuscitation effort- but as noted above, it may also lead to significant improvement in the efficacy of compressions.

Use of the AED: *Standard Features*

Development of the ***automatic external defibrillator (AED)*** is one of the most exciting advances in the field of cardiopulmonary resuscitation. The key feature of the device is its *automaticity-* which significantly reduces the time period from discovery of a victim in cardiac arrest, until delivery of electrical countershock. *Minimizing this time interval is clearly the single most important factor for improving survival from cardiac arrest.* Additional benefits derived from automaticity of the AED are that it facilitates the process of defibrillation by less experienced medical personnel- and that it even enables lay individuals with no prior medical training to deliver a countershock to a family member in the event that a cardiac arrest occurs in the home.

> Surprisingly, use of an AED will reduce the time interval from arrival at the scene of a cardiac arrest until countershock delivery by an average of one full minute (*or more!*)- even when highly skilled paramedics are operating the device. Thus, regardless of the clinical experience of the user- incorporation of an AED into the protocol for defibrillation will save invaluable time that may make the difference for determining whether a patient recovers- and if so, whether neurologic function will be intact.

Many different brands of AED devices are available on the market. Virtually all share a number of common features- and most devices work in a similar manner. Basic operation is intentionally simple by design, in order to facilitate use by lay individuals. Allowing for minor differences in certain features among the various brands of AEDs, the general procedure for operation can be summarized within the framework of the following four *sequential* steps:

i) ***P****ower* on.
ii) ***A****ttach* cables and pads.
iii) ***I****nterpret* (i.e., *analyze*) the rhythm.
iv) ***D****efibrillate* (if indicated).

> **Note**- The *4 sequential steps* that are common to operation of virtually any AED are conveniently recalled by the acronym " **P** - **A** - **I** - **D** ".

The initial step in operation of an AED is to *turn* ***P****ower on.* This activates the device to record all subsequent events (in the form of a tape recording and/or printed record)- that will then be available for review of what transpired during the code.

All AEDs are equipped with ***patient*** *(defibrillatory)* ***cables*** and *adhesive* ***defibrillator pads***. The two defibrillator *pads* must first be ***A****ttached* to the defibrillatory *cables*- which are in turn connected to the AED unit. The pads are then placed on the patient's chest in two positions (at the right upper sternal border and on the left side of the chest over the apex). These pads serve the *dual* function of sensing the rhythm and conducting the current that will defibrillate the patient.

The cardiac rhythm can now be ***I****nterpreted.* This step is accomplished by pressing the ***analyze control* switch** on the AED. If CPR was being performed (as it might be if more than one rescuer is present)- it should be *stopped* for the 5-15 seconds required for the machine to analyze the rhythm. Momentary cessation of CPR minimizes the chance of introducing artifact from chest compression (that might adversely affect the validity of AED rhythm interpretation). For similar reasons, the device should *not* be operated in a moving ambulance. Fortunately in practice, the likelihood of precipitating an inappropriate shock is exceedingly small- even when abrupt patient movements occur (as might be produced by seizure activity or agonal respirations).

The final step in the process after sensing the rhythm is to ***D****efibrillate* the patient- *if this is appropriate.* If defibrillation is not indicated, the AED will not discharge (with a few possible exceptions as described below).

AED Rhythm Analysis

AED rhythm analysis is performed by a highly sophisticated microprocessor, and is based on assessment of ECG signal characteristics of amplitude, frequency, and slope of the waveform. Incorporation of additional safety features into the rhythm analysis program (i.e., to detect false signals from 60-cycle interference and/or loose electrode leads)- as well as *cessation of CPR* (and elimination of other potential sources of patient movement while rhythm analysis is occurring)- all contribute to the extremely high level of accuracy achieved by most of these devices in clinical practice.

> The AED can be counted on to *reliably* deliver a shock when it determines that the rhythm is V Fib. It will also shock cases of VT in which the ventricular rate exceeds a certain preset value. *The AED will not shock asystole.*

In general, it is quite rare for the AED to make an *error of commission* (i.e., shocking a rhythm that is not V Fib). *Errors of omission* (i.e., failure to shock a rhythm that should be shocked) are more likely to occur- and are most often a result of the machine not distinguishing between very fine V Fib and a flat line recording. Practically speaking, this type of error is usually of little clinical significance- since *realistic* chances for survival are almost as poor when the initial mechanism of cardiac arrest is very *fine* V Fib as when the rhythm is asystole.

An additional "check" against delivery of an inappropriate shock automatically results from the protocol recommended for utilization of the AED- because rescuers are taught to apply the device *only* to unresponsive victims who are breathless *and* pulseless. Considering that the AED will not shock asystole- defibrillation of virtually *any* other rhythm that occurs in this situation will probably not adversely affect prognosis (and defibrillation may convert the rhythm if the pulseless condition is the result of V Fib or pulseless VT).

AED Operating Procedure/Treatment Protocols

The degree of *automaticity* incorporated into the operation of an AED is variable. There are two basic types of devices:

i) *Fully automatic* models.
ii) *Partially (or semi-) automatic* models.

Fully automatic AEDs are ideal devices for lay person use- because they do *not* depend at all on the operator to make any decisions. Instead, they simply require the operator to turn power on and attach the patient cables. *The device does the rest.* If the AED interprets the patient's rhythm as V Fib (or VT at an exceedingly fast rate)- it automatically charges the machine and defibrillates. The operator *never* even sees the rhythm that is analyzed.

Semiautomatic AEDs (i.e., ***SAEDs*** or *"shock-advisory" defibrillators*) differ from fully automatic devices in that one or more additional operator steps are required for defibrillation to occur. More than simply turning power on and attaching patient cables- the operator must *also* activate the rhythm analysis control and physically depress a switch to discharge the electrical energy if defibrillation is indicated. This extra measure of operator control is the reason trained medical personnel generally prefer semiautomatic devices.

> **Note**- Although in theory one might expect semiautomatic AEDs to be safer than fully automatic devices (since the operator retains control of the final step in the decision-making process)- this expectation has *not* been borne out in practice. Clinical performance of both types of AEDs is comparable- and *highly* accurate.

It should be emphasized that *initial* assessment and management of a patient in cardiopulmonary arrest is similar *regardless* of the therapeutic modalities that happen to be available (and *regardless* of whether initial rescue personnel are lay individuals or a highly skilled medical team). Initial priorities are therefore the same as those stated in the ***Universal Algorithm*** for emergency cardiac care:

i) Assessing responsiveness (i.e., *identification* of the cardiopulmonary emergency).
ii) Calling for help.
iii) Opening the ***A****irway* (after positioning yourself and the victim).
iv) Assessing ***B****reathing* (and beginning *rescue breathing* if the victim is breathless).
v) Assessing ***C****irculation.*

It is at *this point* in the process (i.e., right *after* assessing ***C****irculation*) that treatment will differ- depending on which therapeutic modalities are available and the skill of the rescue team. Clearly, once the diagnosis of *pulseless* cardiac arrest has been confirmed (and respiratory obstruction has been ruled out)- electrical *defibrillation* assumes *highest* priority. All other actions (*including* performance of CPR)- become *secondary* compared to the urgent need for *immediate* defibrillation.

In Figure 1A-3 we illustrate the approach recommended by AHA Guidelines for the ***lone rescuer*** who comes upon a victim of cardiopulmonary arrest- and who has ***immediate access*** to an **AED**. Note how the first few steps in Figure 1A-3 are *identical* to the first few steps in the *Universal Algorithm* (that we presented in Figure 1A-1). A difference in the treatment approach occurs only *after* pulselessness is confirmed. If the patient is pulseless and an AED is immediately available- the recommended sequence *omits* chest compressions. Instead, the AED device should be sought, applied to the patient- and set up to ***D****efibrillate* as soon as the diagnosis of V Fib can be confirmed (AHA Text- Pg 1-6).

Note- In the past, intervention by a *lay rescuer* was limited to performing CPR and awaiting arrival of EMS personnel. Development of the AED has added an extra dimension to this treatment approach- since it now enables a single lay rescuer to provide definitive treatment for what might otherwise be a lethal condition.

Figure 1A-3- *Use of the Universal Algorithm by the Lone Rescuer who has Immediate Access to an AED*

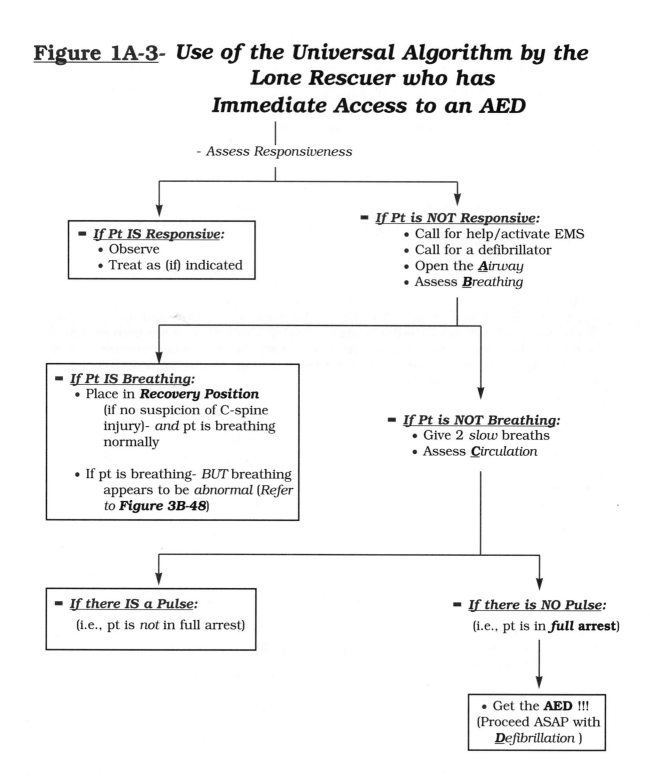

- *Assess Responsiveness*

▬ *If Pt IS Responsive:*
- Observe
- Treat as (if) indicated

▬ *If Pt is NOT Responsive:*
- Call for help/activate EMS
- Call for a defibrillator
- Open the ***A**irway*
- Assess ***B**reathing*

▬ *If Pt IS Breathing:*
- Place in ***Recovery Position*** (if no suspicion of C-spine injury)- *and* pt is breathing normally
- If pt is breathing- *BUT* breathing appears to be *abnormal* (*Refer to* ***Figure 3B-48***)

▬ *If Pt is NOT Breathing:*
- Give 2 *slow* breaths
- Assess ***C**irculation*

▬ *If there IS a Pulse:*
(i.e., pt is *not* in full arrest)

▬ *If there is NO Pulse:*
(i.e., pt is in ***full* arrest**)

- Get the **AED** !!! (Proceed ASAP with ***D**efibrillation*)

Figure 1A-4 is the continuation of Figure 1A-3- in which the AED is used in the treatment of a patient in V Fib or pulseless VT. The overall approach that is outlined in this algorithm will be similar *regardless* of whether one or more rescuers are present- with the exception that extra rescuers may perform CPR while the initial rescuer is activating the AED.

Figure 1A-4- *AED Treatment Algorithm for V Fib/Pulseless VT*

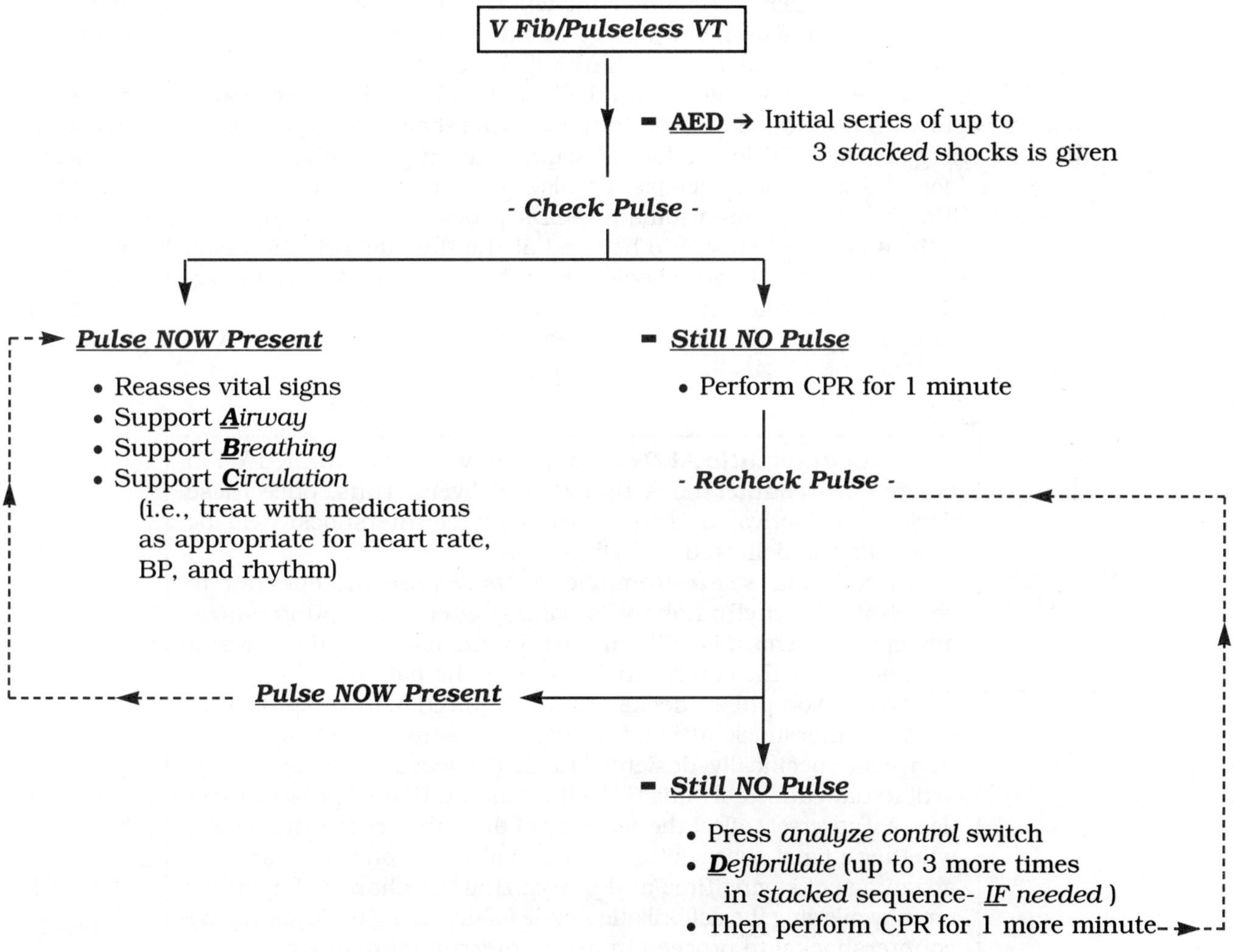

Activation of the AED entails implementation of the 4 *sequential* steps that were discussed earlier:

i) ***P****ower* is turned on.
ii) Defibrillator cables and pads are ***A****ttached.*
iii) The analyze control switch is depressed which allows the machine to ***I****nterpret* the rhythm.
iv) The patient is ***D****efibrillated* if V Fib (or pulseless VT) is sensed. An initial series of 3 *stacked* shocks is given (using an energy level of between **200-360 joules**).

All AEDs inform the operator of the decision they reach from analysis of the patient's rhythm. This *advisory message* is conveyed to the operator in one or more ways such as a statement in writing (that may appear on the AED oscilloscope screen), a visual or auditory alarm, and/or a voice synthesized phrase.

Depending on the type of AED used, charging of the defibrillator and discharge of the electrical energy will either occur *automatically*- or *on command* from the operator. As a safety precaution, a visual and/or auditory warning will be issued to rescuers to stop CPR and stand clear while the machine is charging and defibrillating.

The amount of energy delivered with defibrillation by AED devices varies. Virtually all models begin with 200 joules for the initial countershock attempt. Some automatically increase energy to 300-360 joules for subsequent attempts. Others maintain a constant energy level for all defibrillation attempts- or allow preprogramming of the amount of energy to be used. Finally, some semi-automatic AEDs provide the operator with the option of determining the amount of energy to be used at the time defibrillation is ordered.

As noted above- defibrillatory shocks should be *"stacked"* in groups of three. Pulse checks need *not* be performed after each countershock attempt in a series. However, the rhythm *must* be analyzed after each countershock attempt in order to verify persistence of V Fib.

> ***Fully automatic AEDs*** automatically verify continued V Fib before each countershock that they deliver. Thus, once these devices are activated- three successive countershocks will be *automatically* delivered if V Fib persists.
>
> In contrast, ***semiautomatic AEDs*** require the operator to reactivate the rhythm analysis control after each countershock attempt. If a shock is still "advised" by the machine- the operator then activates the control to defibrillate the patient.
>
> The reason pulse checks are *not* required with the AED after each countershock attempt is that the sensor system of this device is specifically designed to detect loose leads and other artifactual causes of "false" V Fib. Elimination of pulse checks does *not* adversely affect the accuracy of these devices for determining whether a particular rhythm is "shockable". It offers the distinct advantage of saving time and minimizing the chance of operator error by allowing the defibrillation cycle (of delivering three successive countershocks) to proceed in an uninterrupted manner.

After *each* series of three successive countershocks is completed, the patient should be reassessed. *Check for the presence (return) of a pulse.* If there is still no pulse- perform CPR for one minute. Then *reassess* the patient again. If pulselessness persists- activate the *analyze control* switch of the AED to again interpret the rhythm. Subsequent management is then determined by whether the patient is still in V Fib- in which case another *stacked* series (of up to 3 successive countershocks) should be initiated. After this the patient is again rechecked (for return of a pulse)- and the cycle restarted if no pulse is found.

> Although no *end point* (i.e., no maximal number of defibrillations) is specified in the algorithm shown in Figure 1A-4- *realistic* chances for ultimate recovery become exceedingly small if the patient has not responded after nine shocks (i.e., after completion of three series of 3 successive countershocks). How long to continue *beyond this point* is a matter of judgement . . . . .

Special Points in the AED Treatment Protocol

- If at any time during the course of treatment (in Figure 1A-4) the patient *regains* a pulse (and perfusing rhythm)- management priorities should change. In this case, the patient should be *reevaluated,* with attention directed at assessing and supporting the ***ABCs*** (***A****irway*/***B****reathing*/***C****irculation*)- and implementing specific treatment/medication as appropriate for the heart rate, blood pressure, and the cardiac rhythm.
- If V Fib later recurs- restart the treatment protocol sequence.
- If the patient remains persistently pulseless, but the AED does *not* initiate/advise defibrillation- the rhythm is most likely asystole. CPR should be restarted (since the patient is pulseless). Realistic chances for ultimate surival are small.
- Persistent display of a *"No Shock indicated"* message does *not* necessarily mean persistence of a nonshockable, pulseless rhythm of cardiac arrest (such as asystole). ***R****eturn* ***O****f* ***S****pontaneous* ***C****irculation (ROSC) could have occurred in the interim-* despite the fact that the patient may still be unresponsive. Early recognition of ROSC if (and when) it occurs is the reason for inserting *periodic* ***pulse checks*** after each minute's performance of CPR (and after completion of each series of consecutive shocks). Return of a pulse clearly negates the need for subsequent countershock (assuming the pulse persists).
- Once ACLS providers arrive on the scene, they should take over care. Ideally, this will be done in a *coordinated* manner with the AED operators already present who had initiated the resuscitation effort. Shocks already delivered by AED operators count as part of the ACLS protocol. Initially, ACLS providers should continue to use the AED for rhythm monitoring and delivery of any additional shocks that may be needed. Changeover to a conventional defibrillator should only be made if (after) the patient regains a spontaneous rhythm, at the time of transport, and/or if the ACLS provider suspects AED malfunction.

> **Note**- By way of perspective, AHA Guidelines emphasize that *"resuscitation attempts in which AEDs are used are relatively simple- because there are fewer therapeutic options".* That is- only automated defibrillation and basic CPR can be implemented (AHA Text- Pg 4-11).

<u>Section 1B:</u> *V Fib/Pulseless VT*

By far, the most common precipitating mechanism of cardiopulmonary arrest in adults is V Fib/Pulseless VT. Depending on the setting of the arrest (i.e., *inside* or *outside* of the hospital)- and depending on what criteria are used to identify the *precipitating mechanism* (i.e., the initial rhythm documented by hospital or EMS personnel)- ***V Fib*** or ***Pulseless VT*** may be found on arrival at the scene in up to 80% of nontraumatic cardiac arrests in adults.

Overall Perspective on the Initial Mechanism

AHA Guidelines emphasize the following *KEY* points about the *initial* moments (and rhythm responsible) for cardiac arrest in adults:

- In addition to being the most common precipitating mechanism of cardiac arrest in adults- V Fib/Pulseless VT is also a potentially treatable mechanism. In contrast, the finding of bradycardia/asystole as the initial mechanism of out-of-hospital cardiac arrest is almost uniformly associated with a dismal long-term prognosis *regardless* of what interventions are undertaken.

> **Note**- Implicit in defining the ***"initial"*** **mechanism** of arrest for any given patient is the time interval between patient collapse and EMS arrival on the scene. The longer this interval- the greater the chance that the *true* initial rhythm will have already deteriorated to a flat line recording. The figures we cite above for the incidence of V Fib/Pulseless VT imply relatively rapid arrival on the scene by EMS personnel (usually *before* deterioration to asystole has occurred).

- For practical purposes, the finding of either ***V Fib*** or ***Pulseless VT*** as the initial mechanism of arrest has similar prognostic and therapeutic implications. The treatment of choice for both conditions is immediate defibrillation.
- By far, the single *most* important intervention in adult emergency cardiac care is defibrillation. Regardless of the setting in which cardiac arrest occurs (i.e., *home- community-* or in the *hospital*)- successful adult resuscitation depends most often on *early* defibrillation.

> **Bottom Line**- The *sooner* a patient in V Fib/Pulseless VT is defibrillated- the *better* the chance for long-term survival.

- Outside of the hospital setting, it would seem that the most practical (and effective) way to implement *rapid* defibrillation is by increasing emphasis on use of the ***AED***- both by professional rescuers, as well as by the lay public.

Treatment Algorithm: *Initial Actions*

In Figure 1B-1 we illustrate the *initial* approach recommended by AHA Guidelines for the patient who is found in ***V Fib/Pulseless VT***. Note that the algorithm assumes ***the rhythm is real*** (i.e., that the patient is *truly* pulseless- and that the ECG recording is *not* the result of artifact).

- Although not shown in Figure 1B-1- resuscitative efforts routinely begin with the ***Universal Algorithm*** (Figure 1A-1)- in which *responsiveness* of the victim is first assessed and the ***ABCs*** (of *Airway/Breathing/Circulation*) are attended to.
- While CPR is being performed- a defibrillator should be immediately sought. The patient is defibrillated *as soon as* V Fib/Pulseless VT is confirmed.
- All efforts should be directed at *expediting* the process of identifying V Fib/Pulseless VT- and then proceeding immediately with defibrillation. Use of ***quick-look* paddles** facilitates rapid implementation of this process. When available, quick-look paddles should be applied *before* attempts are made either at intubation or at securing IV access. This holds true *not only* for cardiopulmonary arrests that occur in the field- but also for those that take place in the hospital or emergency department when the patient is not being monitored. Immediate application of quick-look paddles by hospital personnel may save precious seconds that ultimately determine whether or not the resuscitation effort will be successful.
- Use of a ***precordial thump*** is *no longer* encouraged when a defibrillator is nearby. AHA Guidelines advise that "it makes more sense to go *directly* to that therapy (i.e., defibrillation)- than to waste even a minimum of time with the thump (AHA Text- Pg 1-15).
- The protocol for treatment of V Fib/Pulseless VT described in Figure 1B-1 is different if rescuers have immediate access to an ***AED***. In this case (as emphasized in Figure 1A-3)- application and activation of the AED is *immediately* indicated *as soon as* rescuers determine that the patient is in full cardiac arrest.

Initial Series of Countershocks

The recommended energy level for the **1st countershock attempt** in adults remains at **200 joules**. If this shock is ineffective in converting the patient out of V Fib/Pulseless VT- a **2nd shock** should be given using using an energy level of between **200-300 joules**. If V Fib/Pulseless VT persists- a **3rd shock** should be given, this time using full energy (i.e., **360 joules**) for this third shock in the series (AHA Text- Pg 1-15).

- AHA Guidelines recommend delivery of countershocks in ***"stacked"* sequence** (i.e., *one right after another*) for the *initial* defibrillation series. Thus, rescuers should *not* pause to check for a pulse between countershock attempts. Minimizing the time between shock attempts in this manner helps to ensure rapid delivery of the initial defibrillation series. It also reduces TTR (*TransThoracic Resistance*) of the victim's chest wall- and therefore allows a greater amount of *current* to pass through the victim's heart with the 2nd shock (*See Section 2D*).

Figure 1B-1- *Treatment Algorithm for V Fib/Pulseless VT (Initial Approach)*

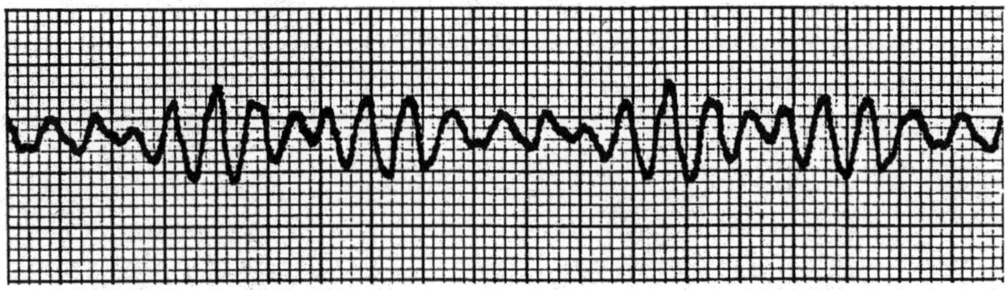

Initial Actions:

- ABCs/Perform CPR until defibrillator attached/Confirm V Fib.
- **Shock** (up to ***3 times*** in *stacked* sequence- *if/as needed*) for persistent V Fib/Pulseless VT:
    - Use energy levels of **200j**- **200-300j**- and then **360 joules**.

> ***NOTE***- *NO pulse check is needed between shocks that are given in stacked sequence!*

If V Fib/Pulseless VT persists:

- Continue CPR/Intubate/Establish IV access.
- **Epinephrine:**
    - Use an **SDE** dose (i.e., **1.0 mg** by IV bolus) initially.
    - May *either* repeat SDE (every 3-5 minutes- if/as needed)-
        - or *increase* the dose (i.e., to **HDE**) if there has been no response, choosing between several HDE regimens:

i) *"Intermediate"* dose Epinephrine = **2-5 mg** IV boluses

- OR -

ii) *Escalating* **1- 3- 5 mg** IV boluses

- OR -

iii) Dosing at **0.1 mg/kg** as an IV bolus.

- **Shock** (within 30-60 seconds after 1st Epinephrine dose):
    - Use *either* **360j** as a *single* shock- *or* may again shock in *stacked sequence* (with another series of 3 successive shocks at 200-360j).

> ***NOTE***- *Use of stacked shocks would be especially appropriate at this time- IF administration of medication is delayed.*

- AHA Guidelines now allow for *continued* delivery of shock attempts in *stacked* sequence- even *after* delivery of the first three shocks. Continued use of *stacked* shocks in "sets" of three (with energies from 200-360 joules) might be especially appropriate for treatment of patients with persistent V Fib when administration of medication is delayed (AHA Test- Pg 1-18).

- Although AHA Guidelines allow for a ***range*** (i.e., *between* 200-300 joules) as the accepted energy for the **2nd shock**- we generally prefer to use the higher level (i.e., **300 joules**). Routinely increasing the energy level within a given series of shocks provides the advantage of a "greater and more predictable increase in current" (AHA Text- Pg 4-6). The reason for increasing energy further (i.e., to 360 joules) for the 3rd shock attempt is that some patients only respond to defibrillation with maximal energy.

- As noted above, ***pulse checks*** are *no longer recommended* in between shocks of a stacked series- provided that rescuers can be *confident* that the monitor is correctly hooked up, and that the rhythm being displayed is *truly* V Fib (AHA Text- Pg 1-15). Instead of inserting pulse checks, all efforts should be directed at confirming that the rhythm displayed *continues* to be V Fib- and then delivering *successive* shocks in a series *as rapidly as possible.*

Use of a *"Clearing Chant"*

AHA Guidelines emphasize the importance of having rescuers call out (in a loud, firm voice) some form of ***"Clearing Chant"*** prior to each defibrillation attempt. An example of an appropriate chant might consist of the following (AHA Text- Pg 1-8):

"I am going to shock on the count of three.
One- I'm clear . . .
Two- you're clear . . .
Three- everybody's clear." At this point the shock is delivered.

Ensuring the safety of everyone involved in the resuscitation effort is essential- and a primary responsibility of the team leader. Routine use of a clearing chant (as suggested above)- in which defibrillation is *not* carried out until the rescuer with the paddles makes absolutely certain that no one is in contact with the patient, the bed, or the equipment- will greatly assist in achieving this goal.

If V Fib/Pulseless VT Persists- *Use of Epinephrine*

If V Fib persists after the 3rd countershock attempt, other measures should be tried. These include resumption of CPR- attempting to *intubate* the patient and establish *IV access*- and hooking the patient up to a monitor. *A trial of medications is now in order.*

- ***Epinephrine*** is the drug of first choice for treatment of cardiac arrest. It is important to emphasize that the most important action of this drug during cardiopulmonary resuscitation is *not* a result of its potent chronotropic and inotropic (beta-adrenergic) effects- but rather from its vasoconstrictor (or alpha-adrenergic) effect, that leads to enhancement of coronary and cerebral flow in the arrested heart.

- Epinephrine may be administered either *intravenously* ***(IV)*** or *endotracheally* ***(ET)***- depending on which route of access is established first. Although IV administration of drug is preferable- one should *not* hesitate to use the ET route if this is the only access available for drug delivery.

- Use ***S**tandard-**D**ose **E**pinephrine (SDE)* first- giving **1.0 mg** of drug (or 10 ml of a 1:10,000 soln.) by **IV bolus**.

- The effect of an IV bolus of Epinephrine peaks in about 2-3 minutes. As a result, the drug should probably be repeated *at least* every 3-5 minutes- for as long as the patient remains in cardiac arrest.

- AHA Guidelines allow for *flexibility* in Epinephrine dosing if the patient fails to respond to the initial SDE dose (AHA Text- Pg 1-16). One may therefore *either* repeat the 1 mg SDE dose in 3-5 minutes (and continue thereafter as needed with 1 mg doses)- ***or** choose between several **H**igh-**D**ose **alternative** regimens.* These include:

i) Administration of **2-5 mg** IV boluses (which AHA Guidelines describe as *"intermediate"* dose Epinephrine)

- OR -

ii) *Escalating* **1- 3- 5 mg** IV boluses

- OR -

iii) Dosing at **0.1 mg/kg** as an IV bolus.

Flexibility in Epinephrine dosing is best illustrated by the AHA statement that- *"Use of higher doses of Epinephrine **(HDE)** can NEITHER be recommended NOR discouraged"* (AHA Text- Pg 7-4). Thus, after the initial SDE dose is given- the amount of Epinephrine for subsequent dosing is at the discretion of the treating clinician(s).

- If Epinephrine is given by the ***ET route***- AHA Guidelines advise using 2-2.5 times the recommended IV dose (i.e, **2-2.5 mg** of 1:10,000 soln). This amount of drug is instilled down the ET tube- and then followed with several forceful insufflations of the Ambu bag.

Additional Defibrillation Attempts

Following administration of Epinephrine- another (i.e., **4th**) **shock** should be given in an attempt to convert the patient out of V Fib/Pulseless VT. Maximal energy (i.e., **360 joules**) should be used for this 4th countershock attempt.

- In general, rescuers should wait about 30-60 seconds (at least) following administration of medication (such as Epinephrine or Lidocaine) *before* proceeding with defibrillation. During this time CPR is performed in the hope of circulating the medication for optimal effect prior to defibrillation.

- As noted earlier, AHA Guidelines now allow for *continued* delivery of shock attempts in *stacked* sequence- even *after* delivery of the first three shocks. Thus, the team leader might either decide on delivery of a 4th shock (with 360 joules) at this time- or on delivery of a *second* set of three more shocks (with 200-360 joules) *without* any pause between shock attempts for a pulse check.

Refractory V Fib: *Medications of Probable Benefit*

V Fib/Pulseless VT that fails to respond to the measures described in Figure 1B-1 is referred to as ***"refractory"***. Lack of response to an initial defibrillation series (of 3 successive shocks), intubation and ventilation, administration of Epinephrine, and a 4th (or 4th, 5th, and 6th) shock is indication for a trial of ***antifibrillatory* therapy** (Figure 1B-2).

- ***Lidocaine*** is generally accepted as the *initial* antifibrillatory agent of choice for medical treatment of refractory V Fib. The recommended dose is **1.0-1.5 mg/kg** (≈50-150 mg) as an *initial* IV bolus- which may then be repeated in 3-5 minutes. Alternatively- AHA Guidelines now allow for administration of a ***single* IV dose** of **1.5 mg/kg** (or ≈100-150 mg) in cardiac arrest.

- Following administration of Lidocaine- *defibrillation* should be repeated (using 360 joules). Wait at least 30-60 seconds after giving the drug before shocking- during which time CPR is performed (in the hope of allowing the drug adequate opportunity to reach the central circulation).

- If V Fib persists after giving Lidocaine- consider the use of ***Bretylium***. Although administration of Bretylium rarely results in spontaneous conversion of V Fib to sinus rhythm- the drug *is* effective as an antifibrillatory agent, and its use may facilitate conversion to sinus rhythm with subsequent countershocks.

- The recommended *initial* IV dose of ***Bretylium*** for treatment of refractory V Fib is a bolus of 5 mg/kg. Considering the empiric nature of dosing in the setting of cardiac arrest (and in the interest of facilitating calculations in this situation)- we favor administration of one complete ampule (= **500 mg**) for the initial **IV bolus** (rather than strict calculation on a bodyweight basis). Circulate the drug (by performing CPR) for 30-60 seconds after giving Bretylium- and then *defibrillate* the patient again.

- If the initial bolus of Bretylium fails to convert the rhythm- a *second* IV bolus of ***Bretylium*** (now using 10 mg/kg- or ≈1-2 ampules) may be tried several minutes later. Additional (10 mg/kg) boluses of Bretylium may be given as needed (up to a total dose of 30-35 mg/kg).

> **Note**- Lidocaine and Bretylium appear to be of *comparable* clinical efficacy as antifibrillatory agents for the treatment of refractory V Fib. The reason why Lidocaine is listed first by AHA Guidelines is that emergency personnel are generally more familiar (and comfortable) with use of this drug. In addition, Lidocaine is faster acting (and probably safer) than Bretylium when used in the setting of cardiac arrest (AHA Text- Pg 1-19).

Figure 1B-2- *Treatment Algorithm for Refractory V Fib* *(Continued from Figure 1B-1)*

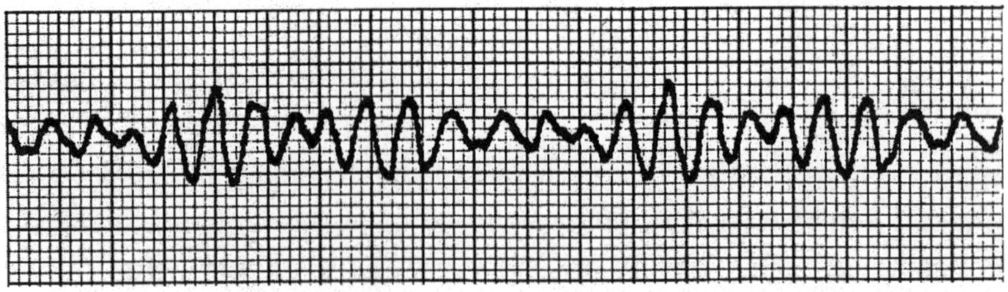

Persistence of V Fib/Pulseless VT

- The patient has *not* responded to:

  - *Shock* (X3)- *Intubation* (and ventilation)-
  - *Epinephrine*- and *shock* again

> This defines the condition as ***refractory* V Fib**. A trial of ***antifibrillatory* therapy** is now in order.

❖ Consider ***Medications*** *of* ***Probable Benefit***:

- **Lidocaine:**
  - Give **1.0-1.5 mg/kg** (≈50-150 mg) as an initial bolus by IV push. May repeat in 3-5 minutes- *although a single dose* (at 1.5 mg/kg) *IS acceptable in cardiac arrest.*
  - Resume CPR for 30-60 seconds after giving Lidocaine- *then shock again.*

> AHA Guidelines recommend ***Lidocaine*** as the *antifibrillatory agent of choice* for treatment of refractory V Fib. The drug need *not* be given as a continuous IV infusion- *until* the patient is converted out of V Fib (at which time a ***prophylactic* IV infusion** should be started).

IF Lidocaine is ineffective- then consider:

- **Bretylium:**
  - Give 5 mg/kg (*or* a single **500 mg** IV bolus ≈**1 amp**)- resume CPR for 30-60 seconds- *and then shock again.*
  - A 2nd IV bolus (of 10 mg/kg- *or* ≈1-2 amps) may be given in 5 minutes if V Fib persists (up to a total dose of 30-35 mg/kg).

- May also use **Magnesium**:
  - Give **1-2 gm** by IV push- especially for patients with *known* (or suspected) *hypomagnesemia* and/or *Torsade de Pointes.*

- Search for a ***Cause*** of the Arrest (i.e., ***D****ifferential* ***D****iagnosis*)
- Consideration of ***Other Measures*** (See text)

- When ***Lidocaine*** is used to treat refractory V Fib- if a single IV bolus fails to work, in most cases a second IV bolus will *not* fare much better. As a result, despite allowance by AHA Guidelines for repetition of the Lidocaine dose- we generally prefer to limit Lidocaine administration to a *single* IV bolus while the patient is in V Fib. Instead of additional Lidocaine, we favor consideration of *other* therapeutic measures (i.e., a trial of Bretylium and/or Magnesium) at this time. Another reason to move on to Bretylium if a single IV bolus of Lidocaine fails to convert V Fib is that *combined* use of these drugs may result in a *synergistic* antifibrillatory effect (AHA Text- Pg 7-7).

- Remember when using ***Bretylium*** that the onset of action of this drug may be *delayed* for at least a few minutes if treating V Fib- and for *up to* 10-20 minutes if treating VT! It is therefore important *not* to abandon resuscitative efforts until the drug has adequate opportunity to work.

> **Note**- Because clearance of Lidocaine is markedly decreased in the arrested heart- continuous IV infusion of the drug need *not* be started for as long as the patient remains in V Fib. However, *as soon as* the patient is converted *out of* V Fib- Lidocaine pharmacokinetics will change. As a result, a ***prophylactic*** IV infusion of ***Lidocaine*** (and/or Bretylium) should be started as soon as possible in the hope of preventing recurrence (*See Page 43*).

Use of *Magnesium* for Refractory V Fib

The role of Magnesium Sulfate in the treatment of cardiac arrest has not been completely clarified. As a result, use of the drug in this setting is still largely empiric. Although one might intuitively expect patients with low serum magnesium levels to benefit most from this form of therapy- serum levels do *not* necessarily correlate with body stores of this cation. Moreover, a beneficial antiarrhythmic effect has clearly been shown to occur in some patients *despite* normal serum magnesium levels at the time of administration. We therefore suggest consideration of the following *KEY* points with regard to ***Magnesium*** administration:

- Magnesium should clearly be given to patients in cardiac arrest who are *known* to be hypomagnesemic (AHA Text- Pg 1-20). It should also be given to hypomagnesemic patients who have cardiac arrhythmias- especially when these arrhythmias have been refractory to other treatment.

- Magnesium is the medical treatment of choice for Torsade de Pointes.

- Serum magnesium levels do *not* tell the whole story. Serum levels merely reflect *extracellular* magnesium. Because the overwhelming majority of body magnesium stores are contained within the *intracellular* compartment- the serum level may sometimes be normal despite significant *intracellular* (and *intramyocardial*) magnesium depletion.

- Certain clinical conditions are commonly associated with *intracellular* magnesium depletion- *regardless* of whether or not the serum magnesium level falls within the normal range. These conditions include:

  - *other electrolyte abnormalities* (especially hypokalemia, hyponatremia, hypocalcemia, and hypophosphatemia)
  - acute myocardial infarction and cardiac arrest
  - patients receiving Digoxin or diuretic therapy
  - patients with a history of alcohol abuse or renal impairment

- Practically speaking, the risk of toxicity from giving Magnesium Sulfate to a patient in cardiac arrest is *minimal* (if not negligible)- even if prearrest serum magnesium levels are normal. As a result, we feel that ***empiric* administration** of this drug *is reasonable* in life-threatening clinical situations- especially if standard measures have already been tried and failed. Empiric administration of Magnesium is reasonable when the serum level of this cation is *either* unavailable or normal in such situations.

- Empiric administration of Magnesium is also reasonable (and should be strongly considered) for treatment of potentially life-threatening conditions in which *suspicion* of hypomagnesemia may be high (AHA Text- Pg 1-20). This includes those clinical conditions listed above that are commonly associated with intracellular magnesium depletion.

- Dosing of ***Magnesium Sulfate*** is largely empiric. When used to treat V Fib- AHA Guidelines recommend giving **1-2 g** of the drug by **IV push** (AHA Text- Pg 1-20). This dose may be repeated in 5-10 minutes if there is no response. More gradual dosing (i.e., giving 1-2 g over several minutes, or longer) is suggested for treatment of cardiac arrhythmias with less immediate hemodynamic consequences. This may be followed (if/as needed) by continuous IV infusion of 500-1,000 mg per hour for up to 24 hours. AHA Guidelines emphasize the point that *higher* doses of Magnesium (of up to 5-10 grams!) have been used with success in the treatment of some patients with Torsade de Pointes (AHA Text- Pg 7-14).

Search for a *Potentially Correctable* Cause of V Fib

Persistence of V Fib at this point in the code should prompt consideration of other factors that could account for the patient's refractory condition. This might include a problem with the ***ABC*s** (i.e., a nonpatent airway, asymmetric or absent breath sounds, lack of a pulse with CPR)- and/or some other predisposing cause.

- ***Potentially correctable*** predisposing causes of refractory V Fib were discussed in Section 1A under the "**D**" component (i.e., ***D**ifferential **D**iagnosis*) of the ***Secondary Survey***. Important causes to consider include underlying metabolic disturbance (such as diabetic ketoacidosis or hyperkalemia), hypothermia, hypovolemia, drug overdose (especially of cocaine, tricyclic antidepressants, or narcotics)- and/or development of a complication of CPR (such as tension pneumothorax or pericardial tamponade).

- V Fib may also be the end result (i.e., *caused* by) many other kinds of processes- such as cardiogenic shock (from extensive myocardial infarction), massive pulmonary embolism, ruptured aortic aneurysm, or severe trauma with exsanguinating hemorrhage. Practically speaking- specific diagnosis of these types of conditions is much *less* important clinically because of the *improbability* that V Fib resulting from *any* of these conditions will be amenable to *any* form of treatment at this point in the code.

> **<u>Bottom Line</u>-** Although a predisposing, potentially correctable cause of refractory V Fib will *not* be found in most cases of cardiac arrest- it is still important to *always* keep this possibility in mind because:
>
> i) Cardiac arrest *may be* potentially reversible if it is caused by a predisposing factor that can be corrected.
>
> ii) If a predisposing cause does exist- standard treatment measures are *unlikely* to be successful unless (and *until*) that predisposing cause can be identified *and* corrected.

<u>Refractory V Fib: *Other Measures to Consider*</u>

Clinically, it may be helpful to realize that if V Fib persists *despite* implementation of the actions listed in Figures 1B-1 and 1B-2- that remaining therapeutic options are relatively limited. *There simply is not that much more that can be done.* At this point in the process, we suggest consideration of the following measures:

- *Continuing* ***Epinephrine.*** Recovery from prolonged cardiopulmonary arrest is unlikely unless coronary perfusion pressure (CPP) is adequate (i.e., ≥15 mm Hg). In the arrested heart- it appears that Epinephrine is needed in *sufficient amount* to achieve such pressures. As a result, the drug should be repeated *at least* every 3-5 minutes for as long as the patient remains in cardiac arrest. Consideration might also be given to the use of *higher* doses of drug (i.e., ***HDE***) if the patient fails to respond to SDE doses (*See Section 2B*).

- *Considering* **Sodium Bicarbonate.** Although Sodium Bicarbonate has been freely used in the past for the treatment of cardiac arrest, recent data strongly question this practice. In fact, a strong case could be made for *never* administering any Sodium Bicarbonate at all during cardiopulmonary resuscitation- *regardless* of what the pH value happens to be. Instead, efforts at correcting acidosis are probably better directed at *optimizing ventilation-* especially during the early minutes of a code when the major component of acidosis is likely to be *respiratory* in nature (from ***hypo****ventilation*). Practically speaking, acceptable indications for use of Sodium Bicarbonate in the setting of cardiac arrest are limited. They include:

  - Severe *metabolic acidosis* (usually to a pH value of *less* than 7.20)- that persists beyond the initial phase (i.e., *beyond* the first 5-15 minutes) of the arrest.
  - Cardiac arrest in a patient *known* to have a severe *preexisting* metabolic acidosis *prior* to the arrest-

    - *<u>IF</u> any Bicarb is indicated at all during cardiac arrest . . . .*

> **<u>Note</u>-** A number of *special* resuscitation situations exist in which use of Bicarb is both appropriate and *likely* to be helpful. These include hyperkalemia and drug overdose with tricyclic antidepressants or phenobarbital (AHA Text- Pg 7-15).

- ***Repeat Countershock** as Needed.* Practically speaking, there is *no limit* to the number of times that a patient can be defibrillated. As long as V Fib persists- a *potentially treatable* situation is present. After every intervention, CPR should be performed (for a period of at least 30-60 seconds) to allow time for drug to reach the central circulation- and this should then be followed by *repeat countershock* (at an energy level of between 200-360 joules)- until there is conclusive evidence of cardiovascular unresponsiveness.

> It is essential to *always* check for a pulse after *every* intervention- and/or *whenever* the rhythm changes on the monitor. Forgetting to do so may result in iatrogenic defibrillation of the patient in sinus rhythm whose monitor leads fell off. (*It will probably also result in your failure of the ACLS course!*) The *only* exception to this rule is between shocks in a given *stacked* defibrillation series.

- *IV **Beta-Blockers**.* The most difficult part about suggesting recommendations for the use of IV beta-blockers in the setting of cardiopulmonary arrest is knowing when to administer these drugs. Clearly, most resuscitation attempts will *not* need IV beta-blockers. However, there *may* be times when all other treatment measures will fail- and *only* IV beta-blockers will save the patient.

  Situations in which the use of an IV beta-blocker is most likely to be potentially lifesaving are those in which excessive *sympathetic* tone is implicated as an important etiologic factor in the arrest. Such situations include a *prearrest* setting of known ischemia and/or acute *anterior* infarction (especially when cardiac arrest is preceded by a period of tachycardia or hypertension); cardiac arrest that occurs in association with drug overdose from either cocaine or amphetamines- and/or a period of severe stress or anxiety during the prearrest period. Empiric use of an IV beta-blocker should be strongly considered if *refractory* V Fib occurs in association with any of these factors- especially if other antiarrhythmic agents have failed (and/or sinus tachycardia appears to precede each recurrence).

  Because of ease of administration and familiarity with its use- ***Propranolol*** is the IV beta-blocker most commonly selected for treatment of patients in cardiac arrest. The recommended dose of this drug is to give **0.5-1.0 mg** by ***slow* IV** administration (i.e., *not to exceed 1 mg/minute!*). This dose may be repeated (if/as needed)- up to a total dose of 3-5 mg. Alternatively- *other* IV beta-blockers could be used instead of Propranolol (*See Section 2B*).

- ***Procainamide**.* AHA Guidelines list Procainamide as a medication "of probable benefit for treatment of persistent/recurrent V Fib". However, they also acknowledge that Procainamide is *rarely* used for this purpose *"because of the prolonged time required to administer effective doses"* (AHA Text- Pg 7-8). We share these reservations about the use of Procainamide as an antifibrillatory agent, and question its efficacy in this setting. *Other* measures should probably be considered first.

- ***Amiodarone**.* Amiodarone is a class III antiarrhythmic agent. Although the drug is remarkably effective as an oral agent in the long-term management of supraventricular and ventricular arrhythmias- experience with use of IV Amiodarone in the setting of cardiac arrest is limited. However, initial experience is encouraging, and it appears that IV Amiodarone may provide a more effective alternative than either Lidocaine or Bretylium for antifibrillatory therapy in this setting.

IV Amiodarone has recently been approved by the FDA for general use. Although *not* yet included in AHA Guidelines- the drug holds promise of fulfilling an important role in the treatment of *refractory* V Fib that has *not* responded to other measures, as well as for the patient in cardiac arrest from recurrent VT who is not able to maintain sinus rhythm with conventional therapy. Time will determine the ultimate role of this newly approved drug (*See Section 2E*).

IF (*As Soon As*) the Patient is Converted *Out of* V Fib

It is important to emphasize the need to *immediately* start a ***prophylactic* IV infusion** of an ***antiarrhythmic* agent** as soon as the patient is converted out of V Fib/Pulseless VT. Failure to do so may result in recurrence of the cardiac arrest. AHA Guidelines advise beginning IV infusion with *that* antiarrhythmic agent *"that appeared to aid in the restoration of a pulse"* (AHA Text- Pg 1-20).

In most cases, the appropriate antiarrhythmic agent to use will be ***Lidocaine***. If bolus therapy has *not* yet been given (and/or if more than 5 minutes have elapsed since the time of the last Lidocaine dose)- then an **IV bolus** (of **50-100 mg**) should also be administered when the IV infusion is started.

- For the patient with a spontaneous rhythm- the usual *range* for an IV infusion of Lidocaine is between 0.5-4 mg/minute. Practically speaking, most patients will be adequately treated at infusion rates of between 1-2 mg/minute.

- Lower infusion rates (of 0.5-1 mg/minute) are advised for patients at greater risk of developing Lidocaine toxicity. Such patients include the elderly and patients with heart failure, liver disease, or shock. In the *absence* of these factors- we suggest ***beginning*** the ***prophylactic* IV infusion** of ***Lidocaine*** at a rate of **2 mg/minute**. To minimize the risk of developing Lidocaine toxicity, we suggest avoidance of higher infusion rates if at all possible (*See Section 2B*).

Lidocaine pharmacokinetics are markedly altered in the arrested heart. As already noted, clearance of the drug is significantly *decreased* in this situation- so that as little as one (or *at most* two) boluses of Lidocaine will usually be enough to maintain adequate therapeutic levels *without* the need for continuous IV infusion. As a result, AHA Guidelines recommend *withholding* initiation of a maintenance IV infusion until *after* the patient is converted out of V Fib (AHA Text- Pg 1-19).

Our practice differs slightly from that recommended by AHA Guidelines. Instead of delaying IV infusion of Lidocaine until after the patient is converted out of V Fib- we prefer to initiate an IV infusion while the patient is *still in* cardiac arrest. Our reason for doing so is that we feel it far simpler to *always* initiate the maintenance infusion *at the same time* the decision is made to administer IV loading boluses- even during the low-flow state of cardiac arrest. Pharmacokinetically, this practice should *not* pose a significant risk of developing drug toxicity- since the amount of drug administered at an infusion rate of 2 mg/minute during a 15- to 30-minute resuscitation effort will not exceed 30 to 60 mg. On the other hand, stopping (or never starting) the Lidocaine infusion during the period of cardiac arrest makes it all too easy to forget to immediately start (or restart) the infusion after conversion out of V Fib- which would substantially increase the risk of recurrence.

> **Bottom Line**- It should be equally acceptable to *either* begin the IV infusion of Lidocaine *while* the patient is still in V Fib- or to *defer* this action until *after* the patient is converted out of V Fib. The point to emphasize is that Lidocaine clearance will markedly increase as soon as the spontaneous circulation has been restored. Therefore, if you choose *not* to begin the Lidocaine maintenance infusion at the time you administer one or more loading boluses of the drug- it is *imperative* to remember to do so *as soon as* the patient is converted *out of* V Fib.

Lidocaine is clearly the most commonly used antifibrillatory agent in the setting of cardiac arrest- as well as the drug most commonly selected for prophylactic IV infusion to prevent V Fib recurrence. However, it should be realized that this drug is *not* necessarily the optimal agent for this purpose in all patients. Although it will often be admittedly difficult in the setting of cardiac arrest to determine which drug(s) or actions are directly responsible for a beneficial (or detrimental) clinical response by the patient- there are times when Lidocaine will fail, and the patient will seemingly *only* be converted out of V Fib after use of ***Bretylium***. In such cases, the *prophylactic* approach to prevent V Fib recurrence may differ from that stated above. We suggest consideration of the following points:

- Because the duration of action from an **IV bolus** of ***Bretylium*** is relatively prolonged (usually lasting 2-6 hours)- some protection against immediate recurrence of V Fib is automatically provided by this form of administration.
- Additional protection against V Fib recurrence may be afforded by starting an IV infusion of ***Lidocaine*** (after appropriate bolus therapy)- *as suggested above.*
- *Alternatively*- selecting a prophylactic **IV infusion** of ***Bretylium*** (at a rate of between **1-2 mg/minute**) may be preferred to Lidocaine when this antifibrillatory agent is effective in converting V Fib after Lidocaine has failed. Rarely, IV infusion of both agents may be needed. As already noted- AHA Guidelines advise use of *that* antiarrhythmic agent *"that appears to aid in the restoration of a pulse"*.

Post-Resuscitation Care

AHA Guidelines use the term ***Post-Resuscitation Care*** to refer to the period *between* ***ROSC*** (*Return Of Spontaneous Circulation*)- and transfer of the patient to the ICU (AHA Text- Pg 1-25). They emphasize that although this period is usually quite brief (ideally *less* than 30 minutes)- proper care during this time is a *critical* determinant of long-term outcome.

> **Note**- By definition, the term ***"Post-Resuscitation" Period*** means that the patient is *no longer* in cardiac arrest. As a result, some recommendations in the ACLS algorithms for treatment (that were designed for patients who are *in* cardiac arrest) may need to be *modified* (AHA Text- Pg 1-25).

- *The algorithms should not be applied in reverse.* That is- tachycardia, bradycardia, and hypotension should *not* be treated the same *after* successful resuscitation (in the postresuscitation state) as is indicated for a patient with imminent cardiac arrest. AHA Guidelines emphasize the point that *most* resuscitation arrhythmias "should be left untreated for the immediate postresuscitation period" (AHA text- Pg 1-25).

The most important actions to implement during the post-resuscitation period involve the ***ABCDs*** of the ***Primary*** and ***Secondary* Surveys**. These actions (discussed in detail in Section 1A) are briefly summarized below:

- ***A**irway-* verify ET tube placement; check for equal bilateral breath sounds; obtain chest X-ray, etc.
- ***B**reathing-* ensure that ventilation is adequate; provide supplemental oxygen; monitor oxygen saturation, and obtain ABGs; etc.
- ***C**irculation-* assess vital signs and clinical parameters of adequate perfusion (i.e., blood pressure, skin color, mental status, etc.); implement ECG monitoring (if not already done); obtain a full 12-lead tracing.
- ***D**ifferential **D**iagnosis-* search for an *identifiable* (and hopefully *correctable*) precipitating *cause* of the arrest.

Additional actions to implement in the post-resuscitation period include:

- Insertion of a Foley catheter; monitoring urine output.
- Insertion of an NG tube; ensuring proper IV access.
- Infusion of IV fluid (as appropriate for the clinical situation).
- Checking essential lab work (i.e., serum electrolytes including magnesium, complete blood count, renal profile, etc.).
- Check the chest X-ray (for assessment of hemodynamic status- as well as ET tube and central line placement).

Additional issues/questions to address in the post-resuscitation period include:

i) Is the patient on a continuous ***prophylactic* IV infusion** of ***Lidocaine*** (or other antiarrhythmic agent) to *prevent* recurrence of VT/V Fib?
ii) What *other* **IV infusions** (that were started *during* the code) are still currently running? *Are these infusions still needed* ?
iii) Is the patient a *candidate* for ***thrombolytic* therapy**? This question is usually answered by review of the patient's 12-lead ECG- looking for evidence of acute infarction with new ST segment elevation. Keep in mind that thrombolytic therapy *may* still be administered even if the patient has received CPR- provided that the period of chest compression was not prolonged (usually 10 minutes or less).

Complete the process. Components of this last step include the following:

i) Being sure the patient's family has been talked to (and that they are satisfied with the explanation of events of the code that was given to them).
ii) Acknowledging the efforts of your co-workers.
iii) Writing a note in the chart.
iv) Notifying the patient's attending physician (if this is not you).
v) Spending a moment to reflect on how things went during the code- *how things might have gone better-* and what you might do differently (if anything) next time.
vi) Updating the patient's code status (in the event that they arrest again).

Note- The items we list above should be performed *regardless* of whether or not the resuscitation effort was successful.

V Fib/Pulseless VT: *Special Situations* in Resuscitation

Special considerations are needed for treatment of cardiac arrest that occurs in association with the following situations (AHA Text- Pg 1-16):

- If a ***Nitroglycerin patch*** is on the victim's chest- remove it *prior* to defibrillation (or at least make sure the defibrillator paddle does *not* touch the patch). Practically speaking, the nitroglycerin in the patch will not "explode"- although it may *smoke*, produce *visible arcing*, or *burn* the patient if it comes in contact with the electrical discharge.
- If the victim has either an *implanted* ***pacemaker*** or ***ICD*** *(Implanted Cardioverter-Defibrillator)*- *avoid* placement of the defibrillator paddles or pads directly over (or close to) the generator unit. Passage of current in close proximity to the unit may severely damage or lead to misprogramming of the device.
- If the victim is ***hypothermic***- continued defibrillation (i.e., *after* the initial series of the first 3 shocks) is *not* indicated. Instead, the hypothermic victim who remains in V Fib/Pulseless VT should be **rewarmed** *before* delivery of additional shocks.

> In our experience- body temperature is the most *neglected* vital sign in the setting of cardiac arrest. Typically, no mention at all is made in the resuscitation record of the patient's body temperature either before or during the arrest. Be aware that ***hypothermia*** occurs more often than is commonly appreciated- and may be unsuspected. Hypothermia may occur even in warm weather states during warm weather months- especially if the patient is predisposed to developing hypothermia (because of being elderly, debilitated, alcoholic, and/or septic).

Addendum: ECC for the Adult who is *NOT* in *full* Cardiac Arrest

Cardiopulmonary conditions that are considered within the category described by the heading of this paragraph are those in which the patient is *not* yet in full cardiac arrest- but which *"if not diagnosed and managed correctly- could lead to cardiac arrest within 30 to 60 minutes"* (AHA Text- Pg 1-27). Examples include certain problematic *cardiac arrhythmias* (that may either be *"too fast"* or *"too slow"*)- *Acute MI- hypotension* (from *whatever* cause)- *cardiogenic shock*- and *pulmonary edema.* The suggested initial approach to evaluation and management of these conditions is reflected in the ***left-sided*** **branch** of the ***Universal Algorithm*** (*See Figure 1A-1*).

> **Note**- The ***Universal Algorithm*** is an invaluable tool for assessing the patient with an acute cardiopulmonary emergency. As emphasized in Figure 1A-1- ***If a pulse IS present***- then by definition, the patient is *not* in full cardiac arrest! Management decisions now follow the *left-sided* branch of this algorithm:

- ***Ventilation*** *may or may not be adequate.* The *KEY* is to *immediately* assess the adequacy of breathing and ventilation- *to provide whatever support is needed* (i.e., rescue breathing, intubation, etc.)- and then to *reassess* the patient on a frequent basis.

- Additional ***Critical Actions*** to consider/perform include:

  - **O**xygen-**I**V-**M**onitor.
  - Obtain and closely follow vital signs (for stability or changes).
  - Review the patient's history/medical chart.
  - Perform targeted physical exam.
  - Obtain 12-lead ECG.

- Attempt to determine the ***Suspected Cause*** of the cardiopulmonary emergency (based on the above initial evaluation). Realize that causal conditions are often complex and may overlap.

  - Arrhythmia- *"Too FAST"* (*See Section 1C*).
  - Arrhythmia- *"Too SLOW"* (*See Section 1D*).
  - *Acute MI/hypotension/shock/acute pulmonary edema.*
  - *Other* condition (i.e., a *non-cardiac* cause).

Section 1C: *Tachycardia*

The goal of this section is to present an overall approach to evaluation and management of the patient with ***tachycardia.*** Although *supraventricular* and *ventricular* tachyarrhythmias are *not* usually grouped together- doing so allows the broadest overview of the clinical situations that are likely to be encountered.

Simplified Rhythm Classification

AHA Guidelines suggest that for practical purposes, rhythm interpretation in the emergency care setting can be simplified by separating cardiac rhythms into *two* basic types: 1) rhythms that are considered as ***"lethal"*** ; and 2) rhythms that are ***"not lethal"*** (AHA Text- Pg 1-28). An advantage of this simplified classification is that a total of *only* six basic cardiac rhythms need be considered (Table 1C-1):

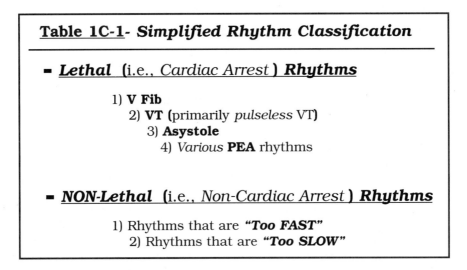

Table 1C-1- *Simplified Rhythm Classification*

- ***Lethal*** (i.e., *Cardiac Arrest*) ***Rhythms***

1) **V Fib**
2) **VT** (primarily *pulseless* VT)
3) **Asystole**
4) *Various* **PEA** rhythms

- ***NON-Lethal*** (i.e., *Non-Cardiac Arrest*) ***Rhythms***

1) Rhythms that are ***"Too FAST"***
2) Rhythms that are ***"Too SLOW"***

As can be seen from Table 1C-1, there are *four* basic types of ***lethal rhythms*** (i.e., rhythms *associated* with cardiac arrest)- and *two* basic types of ***non-lethal rhythms*** (i.e., rhythms *not* associated with cardiac arrest).

Note- According to the simplified rhythm classification- AHA Guidelines describe a rhythm as ***"too FAST"*** if the rate *exceeds* **120 beats/minute** (*regardless* of whether or not the QRS complex is wide). In contrast, a rhythm is described as ***"too SLOW"*** if the rate is *less* than **60 beats/minute.**

Semantics/Definitions of *KEY* Terms

A word on clarification of the terms ***"tachycardia"*** and ***"bradycardia"*** is in order- especially with regard to understanding the correlation between these terms and designation of a rhythm as being either *"too FAST"* or *"too SLOW"*.

- Technically- the term ***"tachycardia"*** refers to rhythms in which the heart rate is **100 beats/minute** or greater. Note that this definition allows for a range of rates *between* 100-119 beats/minute within which a rhythm technically qualifies as being a "tachycardia" (in that it is *faster* than 100 beats/minute)- but at a rate that should *not* be ***"too FAST"*** (i.e., *below* 120 beats/minute) according to the simplified system that we have just introduced.

> We emphasize that even if a rhythm is *"too FAST"* according to this system (i.e., *more* than 120 beats/minute)- that specific treatment (for rate control or conversion of the rhythm) will *not* necessarily be needed in all cases. AHA Guidelines suggest that a major reason for thinking about a rate "cutoff" point is that rhythms *below* this rate (i.e., *less* than 120 beats/minute) are clinically *unlikely* to require *emergent* medical therapy for rate control.

A commonly occurring arrhythmia that illustrates the above principle is *AIVR* (*Accelerated IdioVentricular Rhythm*). Despite the fact that this is a *ventricular* rhythm- the ventricular rate with AIVR generally does *not* exceed 100-110 beats/minute. Clinically, most patients with this rhythm are hemodynamically stable- *and no specific treatment is needed.*

- The term ***"bradycardia"*** technically refers to rhythms in which the heart rate is *below* **60 beats/minute**. Note that this is the same rate cited in the *simplified* classification for describing a rhythm as ***"too SLOW"*** .
- An additional term- ***"relative bradycardia"*** - is used to refer to those rhythms that are faster than 60 beats/minute but still *inappropriately SLOW* for the clinical situation at hand. For example, a patient in shock will normally develop a tachycardia in an attempt to compensate for the drop in blood pressure. Although a heart rate of 70 beats/minute does *not* technically qualify as "bradycardia" in such a patient- this rate is still *inappropriately* slow (i.e., a *"relative"* bradycardia)- given the clinical setting of shock and marked hypotension.

Assessing the Clinical Significance of an Arrhythmia

Even more important than the rate parameters cited above is the ***clinical condition*** of the patient. Thus, the most *critical* question to ask after determining the rate of a *non-lethal* rhythm is the following:

> *Is the rhythm causing the patient problems as a* ***direct result*** *of the rate ?*
>
> In other words-
>
> - *Is the rhythm* ***hemodynamically*** **significant** ?

A brady- or tachyarrhythmia *becomes* hemodynamically significant- IF the rhythm produces *serious* ***signs*** or ***symptoms*** as a *direct result* of the reduction (or increase) in heart rate. For the purpose of this definition:

- ***Signs of Concern***- include hypotension (i.e., systolic BP ≤80-90 mm Hg), shock, heart failure/pulmonary edema, and/or Acute MI.

- ***Symptoms of Concern***- include chest pain, shortness of breath, and/or decreased mental status.

It is important to emphasize that the definition of *hemodynamic stability* is equally applicable for *SUPRAventricular* tachyarrhythmias- as it is for VT. Thus, a patient with tachycardia who is hypotensive, having chest pain, and mentally confused is probably in need of immediate cardioversion- *regardless* of what the rhythm happens to be. On the other hand, if the patient with tachycardia is *asymptomatic* (i.e., normotensive and *without* chest pain, shortness of breath, or mental confusion)- then there probably is time for more careful evaluation and a trial of medical treatment.

> ***KEY***- *Not all patients with sustained ventricular tachycardia are (or immediately become) hemodynamically unstable* ! In fact, some patients with VT are able to remain alert and maintain an adequate blood pressure for minutes, hours (*and even days!*)- *without* showing any signs of decompensation.

With this as an introduction, we delve into the various tachycardia rhythms and specific algorithms for evaluation and treatment . . . .

The *Overview* Algorithm for Tachycardia

In Figure 1C-1 we illustrate the initial *overall* approach recommended by AHA Guidelines for the patient who is found in ***Tachycardia.*** Note that this algorithm assumes that the tachycardia *IS* associated with a pulse!

- ***If there was NO Pulse***- then the rhythm shown in Figure 1C-1 would have to be interpreted as *pulseless* VT. As emphasized in Section 1B- ***Pulseless VT*** should be treated in the identical manner as ***V Fib*** with *immediate* defibrillation (i.e., *unsynchronized* countershock).

> **Note**- Although *not* specifically shown in Figure 1C-1, evaluation of the patient routinely begins with the ***Universal Algorithm*** (Figure 1A-1)- in which *responsiveness* of the victim is first assessed and the ***ABCs*** are attended to. Other ***Supportive Actions*** listed are implemented at the earliest appropriate opportunity (depending on resources and the number and skills of available rescuers).

- Given that a pulse *is* present in association with the rhythm shown in Figure 1C-1- the patient (by definition) is *not* in full cardiac arrest. The *KEY* to management now lies with determining if the patient is hemodynamically stable.

Figure 1C-1- *Overview Algorithm for Tachycardia*

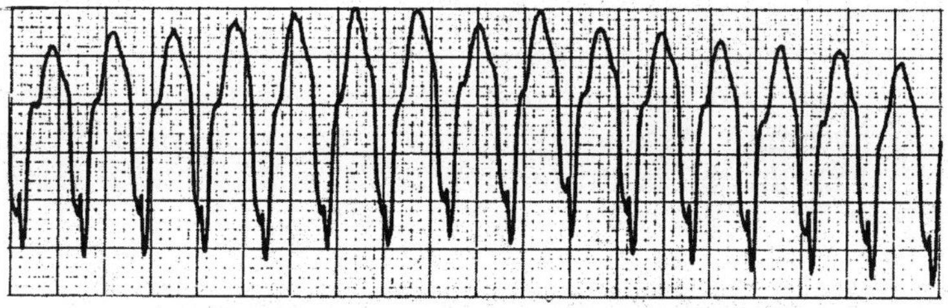

The Algorithm below assumes that the tachycardia *IS* associated with a pulse. (***Pulseless VT*** would be treated as ***V Fib***- *See Figure 1B-1 on page 34*).

- *Supportive Actions*
  - Assess the ABCs/Secure airway/Ventilate/Intubate if needed
  - **O**xygen-**I**V-**M**onitor/Attach pulse oximeter
  - Review the pt's history/medical chart
  - Perform targeted physical exam
  - Obtain 12-lead ECG/Obtain portable chest X-ray

Is the Pt ***Hemodynamically UNSTABLE*** *?*

- Is the rhythm producing *serious* ***signs*** or ***symptoms*** as a *direct result* of the increase in heart rate ?

No

NO Serious Signs or Sx

- Subsequent management depends on the ***specific diagnosis*** of the tachyarrhythmia

Yes

Serious Signs/Sx ARE Present !

- Consider the need for *immediate* ***Synchronized Cardioversion*** !

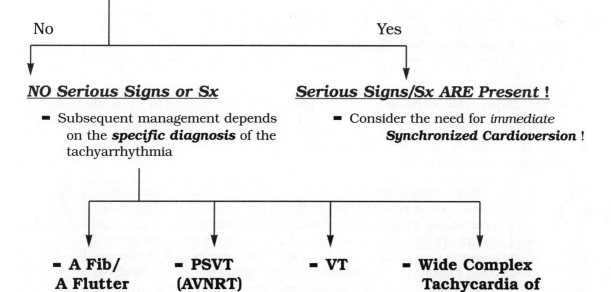

- A Fib/ A Flutter

- PSVT (AVNRT)

- VT

- Wide Complex Tachycardia of *Uncertain* Type

- ***If the patient IS hemodynamically STABLE***. If the rhythm is *not* producing any serious signs or symptoms as a result of the rapid rate- then the patient is said to be hemodynamically stable. In this situation it is reasonable to initiate a trial of antiarrhythmic therapy. Subsequent management will depend on ***specific* diagnosis** of the tachyarrhythmia. As shown in Figure 1C-1- the principal entities to consider include atrial fibrillation or flutter, PSVT, VT, and the *WIDE-complex* tachycardia of *uncertain* type.

> **Note**- AHA Guidelines do *not* include *sinus tachycardia* in the algorithm for treatment of *Tachycardia* (AHA Text- Pg 1-33). This intentional omission emphasizes the point that the treatment of choice for ***sinus tachycardia*** is *NOT* drugs or cardioversion- but rather to *identify* and *correct* the underlying *cause* the tachycardia.

- ***If the patient is NOT hemodynamically STABLE***. Hemodynamic instability is said to be present if the rhythm produces *serious signs* or *symptoms*- and is doing so as a *direct result* of the increase in heart rate. In this situation the need for *immediate* treatment is much more pressing. As a result- *immediate* **synchronized cardioversion** takes precedence over antiarrhythmic therapy. Treatment should *not* be delayed for the time that it takes to draw up and administer medication.

> **Note**- AHA Guidelines allow that even when the decision to cardiovert *"immediately"* has been made, medical therapy *may* still be tried- *IF* drugs are *immediately* available- and provided that giving these drugs does *not* result in delay of cardioversion (AHA Text- Pg 1-35). Clearly- *clinical judgement is needed at the bedside* in the decision making process.

- The ***Supportive Actions*** listed in Figure 1C-1 are similar to those that should be implemented in virtually *all* of the ACLS algorithms for treatment. As already noted, these actions are implemented at the earliest appropriate opportunity.

> **Note**- AHA Guidelines fully acknowledge that "astute clinicians" *cannot* progress slowly (i.e., *step-by-step*) through every intervention in each recommended sequence for the brady- and tachyarrhythmias (AHA Text- Pg 1-30). Thus *despite* being listed separately- many interventions are really performed *simultaneously* in practice, and sometimes in a sequence that is *modified* from that given in the algorithms. For example, synchronized cardioversion may *need* to be performed *before* some of the *Supportive Actions* that are listed in Figure 1C-1- *especially* if the patient is hemodynamically unstable!

- Many of the ***Supportive Actions*** listed in Figure 1C-1 have already been commented on in our discussion of the steps and actions in the ***Universal Algorithm*** (Figure 1A-1). Some of these interventions relate to initial stabilization of the patient (i.e., assessing the ABCs; securing the airway, providing supplemental oxygen and ventilating the patient; and intubating as needed). Other *Supportive Actions* relate to additional treatment measures that should be appropriate for virtually *any* patient who presents with a cardiopulmonary emergency (i.e., establishing IV access, use of pulse oximetry, etc.). Remaining interventions primarily address assessment of the patient's clinical condition (i.e., use of pulse oximetry, performance of a *targeted* physical exam)- and/or are aimed at uncovering the precipitating *cause* of the emergency situation (i.e., review of the patient's history and medical chart, obtaining a 12-lead ECG, portable chest X-ray, etc.).

- ***If at ANY time the patient decompensates***- *STOP* treatment. *Immediately* **cardiovert** the patient. Administration of drugs is of *secondary* importance if the patient is (or at *any* time becomes) hemodynamically unstable.

Is Synchronized Cardioversion *Acutely* Needed?

The purpose of *synchronization* is to deliver the electrical impulse at a point in the cardiac cycle (i.e., at the peak of the QRS complex) when the heart is *least "vulnerable"* to precipitation of V Fib. Cardioversion of *organized* tachyarrhythmias is generally *much safer* when synchronization is used.

The principal indication for use of *synchronized* cardioversion is in the treatment of ***tachyarrhymias*** (including *both* VT and *SUPRAventricular* rhythms) that are either hemodynamically *unstable*- and/or which fail to respond to other measures. Clinically, cardioversion is needed *emergently* only if the patient *is* (and/or *becomes*) acutely unstable. If the patient with tachycardia is *not* acutely unstable- then an initial trial of antiarrhythmic therapy is often preferred. Cardioversion may still be needed *later* in some of these patients (i.e., if medical therapy fails to control the rhythm)- but in such cases it can usually be performed under less urgent conditions (i.e., there should at least be time to *sedate* the patient and call anesthesia to the bedside).

- The decision of whether or not to *immediately* cardiovert a patient may sometimes have to be made *before* determining the specific diagnosis of the tachyarrhythmia! Practically speaking, if the patient is *hemodynamically unstable*- knowing what the specific arrhythmia diagnosis is *no longer matters.* This is because *immediate* synchronized cardioversion now becomes indicated *regardless* of whether the tachycardia is *SUPRAventricular* or *ventricular* in origin.

- AHA Guidelines emphasize that although determination of the *specific* diagnosis of a tachycardia *is* important- "the *critical* therapeutic question to ask first is *whether to perform* synchronized cardioversion" (AHA Text- Pg 1-32).

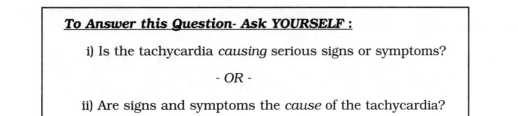

To Answer this Question- Ask YOURSELF :

i) Is the tachycardia *causing* serious signs or symptoms?

- OR -

ii) Are signs and symptoms the *cause* of the tachycardia?

- Synchronized cardioversion is *not* indicated when the tachycardia is simply a reflection of the underlying condition. For example, sinus tachycardia that develops in response to severe hypotension, acute infarction, or pulmonary edema should *not* be cardioverted. As already noted, the treatment of choice for sinus tachycardia is to identify and treat the underlying cause.

- AHA Guidelines emphasize that it is highly *unlikely* for synchronized cardioversion to be needed on an *emergent* basis- IF the heart rate of the tachycardia is *less* than **150 beats/minute** (AHA Text- 1-33). Tachycardias at relatively "slower" rates (i.e., of *less* than 150 beats/minute) are much *less likely* to produce serious signs or symptoms- especially in patients who have normal ventricular function. Cardioversion might still be needed in some of these patients at a *later* time (i.e., *non-emergently* under more stable conditions)- IF medical therapy fails to control/convert the tachyarrhythmia.

- Remember that some patients with *sustained* VT may be hemodynamically stable- and that they may *remain* in VT for surprisingly long periods of time (of minutes, hours- *and even days!*). Thus the first thing to do when confronted with a patient who presents in a worrisome looking tachycardia is to:

  i) *Take a DEEP breath!*
  ii) Remember to assess the patient in the manner suggested in Figure 1C-1.

- Finally- although certain parameters are frequently cited for defining hemodynamic stability (such as a systolic BP of ≥80-90 mm Hg)- *bedside* clinical evaluation is often the *best* way to determine the true need for specific treatment. Simply stated- sometimes *"you just have to be there"*- to make an adequate assessment. For example, a patient in VT may *not* necessarily require immediate cardioversion *despite* an extremely low blood pressure reading (i.e., of 70 systolic)- IF they are *otherwise* alert, comfortable, and asymptomatic.

If Synchronized Cardioversion *IS Immediately* Needed

AHA Guidelines recommend use of the following ***Standard Sequence of Energy Levels*** for *synchronized* cardioversion of the various tachyarrhythmias (AHA Text- Pg 1-35):

- *1st Attempt*- **100 joules**
  - *IF unsuccessful*- increase energy to **200 joules-** - then to **300-** and finally to **360 joules**.

Several ***exceptions*** exist to the above general recommendations (i.e., when a different energy selection might be preferable for cardioversion of certain arrhythmias). These exceptions include:

- ***Polymorphic VT*** (i.e., VT with an *irregular* morphology and rate)- which often requires a *higher* energy level for successful cardioversion. AHA Guidelines suggest *starting* with **200 joules**- which may then need to be increased if the rhythm persists.

- ***Atrial Flutter***- which often responds to *lower* energy levels (probably because it is a very *organized* arrhythmia with rapid but very regular atrial activity). AHA Guidelines therefore allow for selection of **50 joules** as the *initial* energy level for attempts at converting A Flutter.

- ***Atrial Fibrillation***- which in our experience is also often a relatively difficult rhythm to successfully cardiovert when lower energy levels are used. *We* therefore prefer to *start* with **200 joules** for our *initial* attempt at cardioverting A Fib- and to increase this to 360 joules if a second attempt is needed. Other associated clinical factors (i.e., left atrial size, duration of time that the patient has been in A Fib, persistence or correction of the precipitating cause, etc.)- often determine whether or not the patient with A Fib will respond to cardioversion.

> ***KEY***- When attempting to cardiovert a patient- *be sure* that the *SYNCH Mode* is properly engaged- that the machine is *sensing* QRS complexes of the tachycardia (usually indicated by a marker on each R wave that is sensed)- and that both discharge buttons are *simultaneously* depressed by the person who is cardioverting (and *maintained depressed*) until the electrical discharge occurs.

What if *Synchronized* Cardioversion Produces V Fib?

Although *synchronization* to the upstroke of the R wave minimizes the chance that the electrical impulse will be delivered during the "vulnerable period"- it does *not* eliminate this possibility. Thus despite the most appropriate of precautions, synchronized cardioversion may occasionally precipitate deterioration of a tachycardia to V Fib.

Comfort can at least be taken in the fact that even if V Fib is produced by cardioversion, the chance for converting the patient out of this rhythm is excellent. This is because you are right on the scene- and the time from recognition of this complication until action (i.e., defibrillation) should be minimal. *Anticipate this possibility.* Know that even if synchronized cardioversion precipitates development of V Fib- you will probably be able to save the patient by *immediately* deactivating the synchronizer mode and defibrillating the patient (with 200-360 joules). Modern defibrillators facilitate defibrillation in this situation because they *automatically* deactivate the synchronizer mode after electrical discharge.

What if the Cardioverter *Won't* Work?

There are numerous cardioverter/defibrillators on the market. Each features nuances in operation that distinguish one particular model from the next. In many hospitals, different types of defibrillators are present in different patient care areas. The point to emphasize is that the time to learn about operation of all of the various types of defibrillators that are used in your hospital is *not* in the middle of a code.

- If you do find yourself confronted with a patient in *sustained* VT who is in need of electrical therapy- and you are *unable* to get the defibrillator to deliver a synchronized impulse (for *whatever* reason) . . . . - do *not* spend more than a few moments trying to get the device to work. Instead, simply turn off the synchronizer switch- and *defibrillate* the patient.

- Delivery of an *unsynchronized* shock will successfully convert most cases of VT (albeit at a slightly increased risk compared to the use of synchronized cardioversion). The reason for not delaying defibrillation for more than a few moments is that delivery of an unsynchronized countershock to a hemodynamically unstable patient in VT is far preferable to delivery of no electrical energy at all.

The Patient with Tachycardia: *Differential Diagnosis*

Perhaps the greatest challenge faced by the ACLS provider during cardiopulmonary resuscitation and emergency cardiac care situations- is the task of *interpreting* tachyarrhythmias. Management decisions (and the ultimate fate of the patient) often depends on the accuracy of this interpretation.

The importance of determining the ***specific diagnosis*** of the tachyarrhythmia is evident from inspection of Figure 1C-1 (page 51). As shown in this algorithm, once it is established that the patient with ***Tachycardia*** is hemodynamically stable- diagnosis of the *type* of tachycardia becomes the major determinant of what treatment course to follow.

Detailed description of all of the intricacies of arrhythmia analysis clearly extends beyond the scope of this book. Nevertheless, awareness of the *KEY* points we list below should go a long way toward improving the diagnostic process- and facilitating optimal treatment decisions.

- As already emphasized- evaluation of virtually all patients with emergency cardiopulmonary conditions should begin with the ***Universal Algorithm*** (Figure 1A-1).

- ***Supportive Actions*** (as listed in Figure 1C-1) should be implemented at the *earliest* appropriate moment (as feasible, depending on resources and the number and skill of available rescuers). Information obtained from carrying out these *Supportive Actions* will often provide *invaluable* assistance for determining the most likely etiology of the tachycardia (*See below*).

- By far- the *MOST important* facet of evaluation and management to assess for *any* patient with tachycardia (*before* you even *begin* to think about the possible etiology of a particular arrhythmia)- is the ***hemodynamic status*** of the patient:

    - *If the Patient with Tachycardia is Pulseless*- then the rhythm is almost certainly VT. Treatment should be the same as for V Fib (i.e., with immediate *unsynchronized* countershock).

    - *If the Patient with Tachycardia HAS a Pulse*- then the next priority is to determine if serious signs or symptoms are being produced as a *direct result* of the increase in heart rate. If they are- consider the need for *immediate* ***synchronized*** **cardioversion** (Figure 1C-1).

      On the other hand, if the patient with tachycardia has a pulse and is *hemodynamically STABLE*- then there may be time to attend to the diagnostic process of rhythm analysis. Optimal treatment decisions from this time forth will depend on continued assessment of the patient's hemodynamic status and ***specific diagnosis*** of the tachyarrhythmia.

> ***KEY***- It should be emphasized that if the patient's hemodynamic condition deteriorates at *any* time during the evaluative or treatment process- then synchronized cardioversion becomes *immediately* indicated (and it *no longer* matters what the specific diagnosis of the rhythm happened to be).

- *For the Patient who IS Hemodynamically STABLE*- knowing the most commonly encountered diagnostic possibilities will greatly simplify the task of identifying the *type* of tachycardia. Practically speaking, there are *six* principal entities to consider:

  1. Sinus Tachycardia
  2. Atrial Fibrillation
  3. Atrial Flutter
  4. PSVT
  5. Ventricular Tachycardia (VT)
  6. *Wide-Complex* Tachycardia (WCT) of *Uncertain* Etiology

- Differentiation between these six clinical entities can usually be made with surprising accuracy by attention to the following *five* factors:

  i) The ***rate*** of the tachycardia.
  ii) The pattern of ***regularity*** of the rhythm.
  iii) The ***width*** of the QRS complex.
  iv) The presence (and nature) of ***atrial activity***- and its relation (if any) to the QRS complex.
  v) The ***clinical setting*** in which the arrhythmia occurs (which will usually be defined by information obtained from the ***Supportive Actions*** that are listed in Figure 1C-1).

- A *KEY* clinical distinction to make is determination of whether the tachycardia is ***ventricular*** or ***SUPRAventricular*** in etiology. Assessment of the ***width*** of the **QRS complex** provides the most helpful clue in this determination:

> *Regarding* ***QRS Duration***- The QRS complex may normally measure *up to* **0.10 second** in adults. Since one *large* box on ECG grid paper corresponds to a duration of 0.20 second- this means that a QRS complex may normally be *up to* half a large box in duration. Practically speaking then- the QRS complex is said to be ***wide*** if it measures ***more*** than ***half*** a **large box** in duration.

- If the QRS Complex is ***Narrow***- then the tachycardia *must* be ***SUPRAventricular*** (i.e., originating *at* or *above* the AV node). The first *four* entities that we cite-above should then be considered:

  1. Sinus Tachycardia
  2. Atrial Fibrillation
  3. Atrial Flutter
  4. PSVT

  } The most common causes of ***S****upra****V****entricular* ***T****achycardia* (***SVT***)

- If the QRS Complex is ***Wide***- then it is much more likely that the rhythm is of ***ventricular*** etiology (i.e., ventricular tachycardia). Compared to the various SVTs- VT is far more likely to be a potentially *life-threatening* arrhythmia.

> **Note**- Although the presence of QRS widening should always suggest VT as the *probable* diagnosis- this finding by itself does *not* rule out the possibility of a supraventricular etiology (*See caveats below*).

- Four important ***caveats*** should be kept in mind regarding ECG interpretation of the patient with tachycardia. They are:

  i) That a portion of the QRS complex may sometimes lie *on the baseline* in a particular monitoring lead. In such cases, the QRS complex may appear to be narrow- *when in fact it is not.* Viewing the tachycardia from *more* than one perspective (i.e., use of additional leads- and ideally obtaining a 12-lead ECG *during* the tachycardia) should facilitate determining what the *true* width of the QRS complex happens to be .

  ii) That a rhythm *may* be *SUPRAventricular* in etiology *despite* QRS widening- if *either* ***aberrant* conduction** or ***preexisting* bundle branch block** is present. Availability of a prior ECG on the patient may provide an invaluable clue to this possibility (i.e., by revealing *preexisting* widening of the QRS complex while the patient was in sinus rhythm).

  iii) That the patient's hemodynamic status is *not at all helpful* in the diagnostic process. For example, some patients in VT may be normotensive and asymptomatic (and *remain* so) for surprisingly *long* periods of time!

  iv) That *regardless* of the patient's hemodynamic status- VT is (*by far!*) the most common cause of a regular wide-complex tachycardia. Therefore, if the QRS complex is wide- *always* assume VT until *proven* otherwise! *Treat the patient accordingly.*

We now illustrate and briefly describe the six most commonly encountered tachycardias. We then follow in this Section with the corresponding algorithms for treatment.

---

1. Sinus Tachycardia

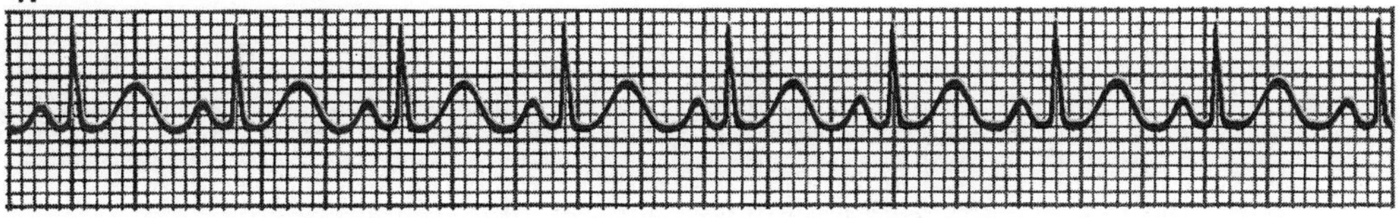

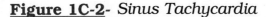

Figure 1C-2- *Sinus Tachycardia*

- ECG Recognition- Sinus Tachycardia is usually easy to recognize by the presence of its normal appearing (i.e., *upright* in lead II) P waves. Each QRS complex is preceded by a P wave that is "married" to it (i.e., the PR interval preceding each QRS complex is fixed- as seen in Figure 1C-2).

- Pitfalls in Diagnosis- Sinus tachycardia can *only* be diagnosed with certainty when you are able to discern a distinct *upright* P wave in lead II. If regularly occurring atrial activity is seen in *other* leads, but *not* in lead II- it is likely that the rhythm is something *other than* sinus.

> ***KEY***- With the exception of lead misplacement and dextrocardia (both of which are rare)- if the P wave in lead II is *not* upright- then the mechanism of the rhythm is *not* sinus!

Another potential problem in the diagnosis of sinus tachycardia may arise when the rate of the rhythm is particularly rapid. In such cases, sinus P waves may not be evident (since because of the rapid rate they may become hidden *within* the preceding T wave).

- Comment- Sinus tachycardia is defined as a sinus mechanism rhythm at a rate of 100 beats/minute or more. An invaluable "pearl" for facilitating ECG diagnosis is that the *upper* rate limit of this rhythm will rarely exceed 150-160 beats/minute- provided that the patient is an adult who is lying in bed. Faster rates may be seen for sinus tachycardia in adults after exercise- or in *children* at rest (for whom the rate of sinus tachycardia may exceed 200 beats/minute!). However, for a *hospitalized* adult (i.e., one who is lying in bed)- the presence of a tachycardia at a heart rate substantially greater than 160 beats/minute makes it highly *unlikely* that the rhythm is sinus tachycardia.

> **Note**- Mention of sinus tachycardia is omitted from the AHA ACLS algorithms. The reason for this omission is probably twofold:
>
> i) That the rhythm is usually easy to recognize.
>
> ii) That there is no specific treatment for sinus tachycardia. The treatment of choice is correction of the *underlying* disorder that is *causing* the tachycardia. For example, if the reason for sinus tachycardia is hypotension from intravascular volume depletion- then the treatment of choice is IV fluid infusion (and *not* administration of rate-slowing drugs!).

2. Atrial Fibrillation

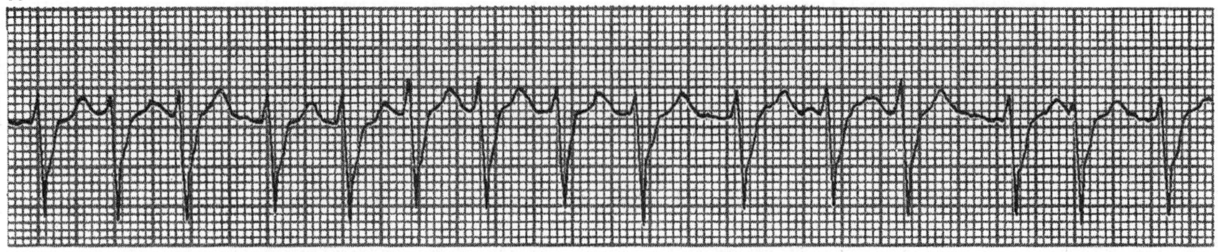

Figure 1C-3- *Atrial Fibrillation*

- ECG Recognition- The hallmarks of A Fib are the *irregular irregularity* of its ventricular response and the *absence* of P waves. Variable undulations in the baseline (known as "fib waves") may be seen- although some patients with A Fib have a perfectly smooth baseline without any evidence at all of atrial activity.

  The ventricular rate with A Fib may vary. Thus, the rhythm may present with a ***rapid* ventricular response** (Figure 1C-3)- as is typically seen in the *untreated* patient with *new-onset* A Fib; with a ***controlled* ventricular response** (after treatment with rate-slowing drugs); or with a ***slow* ventricular response** (as is likely to be seen in patients with sick sinus syndrome or Digoxin toxicity).

- Pitfalls in Diagnosis- An irregularly irregular rhythm that is commonly confused with A Fib is ***M**ultifocal **A**trial **T**achycardia* (***MAT***). The reason that distinguishing between these two clinical entities is so important is that treatment is markedly different. Whereas many clinicians still administer relatively large doses of Digoxin for rate control of A Fib- this drug should only be used with the utmost caution if the rhythm is MAT. This is because patients with MAT have a high propensity to developing Digoxin toxicity, often from relatively low doses of the drug. MAT most often occurs in the setting of severe pulmonary disease. The treatment of choice is correction of the underlying disorder- which most often entails optimizing oxygenation (and *not* antiarrhythmic therapy).

  Electrocardiographically- MAT is recognized (and distinguished from A Fib) by the presence of many different (i.e., ***M**ultifocal*) P waves. Because they arise from multiple ectopic sites- these P waves manifest differing morphologies and variable PR intervals. The problem arises from the fact that the P waves of MAT may not always be evident in all leads. Obtaining a 12-lead ECG is therefore the best strategy for evaluating this possibility when confronted with an irregularly irregular rhythm and uncertain atrial activity in a single monitoring lead- especially if the patient has severe pulmonary disease.

- Comment- A Fib will generally be easy to recognize and distinguish from other SVTs because of its *irregularity* (that will usually be obvious). However, when the rate of A Fib is rapid, it may be much more difficult to detect variability in the R-R interval from one beat to the next- unless *calipers* are used to measure these intervals.

  The QRS complex with A Fib will usually be narrow. On occasion, however- the QRS may be widened (i.e., if there is *preexisting* bundle branch block). This is the case in Figure 1C-3- in which the QRS complex is clearly *more* than half a large box in duration. Despite QRS widening- distinction from VT can still be made in this tracing because of the gross *irregularity* of the ventricular response. Although VT may at times be *slightly* irregular- it should *not* be nearly as irregular as it is in this example.

3. *Atrial Flutter*

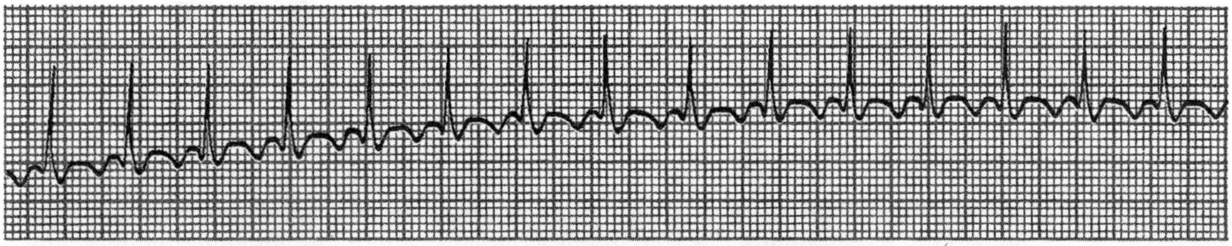

Figure 1C-4- *Atrial Flutter*

- ECG Recognition- The distinctive feature of A Flutter is its regular ***sawtooth* pattern** of atrial activity. The rhythm is unique in that atrial activity in the *untreated* adult almost invariably occurs at a rate that is close to **300/minute** (usual range = 250-350/minute).

  The ventricular response to A Flutter will usually also manifest a characteristic pattern. One to one conduction of each atrial impulse does *not* occur (with rare exceptions)- since the normal AV node is unable to conduct at a rate of 300/minute. This is fortunate because a ventricular rate of close to 300/minute would be far too fast to allow normal ventricular filling with each cardiac contraction. Instead, the most common response of the AV node is to allow conduction to the ventricles of *every other* flutter impulse- which is referred to as **2:1 AV conduction**. Since the atrial rate is close to 300/minute- this means that the most common ventricular response of a patient with *untreated* A Flutter should be *very close* to a rate of **150 beats/minute** (i.e., usual atrial rate ≈300/minute ÷ 2 ≈150/minute). This is precisely the case for the example of A Flutter that is shown in Figure 1C-4 (in which there is 2:1 AV conduction with a ventricular rate of approximately 150 beats/minute).

  The next most common AV conduction ratio for A Flutter is 4:1- which will typically result in a ventricular rate of close to 75 beats/minute (i.e., ≈300 ÷ 4) in the *untreated* patient. Odd conduction ratios (i.e., 1:1, 3:1, 5:1, etc.) are rare. Occasionally flutter may manifest *variable* AV conduction- which produces an irregular ventricular response that resembles the pattern that is seen with A Fib.

- Pitfalls in Diagnosis- The diagnosis of A Flutter is easy to make when regular sawtooth activity is seen at a rate that is close to 300/minute. In practice, however- flutter activity will often be more subtle and difficult to recognize unless *carefully* looked for. For example- it may not be immediately apparent that the negative deflection seen right after the QRS complex in Figure 1C-4 is a flutter wave (and *not* the terminal S wave of the QRS). Sometimes flutter activity will *not* be at all evident in the particular lead being used for monitoring- in which case the diagnosis might be ever so easy to overlook.

When clinically appropriate, application of a ***vagal*** **maneuver** (such as carotid massage) may be an invaluable aid to diagnosis of A Flutter (Figure 1C-5). By temporarily slowing the ventricular response, the maneuver allows "telltale" atrial activity at a rate of 300/minute to become much more evident (*arrows* in Figure 1C-5). We defer more detailed discussion of vagal maneuvers to Section 2D.

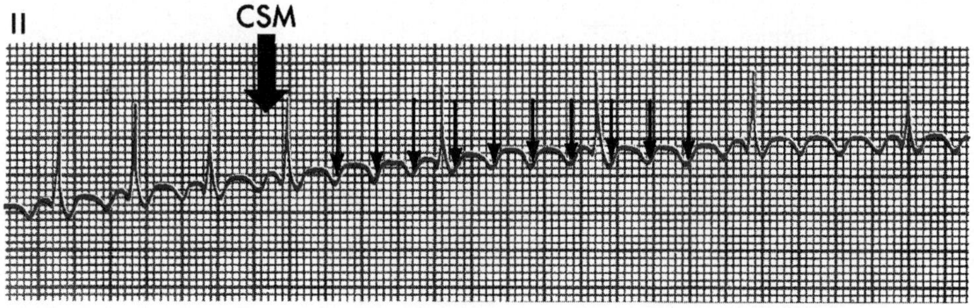

Figure 1C-5- Application of *carotid massage* to the rhythm that was shown in Figure 1C-4.

- Comment- In our experience, A Flutter is (*by far* !) the most commonly overlooked and misdiagnosed arrhythmia. This is because flutter activity will not always be seen in the lead being monitored. The *KEY* to recognizing A Flutter is to always maintain a high index of suspicion for this arrhythmia *whenever* one is confronted with a regular SVT in which the ventricular rate is close to 150 beats/minute. Obtaining a 12-lead tracing (to look for possible flutter waves in other leads), and application of a vagal maneuver are two helpful ways to either rule in or rule out this diagnosis.

  A final caveat to be aware of regarding recognition of A Flutter is that the atrial rate (of 300/minute) holds true *only* for the *untreated* patient. The *atrial* rate may be significantly *slower* than 300/minute if the patient is being treated with antiarrhythmic medication (i.e., Quinidine, Procainamide, Verapamil, etc.)- in which case the *ventricular* rate may *not* necessarily be close to 150 beats/minute.

4. PSVT (Paroxysmal SupraVentricular Tachycardia)

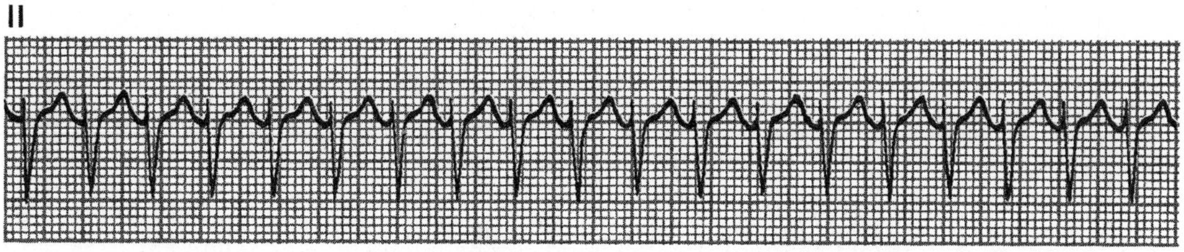

Figure 1C-6- *PSVT*

- ECG Recognition- PSVT is a regular supraventricular tachycardia which lacks normal atrial activity. The rhythm most often begins abruptly- which is why it is called *"paroxysmal"*. Once it begins, the ventricular response tends to be exceedingly regular- most often at a rate of between 140-240 beats/minute. The mechanism of this type of SVT is almost invariably one of *"reentry"* in which at least a portion of the reentry circuit involves the AV Node. As a result of its mechanism, atrial activity is either entirely absent from the surface ECG, or present in the form of subtle retrograde (i.e., *negative* in lead II) deflections that appear in the terminal portion of the QRS complex.

  The rhythm shown in Figure 1C-6 illustrates all of these characteristics. This rhythm is regular at a rate of just under 200 beats/minute. Normal atrial activity appears to be absent (although admittedly it is difficult to rule out the possibility that P waves might be hiding within the T waves seen on this tracing).

- Pitfalls in Diagnosis- When confronted with a ***regular* SVT** in which atrial activity is either absent or uncertain- three clinical entities should be considered:

  1. Sinus Tachycardia
  2. Atrial Flutter
  3. PSVT

  Attention to the ventricular rate will often provide an important clue to the true etiology of the arrhythmia in question. For example, we have already noted that the ventricular rate in Figure 1C-6 is just under 200 beats/minute. Awareness of this rate essentially rules out both sinus tachycardia (which rarely exceeds 150-160 beats/minute) and A Flutter (which almost always presents with 2:1 AV conduction and a ventricular rate that is close to 150 beats/minute). By the process of elimination- this leaves us with PSVT as the most likely diagnosis.

  The pitfall to be aware of is that distinction between sinus tachycardia, A Flutter, and PSVT- may sometimes be extremely difficult when the rate of the regular SVT is close to 150 beats/minute.

- Comment- Many clinicians no longer refer to the rhythm shown in Figure 1C-6 as PSVT. Instead, the newer name for this type of tachycardia is ***AVNRT*** (*AV Nodal Reentry Tachycardia*)- a term that has been selected to emphasize our improved understanding of the usual mechanism of this rhythm (that almost invariably involves *reentry* occurring within or into the AV Node). For the purpose of consistency with AHA Guidelines, we refer to this rhythm as PSVT throughout this book.

5. *Ventricular Tachycardia*

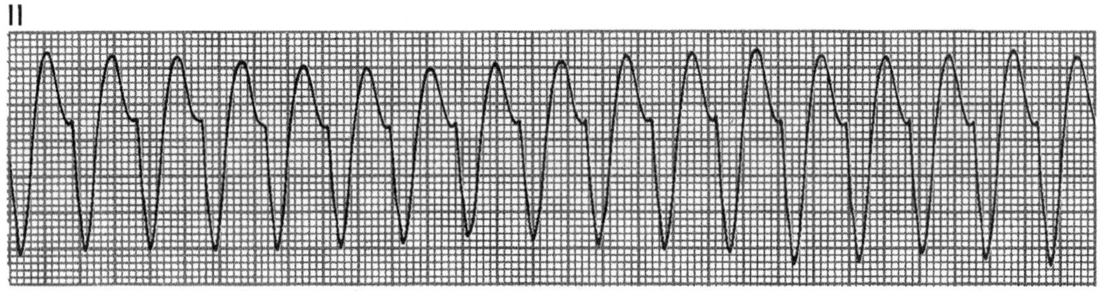

Figure 1C-7- *Ventricular Tachycardia*

- ECG Recognition- VT is a regular (or at least fairly regular) wide-complex tachycardia in which normal atrial activity is absent. Most of the time no P waves at all are seen- although on occasion, AV dissociation or retrograde atrial activity may be present. These features are evident in Figure 1C-7- in which the rhythm is regular (at a rate of about 160 beats/minute), the QRS complex is markedly widened, and P waves are absent.

- Pitfalls in Diagnosis- As we emphasize in discussion of the next arrhythmia (i.e., *WCT* of *Uncertain Etiology*)- SVTs may occasionally present as *wide-complex* tachycardias (if there is preexisting bundle branch block or aberrant conduction)- in which case it may be difficult to distinguish these rhythms from VT. From a clinical standpoint- *always* assume that the rhythm is VT- until *proven* otherwise. *Treat the patient accordingly.*

- Comment- Given the *excessive* amount of QRS widening in Figure 1C-7 (we measure the QRS to be *at least* 0.16 second in duration)- it is hard to imagine that this rhythm could be anything but VT!

6. *Wide-Complex Tachycardia (WCT) of Uncertain Etiology*

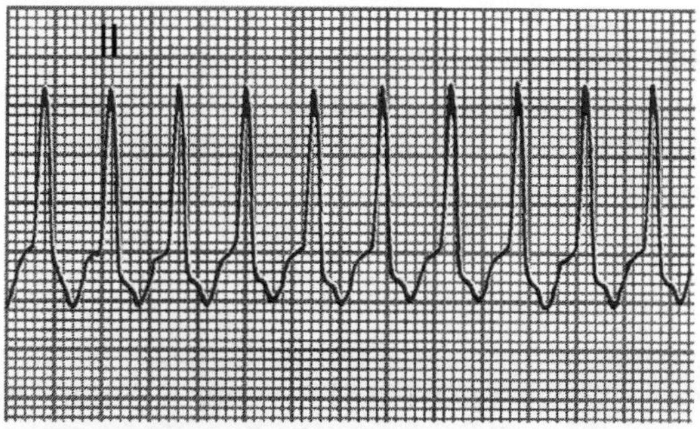

Figure 1C-8- *WCT of Uncertain Etiology*

- ECG Recognition- As implied in its name- the term ***Wide-Complex Tachycardia (WCT)*** of ***Uncertain Etiology*** refers to those rhythms in which the QRS complex is widened, but the reason for this widening is *not* clear. The ventricular rhythm will usually be regular (or at least fairly regular) in this entity- since gross irregularity (as seen in Figure 1C-3) would suggest A Fib. Atrial activity is most often absent.

- Pitfalls in Diagnosis- It is virtually impossible to determine the etiology of the rhythm shown in Figure 1C-8 from examination of this single monitoring lead alone. All one can say is that the rhythm is regular at a rate of just over 200 beats/minute- and that atrial activity appears to be absent. Although we suspect that the QRS complex is widened, it is difficult to be sure of where the QRS complex begins and ends (since transition to and from the ST segment is somewhat indistinct). One is therefore left with the diagnostic dilemma of simply *not knowing* the etiology of this tachycardia.

  - *If the Patient was Hemodynamically UNSTABLE-* then the etiology of this rhythm would no longer matter. This is because synchronized cardioversion would be *immediately* indicated- *regardless* of what the rhythm happens to be (*Refer back to Figure 1C-1 on page 51).*

  - *If the Patient was Hemodynamically STABLE-* then there may be time to further attempt to determine the rhythm. Obtaining a **12-lead ECG** should help clarify if the QRS complex is *truly* wide or not. If the **QRS complex** is ***Wide***- then the cause of the tachycardia could be *either* VT or SVT (in which case QRS widening would be from either bundle branch block or aberrant conduction).

- Comment- The importance of determining the cause of a *WCT* of *Uncertain Etiology* is that VT will require much *different* (and often much *more immediate*) treatment than any of the forms of SVT.

Having stressed the importance of diagnosis of the type of tachycardia- we now move into the algorithms for treatment.

Treatment Algorithm for A Fib/Flutter

The approach we suggest to evaluation and management of the patient in ***Atrial Fibrillation*** or ***Atrial Flutter*** is shown in Figure 1C-9. For practical purposes- the *initial* management of these two arrhythmias in the emergency situation is very similar. That is, the drugs that are used to achieve rate control and/or convert the rhythm are the same- and synchronized cardioversion is the treatment of choice if the patient becomes acutely unstable. Selected special points of interest to keep in mind regarding *differences* between A Fib and A Flutter (that extend *beyond* emergency management and ACLS core material) include the following:

- *Relative Frequency of Occurrence*- In the general population, ***A Fib*** is by far the most common *sustained* cardiac arrhythmia- especially among older individuals. ***A Flutter*** is far less common. Both arrhythmias may occur in the setting of cardiac arrest.
- *Risk of Stroke*- The risk of embolization is high for *chronic* ***A Fib***- especially in patients who have significant underlying heart disease (which is why aspirin and/or anticoagulation should be strongly considered in such individuals). In contrast, because atrial activity is *organized* with ***A Flutter***- the risk of embolization is much less (and anticoagulation is therefore less likely to be needed).

> **Note-** It takes *several days* for clot to form in fibrillating (i.e., *non-contractile*) atria. As a result- anticoagulation is generally *not* felt to be needed in the immediate treatment of *new-onset* (i.e., ≤2-3 day duration) A Fib.

- *Response to Therapy*- Although similar drugs are used to control the rate and convert the rhythm, the response of A Fib and A Flutter to medical therapy is often quite different. In general, it is much easier to control the rate of rapid ***A Fib*** (i.e., with Digoxin, Verapamil/Diltiazem, or a beta-blocker)- than it is to control the rate of A Flutter. Thus, despite even high doses of rate-slowing agents, the ventricular response of ***A Flutter*** often remains unacceptably rapid.

  In contrast- ***A Flutter*** tends to be much more responsive to cardioversion than A Fib (which is why a *lower* initial energy of ≈**50 joules** is usually selected to cardiovert this rhythm). This is as might be expected in view of the fact that A Flutter is an *organized* rhythm. Because ***A Fib*** is *disorganized* (resulting from diffusely chaotic atrial activity)- it is often resistant to cardioversion at lower energy levels. For this reason we favor beginning with **200 joules** when attempting to cardiovert this rhythm.

Look for an *Underlying* Cause

In addition to rate control of the ventricular response, the *KEY* to successful management of A Fib/Flutter is identification and correction of the *precipitating/underlying* condition that is causing the arrhythmia. Outside of the setting of cardiac arrest, the most important underlying conditions to consider in this regard are listed in Table 1C-2.

It is important to emphasize that use of medication and/or cardioversion tends to be much *less* effective in successfully converting A Fib/Flutter to sinus rhythm (and especially in *maintaining* sinus rhythm)- *IF/for as long as* the underlying condition persists.

Figure 1C-9- *Treatment Algorithm for A Fib/Flutter*

(When the patient is hemodynamically stable)

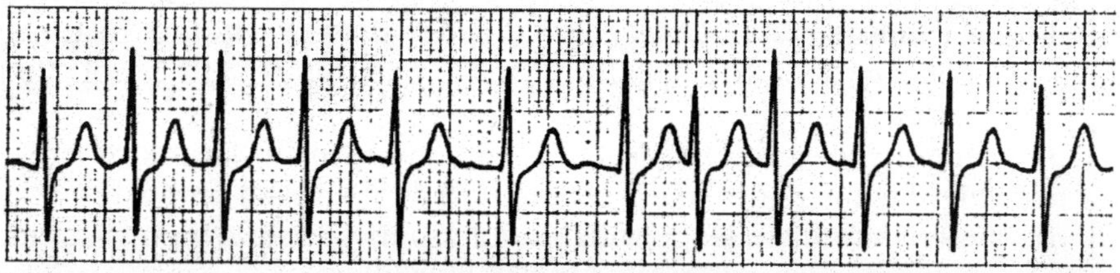

- Supportive Actions
  - as listed on Figure 1C-1 have *all* been accomplished.

Treatment Options:

- Consider possible *Precipitating CAUSES* of the rhythm:
  - *Rule out*- heart failure, Acute MI, hyperthyroidism, hypoxia, pulmonary embolism, alcohol or drug abuse, etc.

- Begin with a *Rate-Slowing* Drug (if the rate is rapid):
  - **Diltiazem**- 0.25 mg/kg (or ≈15-20 mg) initial IV bolus;
    Follow with 0.35 mg/kg (≈25 mg) in 15 min if no response.
    May then follow with IV infusion @ 10 mg/hr (5-15 mg/hr range).

    - or -

  - **Verapamil**- 2.5-5 mg IV initially; then 5-10 mg IV.

    - and/or -

  - **Digoxin**- no longer the first drug of choice.
    Load with 0.25-0.5 mg IV. Then give 0.125-0.25 mg IV q 2-6 hrs (as needed up to 0.75-1.5 mg total).

  - Could also use a ***Beta-blocker*** (i.e., **IV Propranolol**, **Esmolol**)- *but NOT in close association with IV Verapamil/Diltiazem !!!*

- Correct *Electrolyte Disturbance* (if present):
  - *Rule out*- hypokalemia, hypomagnesemia.

- Consider Measures to *Convert* the Rhythm:
  - Spontaneous conversion to sinus rhythm will often occur if a precipitating cause (*See above*) can be found and corrected.
  - *Medical therapy* (usually ***Quinidine*** *or* ***Procainamide***).
  - ***Synchronized Cardioversion*** (performed *non-emergently*).

- Consider the Need for Anticoagulation:
  - Use of Heparin/Aspirin (as appropriate).

> **Note**- If the patient decompensates at *any* time during the process of evaluating/treating the tachycardia- *STOP and immediately cardiovert* !

Table 1C-2: *Important Precipitating (Underlying) Causes of A Fib/Flutter*

i) Heart failure. (*New-onset* A Fib/Flutter may precipitate heart failure- or new heart failure may precipitate either of these arrhythmias).
ii) Ischemic heart disease (especially acute myocardial infarction).
iii) Valvular heart disease (especially "silent" mitral stenosis).
iv) Hyperthyroidism (especially in older patients, in whom there may be no other symptoms of hyperthyroidism).
v) Alcohol use (i.e., the *"Holiday Heart Syndrome"*- although on occasion a single episode of drinking in a nonalcoholic patient may precipitate the arrhythmia).
vi) Acute pulmonary embolus.
vii) Sick sinus syndrome (i.e., *"Tachy-Brady" syndrome*- especially in elderly patients in whom A Fib may be fast or slow).
viii) Acute systemic illness (i.e., pneumonia, sepsis, shock- or other severe illness).
ix) Acute sympathetic "trigger" (i.e., use of cocaine, amphetamines).
x) Atrial myxoma (a rare but potentially curable cause).
xi) *"Lone" A Fib* (i.e., A Fib that occurs in the *absence* of an underlying disorder).

Clinically then, acute care efforts should not only also focus on controlling the ventricular response- but also on *correcting heart failure* (if present); *optimizing the metabolic profile* (i.e., being sure serum electrolytes are normal and that the patient is not hypoxemic); and addressing all *potentially treatable* medical conditions (i.e., sepsis, shock, pneumonia, etc.).

- Reasons why sudden development of rapid A Fib is so likely to precipitate/aggravate heart failure are:

  i) *Loss of the atrial kick* (which accounts for between 5-40% of cardiac output).

  ii) *Reduced filling time*- since the rapid rate of the tachyarrhythmia results in a shortening of the R-R interval (and encroaches most on the period of diastole). Because ventricular filling occurs during diastole, cardiac output may be significantly reduced by the fast rate. Slowing the ventricular response to A Fib (i.e., with Digoxin) may therefore improve cardiac output- *even if A Fib persists.*

Additional concerns in evaluation of the less acutely ill patient who presents with new onset A Fib might be addressed by obtaining an echocardiogram and thyroid function studies. Finally, consideration should be given to the need for *anticoagulation* (which may sometimes be urgent- as in a patient who presents with new-onset A Fib and stroke-in-evolution).

A Fib/Flutter: *If the Ventricular Response is Controlled*

A Fib with a controlled ventricular response is often a stable rhythm (Figure 1C-10A). As a result, no specific treatment may be needed for this condition in the emergency setting. Although A Flutter tends to be a less stable rhythm- it need *not* be treated either if the patient is asymptomatic and the ventricular response is controlled. Such is the case for the example of A Flutter shown in Figure 1C-10B- in which there is 4:1 AV conduction and a ventricular response of approximately 70 beats/minute.

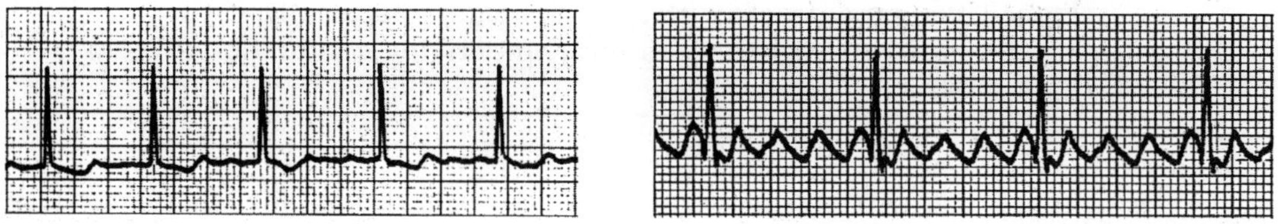

A. *Atrial Fibrillation*

B. *Atrial Flutter (with 4:1 AV Conduction)*

Figure 1C-10- A Fib (**A**) and A Flutter (**B**). The ventricular response for both of these rhythms is controlled. As a result, rate-slowing drugs need *not* be administered in the emergency setting.

If there is a *RAPID* Ventricular Response

Although the ventricular response to A Fib/Flutter may be controlled (as it is in Figure 1C-10)- it will more often be rapid in the acute care setting. In such cases, treatment is needed. If the patient is hemodynamically stable and tolerating the rapid rate- pharmacologic therapy is usually tried first. However, if the patient becomes hemodynamically compromised *at any time* during the treatment process- synchronized cardioversion becomes *immediately* indicated.

For the patient with rapid A Fib/Flutter who is hemodynamically stable- the drugs that are most commonly used to achieve rate control are Diltiazem, Verapamil, Digoxin, and/or use of a beta-blocker. Specific points to keep in mind regarding this ***Rate-Slowing*** **Therapy** include the following:

- ***Diltiazem.*** IV Diltiazem has clearly become a drug of choice for acute rate control of rapid A Fib/Flutter. Onset of action following IV administration of this agent is fast (i.e., usually *within* 3 minutes of giving an IV bolus)- with peak effect most often occurring by 7 minutes. Effects of an IV bolus generally last 1-3 hours.

  Availability for use as a continuous IV infusion allows for ongoing antiarrhythmic effect over the ensuing 24 hours, and offers a decided advantage compared to other antiarrrhythmic agents (such as Digoxin or Verapamil). This is particularly true for *maintaining* rate control over a period of hours when the ventricular response is not readily controlled by intermittent bolus therapy.

  - The recommended dose for the *initial* **IV bolus** of Diltiazem is 0.25 mg/kg (which for an *average-sized* adult is ≈**15-20 mg**). This IV bolus should be given over a 2 minute period.

  - If the desired clinical response is not seen within 15 minutes- a **2nd IV bolus** of approximately **25 mg** (i.e., 0.35 mg/kg) may be given.

- If continued antiarrhythmic effect is desired- a continuous **IV infusion** may be started after bolus administration. The recommended *initial* infusion rate for IV Diltiazem is **10 mg/hr-** which may then be increased to 15 mg/hr (as needed) for clinical effect. IV infusion should generally *not* be continued for more than 24 hours.

> **<u>Note</u>-** It should be emphasized that the above cited doses are for an *average-sized* adult! Significantly *smaller* doses (i.e., of ≈10-15 mg) and *lower* infusion rates (i.e., of 5 mg/hr) should be used for patients of lighter body weight- especially if they are older and/or more likely to have underlying conduction system disease.

- ***Verapamil***. Like Diltiazem- Verapamil is a favored drug for emergency treatment of rapid A Fib/Flutter. Although neither of these drugs are very effective for converting A Fib/Flutter to sinus rhythm- both drugs exert a potent AV nodal blocking effect that reliably *slows* the ventricular response.

  - The recommended dose for the *initial* **IV bolus** of Verapamil is **2.5-5 mg** (to be given over a 1-2 minute period). The *lower* amount should be used first, and the drug given more *slowly* (i.e., over 3-4 minutes) to elderly patients and to those with borderline blood pressure. Cautious dosing in this manner should help to minimize the incidence of hypotension and excessive heart rate slowing that may otherwise be seen.

  - Peak effects from an IV bolus of Verapamil are usually seen within 5 minutes.

  - The dose of IV Verapamil may be ***repeated*** one or more times **after 15-30 minutes** (if/as needed)- up to a *total* dose of ≈30 mg. If the initial dose of 2.5-5 mg is tolerated- then a larger dose (of 5-10 mg) may be given for subsequent IV boluses.

> **<u>Note</u>-** Although *either* Verapamil *or* Diltiazem can be used as *initial* therapy of rapid A Fib/Flutter- recent years have seen an increasing tendency toward selection of IV Diltiazem as the drug of first choice for this indication. Reasons for this trend include a lower risk of producing hypotension and/or exacerbating heart failure with administration of IV Diltiazem. This is because the IV form of Diltiazem produces less vasodilatation and is less negatively inotropic than Verapamil. There also is less potential for drug interaction *with* concommitant use of Digoxin- since Diltiazem does *not* increase serum Digoxin levels to nearly the extent that Verapamil does. The most practical reason for favoring use of IV Diltiazem over Verapamil is availability of an approved formulation for continuous IV infusion (which allows *maintenance* of the rate-controlling effect over a period of hours). In contrast, the rate-slowing effect of repeated IV Verapamil boluses is much more transient and difficult to titrate.

- ***Digoxin.*** Up until recently, Digoxin had been the pharmacologic agent favored by most clinicians for initial treatment of rapid A Fib/Flutter. *No longer.* Both Verapamil and Diltiazem appear to be more effective than Digoxin for initial rate control of the ventricular response to these tachyarrhythmias. Appreciation of this fact is best gained from consideration of the mechanism by which Digoxin works to slow the ventricular response of rapid A Fib/Flutter. The primary action of this drug in this setting is to enhance vagal tone. Conditions that increase the degree of underlying *sympathetic* tone may therefore be resistant to treatment with even high doses of the drug. This is precisely the situation that occurs in the setting of severe acute illness, shock, and/or cardiac arrest- all of which produce a tremendous increase in endogenous catecholamine secretion that may counteract the vagotonic effect of the drug.

  In contrast, the mechanism of action of Diltiazem and Verapamil is quite different than that of Digoxin in the treatment of rapid A Fib/Flutter. Both of these calcium channel blocking agents produce an effect on the AV node that impairs AV conduction regardless of the degree of underlying autonomic tone.

  Regarding the dosing of Digoxin, we emphasize the following points (*See also Section 2E*):

  - When treating a patient who has not previously received Digoxin- one usually begins with an *initial* **IV loading dose** of **0.25-0.5 mg**. This may be followed with additional ***incremental*** **doses** (of **0.125-0.25 mg IV**) that can be given every 2-6 hours as needed (i.e., depending on the ventricular response)- until a *total* loading dose of ≈0.75-1.5 mg of drug has been given.

  - In the *absence* of hyperthyroidism, hypoxemia, Acute MI, and electrolyte disturbance- the ventricular rate response to the above therapy has been used as an indicator of the adequacy of digitalization. According to this practice, persistence of a rapid rate after administration of several boluses suggests that additional Digoxin may still be needed to achieve adequate control of the ventricular response. In the presence of any of the above conditions, however, increased sensitivity to the effects of Digoxin (and a correspondingly increased risk of developing toxicity) augurs for much greater caution (and use of lower doses) in administering the drug.

  - After IV loading is complete, the patient may be placed on a regular daily maintenance dose (that is usually between 0.125-0.25 mg/day).

> **Note**- Combined use of Digoxin and IV Diltiazem/Verapamil may produce a ***synergistic* effect** in controlling the ventricular response to rapid A Fib/Flutter. Combination therapy will also often allow use of lower doses of each agent for achieving adequate rate control than if either of the drugs were used independently.

- ***IV Beta-Blockers.*** Mechanistically, beta-blockers would seem to be ideal antiarrhythmic agents for emergency treatment of the patient with rapid A Fib/Flutter- provided there is no overt heart failure or severe bronchospasm that would contraindicate their use. However, despite their efficacy- beta-blockers appear to be used much less frequently than in the past for this indication. This most likely is a reflection of the preference for using IV Diltiazem/Verapamil (and/or Digoxin) in this emergency situation. Nevertheless, selection of an ***IV Beta-Blocker*** (either **IV Propranolol** or **Esmolol**)- should *not* be forgotten as a potentially effective alternative treatment modality for the patient with rapid A Fib/Flutter.

> **Note-** IV beta-blockers should *never* be administered in close proximity (i.e., within 20-30 minutes) of IV Diltiazem/Verapamil- because combining these agents in this manner could lead to profound bradycardia (and even asystole!).

- ***Synchronized Cardioversion***. As suggested above, pharmacologic therapy (i.e., with IV Diltiazem/Verapamil and/or Digoxin) is often preferred for initial treatment of rapid A Fib/Flutter when the patient is not acutely unstable. If medical therapy is not effective, however, and/or the patient becomes hemodynamically unstable *at any time* during the treatment process- synchronized cardioversion may then be in order.

  - In general, ***A Flutter*** is much more responsive to synchronized cardioversion than A Fib. For this reason, a lower initial energy level (of ≈**50 joules**) is usually selected for cardioversion of this rhythm.

  - In contrast, ***A Fib*** often requires significantly higher energy for successful cardioversion. We suggest beginning with ≈**200 joules** when attempting to cardiovert this rhythm- and then increasing this to 360 joules if the rhythm fails to respond. Realize that A Fib will *not* always respond to synchronized cardioversion (especially if the underlying cause of the rhythm has not been corrected).

  - Synchronized cardioversion is best avoided (if at all possible!) when excessive doses of Digoxin have been administered. Practically speaking, however- the procedure can almost always be performed *safely* if the patient has received *therapeutic* doses of Digoxin and toxicity is not present.

> **Note**- IV Diltiazem/Verapamil, Digoxin, and/or beta-blockers are *all* effective drugs for achieving rate control of the ventricular response to rapid A Fib/Flutter. As a result, these drugs (either alone or in combination) constitute the medical treatment of choice for *emergency management* of these tachyarrhythmias.
>
> Unfortunately- *none* of these agents are more than *minimally* effective for medically converting A Fib/Flutter. Optimal *long-term management* of these arrhythmias entails conversion to (and maintenance of) sinus rhythm. Use of *other* drugs (i.e., Quinidine, Procainamide, Disopyramide, Flecainide, Propafenone, Amiodarone, and/or Sotalol)- and/or *synchronized* cardioversion are clearly far more effective therapeutic interventions for this purpose. (Detailed description of the use of these agents extends *beyond* the scope of this book).

Treatment Algorithm for PSVT

The approach we suggest to evaluation and management of the patient in PSVT is shown in Figure 1C-11. The *KEY* point to emphasize in this approach is the importance of ***reentry*** as the responsible mechanism in almost all cases. As a result of this phenomenon- a *reentry circuit* is set up, whereby the supraventricular impulse gets caught up in a perpetual cycle in which *after* being conducted to the ventricles, the impulse *returns* to the AV node (in *retrograde* fashion)- before it is once again conducted back down to the ventricles. This process continues until it is either interrupted by treatment or spontaneously resolves.

The goal of therapy for PSVT is to *interrupt* conduction over the reentry circuit. Because each part of the cycle is dependent on the integrity of the previous part- even *momentary* delay in conduction over *any* portion of the circuit may be all that is needed to terminate the arrhythmia. This is the reason special maneuvers such as carotid massage (which only act briefly) may be effective in treatment.

PSVT is known as an ***AV nodal dependent*** arrhythmia. This is because at least a portion of the reentry circuit almost always involves the AV node. Drugs that affect conduction *through* the AV node (i.e., AV nodal blocking agents such as Diltiazem/Verapamil, Digoxin, and beta-blockers) are therefore effective in treatment.

In contrast to PSVT- A Fib and A Flutter are *not* AV nodal dependent arrhythmias. This means that even though the same AV nodal blocking agents are used in treatment (Figure 1C-9)- these drugs will usually *not* be effective in converting A Fib/Flutter to sinus rhythm. Instead, the primary function of AV nodal blocking drugs in the treatment of A Fib/Flutter is to *slow* the ventricular response of these arrhythmias.

> **Note**- Although we refer to the rhythms shown in Figures 1C-6 (on page 63) and 1C-11 as PSVT- many clinicians now prefer the newer term- ***AVNRT*** (***AV*** *Nodal* ***R****eentry* ***T****achycardia*)- to designate this arrhythmia. The advantage of this newer term is that it more accurately reflects the *mechanism* of this rhythm- which almost always involves ***reentry*** within (or into) the AV node. For the purpose of consistency with AHA Guidelines, we refer to this rhythm as ***PSVT*** throughout this book.

Initial Approach: *KEY Clinical Questions*

Before discussing the specific interventions described in Figure 1C-11 for the management of PSVT- three *KEY* clinical questions should be considered:

i) Is the patient hemodynamically stable?
ii) Is the QRS complex is *truly* narrow?
iii) Is the diagnosis *truly* PSVT?

The importance of considering these issues is best illustrated by applying the above three questions to the tachycardia shown at the top of Figure 1C-11. The clinical approach to management of a patient with this rhythm will clearly depend first on hemodynamic status. Only if the patient is hemodynamically stable should further evaluation take place. If the patient is *not* hemodynamically stable- then *immediate* intervention with synchronized cardioversion (*rather than* drugs) should be strongly considered (*See Figure 1C-1*).

Figure 1C-11- *Treatment Algorithm for PSVT*

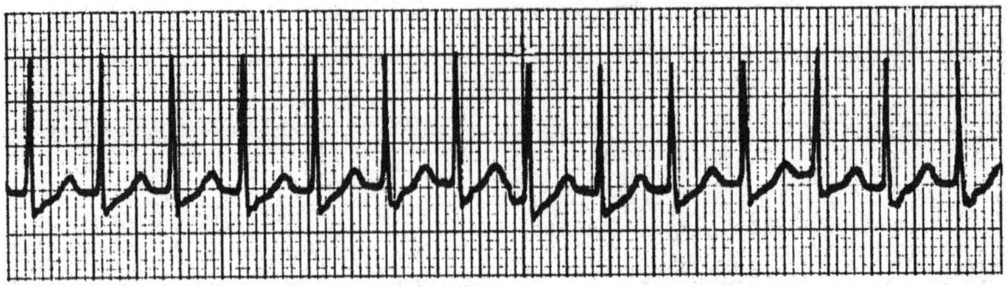

- *Supportive Actions*
  - as listed on Figure 1C-1 have *all* been accomplished.

> **KEY Clinical Questions**
> i) Is the patient hemodynamically stable?
> ii) Is the QRS complex is *truly* narrow?
> iii) Is the diagnosis *truly* PSVT?

Treatment Options:

- Consider the use of a ***Vagal Maneuver***

- **Adenosine:**
  - The drug of 1st choice for PSVT (and the drug of choice for treatment of *SUPRAventricular* tachycardias of uncertain etiology)
  - Begin with **6 mg** by *rapid* **IV push** (i.e., over 1-3 seconds!)- followed by a fluid flush.
  - If no response in 1-2 min, a 2nd dose (of **12 mg**) may be given- and repeated if needed in 1-2 min (for a total dose of 6 + 12 + 12 = 30 mg).

- **Verapamil:**
  - Should only be used if the QRS complex is narrow (or the tachycardia is known with *certainty* to be PSVT)
  - Give **2.5- 5 mg IV** over 1-2 min; may follow 15-30 min later with a 2nd dose of 5-10 mg IV. Give the drug slower (over 3-4 min) to the elderly.

- *Other drugs* that could also be used:
  - **Diltiazem**- comparable effect as Verapamil
  - **Digoxin**- more delayed onset of action
  - **Beta-Blocker-** should *not* be used soon after IV Diltiazem/Verapamil !

> **Note**- If the patient decompensates at *any* time during the process of evaluating/treating the tachycardia- *STOP and immediately cardiovert* !

If the patient is hemodynamically stable- then there *is* time to go further. This brings up the next *KEY* clinical point:

ii) Is the QRS complex is *truly* narrow?

It is easy to get fooled ! Although it certainly *appears* that the QRS complex of the rhythm in Figure 1C-11 is narrow- one can *not* rule out the possibilitity that a portion of the QRS complex in this *single* monitoring lead might be lying *isoelectric* on the baseline:

- Obtaining a **12-lead ECG** while the patient is *still in* the tachycardia would help to confirm that the QRS complex is *truly* narrow in all 12 leads (and that the rhythm is *truly* supraventricular). Obtaining a 12-lead ECG during the tachycardia may also provide *diagnostic* assistance in determining the true mechanism of the arrhythmia, which may be invaluable for optimizing treatment.

- A 12-lead ECG should *not* be obtained if the patient is unstable. As emphasized- the treatment of choice for an unstable patient with tachycardia is *immediate* synchronized cardioversion *regardless* of what the rhythm happens to be.

The *KEY* for deciding on optimal treatment of the various types of SVT lies with determining the ***specific diagnosis*** of the rhythm. This is the message implied with our third clinical point:

iii) Is the diagnosis *truly* PSVT?

As discussed in our section on *Differential Diagnosis*- attention to parameters such as rate, regularity, and the presence and nature of atrial activity will usually provide the clues that are needed for accurate diagnosis *(Pages 56-58)*. Use of a vagal maneuver (*See below*) may provide additional assistance. For example- the narrow complex tachycardia in Figure 1C-11 is regular at a rate of approximately 180 beats/minute. Regularity of this rhythm rules out A Fib as a possibility. The heart rate of 180 beats/minute is too fast to be sinus tachycardia- and not consistent with that expected if the rhythm was A Flutter. This leaves PSVT as the most likely diagnosis. Initiation of treatment based on this diagnosis should now be in order.

Use of a Vagal Maneuver

Vagal maneuvers act by *transiently* increasing parasympathetic tone. This slows conduction through supraventricular and AV nodal tissues. One hopes to delay AV nodal conduction *just long enough* to interrupt the reentry circuit of PSVT and terminate the arrhythmia.

Vagal maneuvers include carotid sinus massage, Valsalva, activation of the gag reflex, facial submersion in ice water, eyeball pressure (which is no longer recommended), digital rectal massage, and squatting (*See also Section 2D*). Patients with recurrent episodes of PSVT have often instinctively learned to perform one of these maneuvers on their own to terminate their arrhythmia.

- In an emergency care setting- ***cartotid sinus massage* (*CSM*)** is the vagal maneuver performed most often for treatment. *Under constant ECG monitoring*- the patient's head is turned to the left and the area of the *right* carotid bifurcation (near the angle of the jaw) is gently but *firmly* massaged for 3-5 seconds at a time. If right carotid massage is ineffective, the left side may be tried. (One should *never* massage both sides simultaneously!)

- If PSVT persists despite application of a vagal maneuver- keep in mind that the maneuver may sometimes work if *reapplied* again *after* administration of antiarrhythmic therapy (since the effect of drugs and the maneuver is often synergistic).

- In addition to its role in treatment, CSM may also be helpful as a *diagnostic* maneuver for distinguishing between the various types of SVT. When CSM is applied to a patient in PSVT- the rhythm will either be converted by the maneuver, or nothing will happen. In contrast, with sinus tachycardia or A Flutter- *transient* slowing of the ventricular response during massage will often allow "telltale" atrial activity to become apparent (*See also Table 2D-1 on page 166*).

> **<u>Note</u>-** CSM is *not* a totally benign maneuver- especially when applied to older individuals. Complications that have been associated with CSM include syncope, stroke, sinus arrest, high-grade AV block, prolonged asystole, and ventricular tachyarrhythmias in patients with digitalis intoxication. As a result- CSM should probaly *not* be attempted in patients with a history of sick sinus syndrome, cervical bruits, or cerebrovascular disease, or when the possibility of Digoxin toxicity exists.

Medical Therapy: *Adenosine and Verapamil*

The two drugs most commonly used for treatment of PSVT are Adenosine and Verapamil. Although AHA Guidelines now favor Adenosine as the drug of first choice for emergency treatment of this arrhythmia- we believe *both* drugs still retain a definite role in therapy.

- ***Adenosine***. One of the most exciting advances in antiarrhythmic therapy has been development of Adenosine for treatment of PSVT. The most remarkable pharmacologic feature of this drug relates to its rapid onset of action and exceedingly short half-life (which is estimated to be *less* than 10 seconds in duration!). A decided advantage of this feature is that the clinician will know within a very short period of time whether or not the drug will work. Side effects such as cough, flushing, and excessive bradycardia may occur- but even if they do, they are likely to be extremely short-lived.

  - The recommended *initial* dose of Adenosine is to administer **6 mg** by **IV push**. If there is no response after 1-2 minutes- a 2nd dose (of **12 mg**) may be tried- and repeated (if needed) after another 1-2 minutes (for a *total* dose of 6 + 12 + 12 = **30 mg**). If this amount is ineffective, it is unlikely that Adenosine will work- and *alternative* therapy (i.e., IV Verapamil or Diltiazem) should be tried.

  - Adenosine is one of the few drugs that *must* be given by ***"IV push"***- injecting the drug *as fast as possible* (i.e., over a period of 1-3 seconds!). Failure to do so may result in the drug breaking down while still in the IV tubing. Drug distribution and absorption may be further facilitated by *immediately* following each dose with a ***saline flush*** (of ≈20 ml of fluid).

- The principal drawbacks of Adenosine are that the drug is ineffective for treatment of other types of SVT that are not dependent on AV nodal reentry (since slowing of the ventricular response with A Fib and A Flutter is so transient)- and that *recurrence* of PSVT is likely to occur in many patients after the effect of the drug wears off.

▪ ***Verapamil***. Up until recently, Verapamil had been the pharmacologic agent of choice for emergency treatment of PSVT. When used appropriately, the drug is usually well tolerated and effective in converting this reentry tachyarrhythmia in more than 90% of cases. Additional advantages of Verapamil include the duration of action of its antiarrhythmic effect (which lasts for up to 30 minutes), availability of an oral formulation of the drug (which facilitates long-term antiarrhythmic control), and its efficacy in treating other types of SVT (including MAT, A Fib, and A Flutter). In contrast- Adenosine has a much shorter duration of action, is not available in an oral formulation, and is only effective in treatment of *reentry* tachyarrhythmias.

> **Note-** Clinical indications, cautions, and adverse effects that we list below for Verapamil are similar for Diltiazem. AHA Guidelines still favor use of IV Verapamil for treatment of PSVT- probably because of greater clinical experience accumulated with this drug (AHA Text- Pg 7-11).

- Dosing considerations for use of Verapamil in the treatment of PSVT are similar to those presented earlier in discussion of A Fib/Flutter. Thus, **2.5-5 mg IV** may be given for the first dose of Verapamil- which may then be increased (to 5-10 mg) for a second IV dose given 15-30 minutes later (if/as needed).

- ***Pretreatment*** with IV infusion of **Calcium Chloride** (infusing 500-1,000 mg over a 5-10 minute period) has been shown to minimize the hypotensive response of Verapamil (or Diltiazem)- *without* diminishing drug efficacy for converting or controlling the ventricular response to supraventricular tachyarrhythmias. Such pretreatment might be considered particularly for patients with borderline hemodynamic status (i.e., systolic blood pressure of *less* than 100 mm Hg).

- The major concern regarding Verapamil (and Diltiazem) is to be sure that these drugs are *never* given to a patient who might have VT. If this were to happen, the vasodilatory and negative inotropic effects of these drugs would be likely to precipitate deterioration of the rhythm to V Fib. Verapamil (and Diltiazem) should therefore *never* be used as a diagnostic/therapeutic trial for treatment of a *wide-complex* tachycardia if the etiology of the rhythm is at all uncertain.

- A decided advantage of Verapamil (and Diltiazem) is that if IV use is successful in converting the rhythm- antiarrhythmic effect can then be maintained (and the chance of recurrence minimized) by continuing the patient on oral therapy.

Other Treatment Options

In almost all cases, use of either a vagal maneuver and/or treatment with Adenosine or Verapamil will be effective in converting the patient with PSVT to sinus rhythm. If it is not- other therapeutic options might be considered. These include:

- ***Sedation***. Although not usually thought of as antiarrhythmic therapy- judicious use of a short-acting benzodiazepine (i.e., 0.5-1 mg of Ativan)- may produce a beneficial effect on the mechanism of PSVT. This is because the degree of autonomic tone at any given moment will directly influence conduction properties in AV nodal reentry pathways. As a result, in addition to relieving the anxiety that so often accompanies PSVT- use of sedation may produce a beneficial *physiologic* effect that significantly contributes to converting the arrhythmia.

- ***Digoxin***. Although frequently used in the past to treat PSVT, the tremendous success of Adenosine and Verapamil have dramatically reduced current use of this drug for this indication. Thus despite the fact that Digoxin is effective for treating PSVT (and is still often used in long-term therapy)- the relatively delayed onset of action of this drug make it a *second-line* agent for treatment of PSVT in the emergency situation.

- ***IV Beta-Blockers***. As is the case for the treatment of rapid A Fib/Flutter, IV beta-blockers seem to be used much less often than Adenosine or Verapamil for emergency treatment of PSVT. The reason for ths is *not* a reflection of drug efficacy, since IV beta-blockers demonstrate comparable success rates for converting PSVT to sinus rhythm. Instead, it is probably because Adenosine is simpler (and perhaps safer) to use than IV beta-blockers- and because most emergency care providers are more comfortable with its use. As a result, Adenosine is usually tried first in the acute treatment protocol. If PSVT persists- IV Verapamil is usually tried next, which essentially precludes subsequent trial of an IV beta-blocker. Because of a cumulative AV nodal blocking effect, IV Verapamil/Diltiazem and IV beta-blockers should *never* be given in close proximity (i.e., within 20-30 minutes) of each other- as the combination of these agents could lead to *marked* bradycardia (and even asystole!).

- ***Synchronized Cardioversion***. Because of the extremely high success rate of medical therapy for treatment of PSVT- synchronized cardioversion is *rarely* needed for treatment of this arrhythmia. In the rare event that it is needed, AHA Guidelines suggest *initial* use of **100 joules** for PSVT- increasing to 200, 300, and 360 joules as needed (*See Section 2D*).

> **Note**- As is the case for treatment of other tachyarrhythmias, immediate synchronized cardioversion is indicated if hemodynamic instability develops *at any time* during the treatment process. Clinically, this is a relatively uncommon occurrence with PSVT.

- ***Diltiazem***. Although AHA Guidelines recommend Verapamil as the drug of second choice for medical treatment of PSVT- use of Diltiazem would seem to provide an equally effective alternative. When dosed appropriately, potential advantages of IV Diltiazem are less myocardial depression and a lower incidence of severe hypotension.

Dosing considerations for IV Diltiazem in the treatment of PSVT are similar to those presented earlier for IV bolus treatment of A Fib/Flutter. Thus, an *initial* IV bolus of 0.25 mg/kg (which for an *average-sized* adult is ≈**15-20 mg**) is recommended- which may then be increased to 0.35 mg/kg (or about **25 mg**) for the second IV bolus that is given 15 minutes later if there is no response. Continuous IV infusion is rarely needed- since once the reentry cycle in PSVT is broken, the arrhythmia will be terminated. Recurrence may be prevented with long-term oral therapy.

Treatment Algorithm for Ventricular Tachycardia

AHA recommendations for emergency treatment of ***sustained*** **ventricular tachycardia (VT)** are summarized in the algorithm we present in Figure 1C-12. Assessment of the patient in *sustained* VT and selection of the optimal course of treatment for this arrhythmia are among the most problematic (and anxiety producing) tasks in emergency cardiac care. In the hope of facilitating the decision making process- we insert three *KEY Clinical Questions* into the earliest part of our approach.

Initial Approach: *KEY Clinical Questions*

Optimal management of sustained VT is best determined by *immediate* consideration of the following three questions:

i) Is there a pulse?
ii) Is the patient hemodynamically stable?
iii) Are you *sure* that the rhythm is VT?

The purpose of these three questions is to hone in on the clinical significance of the arrhythmia, as well as to attempt to confirm the diagnosis. Clinical application of this *Initial Approach* can be illustrated by considering the rhythm shown at the top of Figure 1C-12. Clearly, the *most* important issue to address when confronted with a patient in a rhythm such as this is contained in the first question that we list above- ***Is there a PULSE?*** If the patient does *not* have a pulse, then the approach to the rhythm is simple- shock (*unsynchronized*) as soon as possible. As emphasized in Section 1B (*See Figure 1B-1 on page 34*)- ***Pulseless VT should be treated as V Fib*** (i.e., with immediate *unsynchronized* defibrillation).

Approach to VT: *If a Pulse IS Present*

The approach to management of VT is significantly different when a pulse *IS* present. Highest priority is now given to determining the patient's hemodynamic status. There are two possibilities:

i) *The patient may be* ***hemodynamically UNSTABLE***- in which case the need for immediate action is urgent. As emphasized at the beginning of this section (and illustrated in Figure 1C-1)- *immediate* synchronized cardioversion is indicated if serious signs and/or symptoms are being produced as a *direct result* of the tachycardia.

ii) *The patient may be* ***hemodynamically STABLE***- in which case there should be (by definition) a little more time to reflect on the process. Ideally, the third clinical question can now be addressed and hopefully answered (i.e., ***Are you sure that the rhythm is VT?***). If there is reasonable certainty of the clinical diagnosis- then a trial of medical therapy can be undertaken.

Figure 1C-12- *Treatment Algorithm for VT*

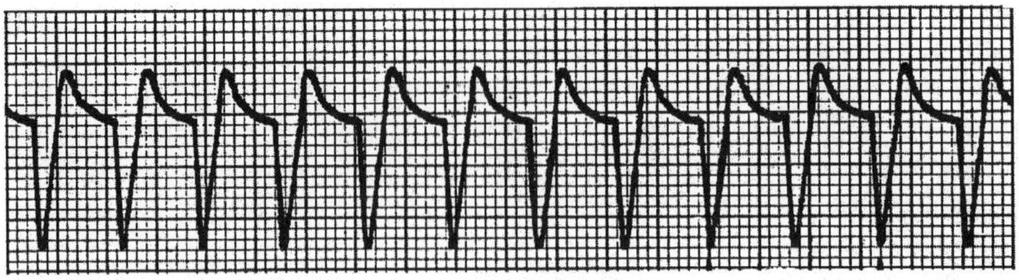

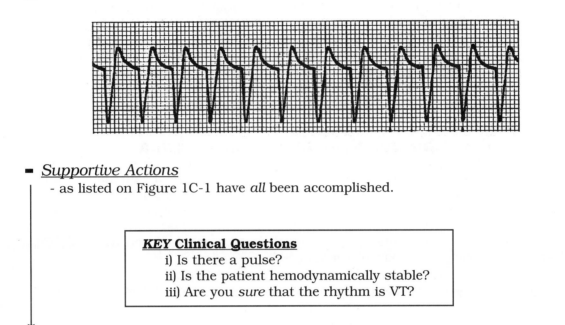

- *Supportive Actions*
  - as listed on Figure 1C-1 have *all* been accomplished.

> ***KEY* Clinical Questions**
> i) Is there a pulse?
> ii) Is the patient hemodynamically stable?
> iii) Are you *sure* that the rhythm is VT?

Treatment Options: (for the pt in VT who *is* hemodynamically stable!)

- **Lidocaine:**
  - Give 1.0-1.5 mg/kg (usually ≈**75-100 mg**) as an *initial* **IV bolus**. Repeat boluses of ≈50-75 mg (i.e., ≈0.5-0.75 mg/kg) may be given q5-10 min up to a total of 3 mg/kg (≈225 mg).
  - If effective, consider a *maintenance* IV infusion @ ≈2 mg/min.

- **Procainamide:**
  - Give in increments of 100 mg IV *slowly* over 5 min (i.e., @ ≈20 mg/min)- up to a total dose of **17 mg/kg IV** (≈1,000 mg). If effective, may follow with a *maintenance* IV infusion @ 2 mg/min (1-4 mg/min range).

- **Bretylium:**
  - Dilute **500 mg** (≈5-10 mg/kg) in 50 ml of D5W- and infuse **IV** over ≈10 minutes. May either repeat this IV loading dose in 10-30 min- and/or begin an IV infusion of Bretylium (@ ≈1-2 mg/min).

- *Other Measures* :
  - **Magnesium**- in a dose of ≈**1-2 gm IV** (over 1-2 minutes)- especially if serum levels are (or are likely to be) low. *May repeat.*
  - Look for a Cause/Other drugs (*See text*).

- *Use of* ***Synchronized Cardioversion*** :
  - May be considered if the pt fails to respond to medical therapy.
  - If time permits, consider premedication- and then begin at **100 joules**.

> **Note**- If the patient decompensates at *any* time during the process of evaluating/treating the tachycardia- *STOP and immediately cardiovert* !

<u>Bottom Line</u>- the *KEY* to management of ***sustained*** **VT** lies with first determining the patient's *hemodynamic* status. One of *three* clinical situations will exist:

i) *The patient will be in VT, but there is* ***NO Pulse.*** Pulseless VT should be treated as V Fib with immediate shock (Figure 1B-1).

ii) *A pulse IS present, but the patient is* ***UNSTABLE.*** Synchronized cardioversion is *immediately* indicated (Figure 1C-1).

iii) *Sustained VT persists, but the patient is (and remains)* ***STABLE.*** In this situation a trial of medical therapy (as suggested below) is reasonable and appropriate.

<u>Hemodynamically Stable VT: *Medical Therapy*</u>

Therapeutic options to consider in the management of hemodynamically stable VT are listed in Figure 1C-12. They include the following:

- ***Lidocaine.*** Lidocaine is generally accepted as the antiarrhythmic agent of choice for medical treatment of sustained VT. AHA Guidelines recommend a dose of 1.0-1.5 mg/kg (usually ≈**75-100 mg**) to be given as an *initial* **IV bolus**. Additional 50-75 mg IV boluses may follow every 5-10 minutes thereafter (either as needed- and/or until a *total* loading dose of *up to* 225 mg has been given). If Lidocaine appears to be effective- then a ***maintenance*** **IV infusion** (at a rate of **2 mg/minute**) should be started.
  - Although many clinicians tend to increase the Lidocaine infusion rate with each additional bolus of the drug that is given- this is *not* essential during the period of Lidocaine loading. On the contrary, routinely increasing the infusion rate (i.e., to 3 and 4 mg/minute) after administration of each Lidocaine bolus may *unnecessarily* increase the risk of developing Lidocaine toxicity. IV infusion at a rate of 2 mg/minute will be adequate for most patients.
  - On the other hand, if the ventricular arrhythmia rapidly resolves after bolus administration- only to recur *after* steady state conditions have been achieved (i.e., at an infusion rate of 2 mg/minute)- then administration of an *additional* 50 mg bolus of Lidocaine *and* an increase in the infusion rate (i.e., to 3 mg/minute) may be warranted.
- ***Procainamide.*** If Lidocaine is ineffective- then Procainamide is generally recommended as the *second-line* agent of choice for medical treatment of sustained VT. The drug is most often given in **IV increments** of **100 mg** (administering each increment *slowly* over a 5 minute period)- until one of the following *end points* is achieved:

  i) The patient receives an adequate loading dose. Although a loading dose of ≈500-1,000 mg is usually given, a total dose of *up to* **17 mg/kg IV** may be administered.
  ii) The arrhythmia is suppressed.
  iii) Hypotension develops.
  iv) QRS widening occurs.

Alternatively, 500-1,000 mg of Procainamide may be diluted in 100 ml of D5W and administered as a loading IV infusion over 30-60 minutes.

An additional advantage of using Procainamide is that even if the drug is not successful in converting the rhythm- it may still *slow* the ventricular response of VT (which may allow the patient to remain hemodynamically stable for a longer period of time).

> **Note**- If either loading regimen of Procainamide achieves the desired clinical effect- a continuous **IV *maintenance* infusion** of the drug may be started at a rate of **2 mg/minute** (range = 1-4 mg/minute).

- ***Bretylium***. Although frequently used in the past, administration of Bretylium Tosylate for medical treatment of PVCs/VT has been deemphasized. Practically speaking, the drug appears to be much more effective as an *antifibrillatory* agent than as an *antiarrhythmic* agent. Moreover, the most common long-term adverse effect associated with Bretylium therapy is hypotension, which further limits its use. As a result, other therapeutic options could be considered if Lidocaine and Procainamide are ineffective (*See below*).

  - If Bretylium is used for treatment of sustained VT- the drug should be given as an **IV loading infusion** rather than as bolus therapy. To do this, one ampule of Bretylium (= **500 mg**) is mixed in 50 ml of D5W- and then infused over a 10 minute period.

  - Following IV loading, a ***maintenance* IV infusion** (at a rate of between **1-2 mg/minute**) may be started to sustain the drug's antiarrhythmic effect.

- ***Magnesium***. The role of Magnesium Sulfate in the treatment of *sustained* VT and cardiac arrest is still not clarified. As a result, use of the drug in this setting is still largely empiric.

  - Consider IV Magnesium if the patient fails to respond to standard therapy- especially if hypomagnesemia is likely.

  - The usual *initial* dose of Magnesium for VT is **1-2 gm IV**. If needed, this amount may be repeated. For life-threatening situations the drug can be administered over a 1-2 minute period. Slower administration, or use of a continuous IV infusion is appropriate when the situation is less urgent.

- ***Other Measures***. Several alternative measures may be considered if the patient with *sustained* VT fails to respond to the above treatment:

  - ***Search for a potentially correctable cause.*** Persistent VT may result from the presence of any of the same factors that predispose to persistence of refractory V Fib (*See Section 1B- and the "D" component of the Secondary Survey*).

- *Use of an **IV Beta-Blocker**.* Although IV beta-blockers are usually *not* considered as first-line agents in the treatment of most tachyarrhythmias- they may be effective, and there clearly *are* times when *all* other treatment measures will fail (and *only* IV beta-blockers may save the patient). This is especially true when excessive *sympathetic* tone is likely to be operative as a cause of the sustained VT.

- *Consideration of **IV Sotalol** or **Amiodarone**.* These drugs are *not* yet included in AHA Guidelines. Experience in the setting of sustained VT and cardiac arrest is still somewhat limited- although initial reports are favorable. Use of these drugs may become more common in the not too distant future.

- ***Synchronized Cardioversion***. In the event that medical therapy (as outlined above) is unsuccessful in converting the patient out of *sustained* VT- cardioversion may be tried. If the patient shows no signs of hemodynamic compromise, this may be attempted under ***"semi-elective"*** conditions. This entails:

  i) Sedation of the patient (i.e., with IV Valium, Versed, or other agent).
  ii) Calling anesthesia to the bedside to assist with intubation if needed (so as to leave you free to concentrate on managing the arrhythmia).

  AHA Guidelines recommend use of the *Standard Sequence of Energy Levels* for synchronized cardioversion of VT. One should therefore *begin* with **100 joules**- and increase to 200, 300, and then 360 joules (if/as needed). An exception to this recommendation is for the patient with *polymorphic VT*- which often requires higher energy levels (of 200 joules or more) for successful cardioversion (AHA Text- Pg 1-35).

If the Patient *Becomes* Hemodynamically Unstable

If at any time during the process of evaluation or treatment the patient *becomes* hemodynamically unstable- *STOP* the process. In this situation- *synchronized* cardioversion should be *immediately* performed.

- The clinical definition of *hemodynamically "unstable"* varies greatly. The *KEY* defining premise of the term is that signs and/or symptoms must be produced in association with the rhythm as a *direct result* of the rapid rate.

- AHA Guidelines emphasize that even when the decision to cardiovert *"immediately"* has been made- that medical therapy (i.e., use of Lidocaine, Procainamide, etc.) may *still* be tried- *IF* these drugs are *immediately* available- provided that giving these drugs *does not* result in delay of cardioversion (AHA Text- Pg 1-35). *Clinical judgement is needed at the bedside.*

Cough Version

If a pulse is present and the patient is alert- consider the use of ***cough version***. Whether the mechanism for cough version is improved coronary perfusion (from the increase in intrathoracic pressure generated by the cough), activation of the autonomic nervous system, or conversion of mechanical energy from the cough (into an electrical depolarization), is unknown. What has been shown is that the cough may effectively convert sustained VT to normal sinus rhythm in a surprising number of cases.

- In practice, cough version appears to be vastly underutilized. The technique should probably be the *first* intervention for treatment of the conscious patient who presents in sustained VT.

- In contrast to cough version, use of the *precordial thump* has been strongly deemphasized as a treatment modality for sustained VT. The problem with the thump is that even though the maneuver may occasionally convert VT to sinus rhythm- it is equally likely (if not more so) to convert this rhythm to V Fib, asystole, or pulseless idioventricular rhythm. Thus, if synchronized cardioversion is readily available, it would seem to be far preferable to delivery of 2-5 joules at a *random* (and possibly vulnerable) point in the cardiac cycle as is provided by the thump.

Treatment Algorithm for WCT of *Uncertain* Type

AHA recommendations for emergency treatment of the patient with a ***WCT*** (***Wide-Complex Tachycardia***) of ***Uncertain Type*** are summarized in the algorithm we present in Figure 1C-13. In many ways, evaluation and management of this problem is similar to that for the patient with VT. The principal difference relates to the fact that *despite* QRS widening- the etiology of this rhythm is *not* quite as certain as it is for VT- hence use of the name, ***WCT*** of ***"Uncertain" Type***. In the hope of facilitating the decision making process, we incorporate the three major diagnostic considerations for WCT into the initial part of our approach in this algorithm.

Differential Diagnosis of WCT: *Key Clinical Points*

For practical purposes, the differential diagnosis of a *WCT* of *Uncertain Type* consists of *three* major entities. They are:

i) VT
ii) SVT with *aberrant* conduction
iii) SVT with *preexisting* bundle branch block

Detailed description of criteria used for distinguishing between VT and these two forms of SVT extends beyond the scope of this book. Nevertheless, the following *KEY* clinical points can be made about the approach we suggest for assessing the patient with ***WCT*** of ***Uncertain Type*** :

- ***Until proven otherwise- always assume that the rhythm is VT.*** Statistically, the etiology of a *WCT of Uncertain Type* is far more likely to be VT than SVT (with QRS widening from either aberrant conduction or preexisting bundle branch block). This dictum holds true *regardless* of whether the patient is alert or not- and *regardless* of what the blood pressure happens to be. ***The patient should be treated accordingly*** (i.e., as if the rhythm was VT- *until proven otherwise*).

- As was the case for evaluating the patient with VT (Figure 1C-12)- the *most* important question to address is ***whether the patient is hemodynamically stable.*** If not- specific diagnosis of the tachyarrhythmia *no longer matters* (since *immediate* cardioversion should now be performed *regardless* of what the arrhythmia happens to be!).

Figure 1C-13- *Treatment Algorithm for WCT of Uncertain Type*

(When the patient is hemodynamically stable)

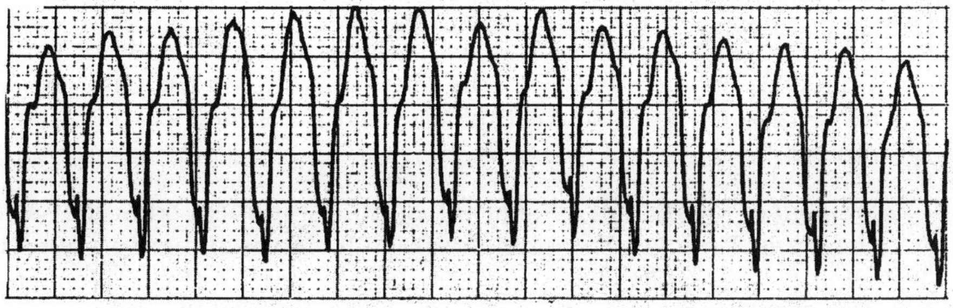

- *Supportive Actions*
  - as listed on Figure 1C-1 have *all* been accomplished.

Consider the Differential Diagnosis
i) VT- *always* assumed until *proven* otherwise
ii) SVT with *aberrant* conduction
iii) SVT with *preexisting* bundle branch block

Treatment Options:

- **Lidocaine:** (*See Figure 1C-12 on page 80.*)

- **Adenosine:**
  - May be considered if the WCT is of *Uncertain* Type (and has *not* responded to Lidocaine)- especially if the rhythm might be supraventricular.
  - -Begin with **6 mg** by *rapid* **IV push** (i.e., over 1-3 seconds!)- followed by a fluid flush.
  - If no response in 1-2 min, a 2nd dose (of **12 mg**) may be given- and repeated if needed in 1-2 min (for a total dose of 6 + 12 + 12 = 30 mg).

- **Procainamide:** (*See Figure 1C-12.*)

- *Other drugs* that could also be used:
  - **Magnesium**- (*See Figure 1C-12 for suggested dosing.*)
  - **Bretylium**- might be used if the WCT was thought to be VT and there was no response to other agents (*See Figure 1C-12 for dosing*).

- *Use of* ***Synchronized Cardioversion*** **:**
  - May be considered if the pt fails to respond to medical therapy.
  - If time permits, consider premedication- and then begin at **100 joules**.

> **Note**- If the patient decompensates at *any* time during the process of evaluating/treating the tachycardia- *STOP and immediately cardiovert* !

- *If the patient IS hemodynamically **STABLE***- then there may be time to evaluate the situation in more detail. Selecting the *most* appropriate therapeutic option for the patient with WCT of *Uncertain* Type will become *far* simpler if the correct diagnosis can be made- at least with *relative* certainty. Clues that may help in this regard (i.e., to distinguish between the three major causes of WCT) include one or more of the following:

  - *Recall of "the facts"*. Given that the overwhelming majority of WCTs of *Uncertain* Type will turn out to be VT- the onus residing on the emergency care provider must *always* be to prove that the rhythm is *not* VT- *and not the other way around.*

  - *Brief review of the patient's medical history*. Statistical odds that a regular WCT of *Uncertain* Type is VT approach 90% (!!!)- *IF* the patient in question is an *older adult* (i.e., >60-70 years old) *and* has a history of *documented* heart disease (i.e., *either* previous infarction, angina, or heart failure).

  - *Use of prior tracings*. A glance through the patient's medical chart to look for prior 12-lead ECGs and/or recent telemetry recordings may sometimes provide invaluable information. Prior tracings may reveal the longterm presence of *preexisting* bundle branch block, or WPW on a baseline ECG. Recent telemetry tracings may reveal other episodes of tachycardia that were *definitely* diagnosed to be VT, A Fib/Flutter, or MAT- and/or PVCs that manifest an *identical* morphologic appearance to that of the QRS complexes in the WCT being assessed.

  - *Obtaining a **12-lead ECG** during the WCT*. If at all feasible, a 12-lead ECG should be obtained while the patient is still in the tachycardia. Atrial activity that might not be evident on a single lead recording may sometimes become *instantly* obvious in other leads obtained as part of the 12-lead tracing. Similarly, *seemingly narrow* QRS complexes in a single monitoring lead may *in reality* be surprisingly wide (if part of the QRS complex in the lead being monitored happens to lie *isoelectric* to the baseline). Finally, use of a few *KEY* (and surprisingly *easy* to remember) clues relating to QRS axis and QRS morphology may dramatically increase the diagnostic reliability of the ECG for those informed/experienced emergency care providers attentive to these findings.

Bottom Line- Assessing the patient *always* comes first! The most important issue to address in evaluating *any* patient who presents with a *WCT of Uncertain Type* is hemodynamic status. Subsequent management depends on this assessment. A 12-lead ECG should *not* be obtained if the patient is acutely unstable. Instead- *immediate* cardioversion is indicated for the unstable patient.

The point to emphasize is that if the patient *is* hemodynamically stable- then optimal management can *only* be selected if the correct ECG diagnosis is known. Appropriate use of a 12-lead ECG obtained *during* the tachycardia will greatly facilitate this determination much of the time. Simply stated, when evaluating a WCT of *unknown* etiology- ***"12 leads are BETTER than one"***.

- <u>*Trial of a diagnostic maneuver.*</u> This may either be in the form of a ***vagal maneuver*** (such as carotid massage or Valsalva)- and/or with use of ***Adenosine*** (i.e., *"chemical Valsalva"*)- <u>*IF*</u> deemed appropriate as determined by assessment of the tracing and the patient's clinical condition!

    Vagal maneuvers are most likely to be helpful in the differential diagnosis of *narrow-complex* tachyarrhythmias (such as A Flutter, rapid A Fib, and rapid sinus tachycardia). They may even be *curative* if the rhythm is PSVT. In contrast, they rarely affect VT (*See Table 2D-1*). Performance of a vagal maneuver may therefore be helpful from a *diagnostic* (as well as *therapeutic*) standpoint- if applied to a patient with a WCT that might well be supraventricular.

> **<u>Note</u>-** The point to emphasize is that vagal maneuvers are *not* completely benign (*See Section 2D*). As a result- they should probably *not* be performed if you strongly suspect that the patient is in VT. Similarly, because Adenosine is *not* a completely benign medication- we prefer *not* to administer this drug to patients with probable VT.
>
> On the other hand- use of *either* a vagal maneuver *and/or* "chemical Valsalva" (with Adenosine) is perfectly appropriate and often of invaluable assistance for evaluating patients with WCT that is at least *somewhat likely* to be of supraventricular etiology.

<u>Treatment Options for WCT</u>

The drugs that are listed in Figure 1C-13 for treatment of a WCT of *Uncertain* Type are virtually the same as those listed in Figure 1C-12 for treatment of VT- with the *exception* of Adenosine. (*Dosing specifics for these drugs is also the same as shown in Figure 1C-12.*)

- ***Lidocaine.*** AHA Guidelines recommend Lidocaine as the drug of 1st choice for medical treatment of *both* VT and WCT of *Uncertain* Type. Their reason for doing so is to emphasize the point that the *most* common cause (*by far!*) of a WCT is VT- for which Lidocaine is the drug of choice.

- ***Adenosine.*** As noted above, AHA Guidelines suggest use of Adenosine as a *diagnostic/therapeutic* trial when the etiology of the WCT is *uncertain* and Lidocaine has *not* been effective. The advantage of using Adenosine in this situation is that <u>*IF*</u> the rhythm turns out to be supraventricular, administration of this drug will usually either *slow* the rate enough to allow correct diagnosis- or convert the rhythm (if the WCT is PSVT). With rare exceptions, Adenosine is unlikely to do anything if the rhythm turns out to be VT. Although use of this drug is *not* completely benign- most of the time administration of Adenosine will *not* be deleterious even if the drug is inadvertently given to a patient who is in VT (since the duration of its action is so short).

    - The recommended *initial* dose of Adenosine is **6 mg** by rapid **IV push** (i.e., given over 1-3 seconds!). If there is no response after 1-2 minutes, a 2nd dose (of **12 mg**) may be tried- and repeated (if needed) after another 1-2 minutes (for a *total* dose of 6 + 12 + 12 = **30 mg**).

> **Note-** Unlike Adenosine (which *may* be used in the treatment of a WCT of *Uncertain* Type)- Verapamil and Diltiazem should ***never*** be used as a diagnostic/therapeutic trial to treat WCT unless it is known *with certainty* that the rhythm is supraventricular. Empiric treatment of a WCT with Verapamil (or Diltiazem) could be a "lethal error" if the WCT turned out to be VT (AHA Text- Pg 1-38).

- ***Procainamide***. AHA Guidelines recommend Procainamide as the 3rd drug to use in the treatment protocol for WCT- if Lidocaine and Adenosine have not been effective. An advantage of Procainamide over other antiarrhythmic agents is that this drug may be effective in treating a WCT- *regardless* of what the rhythm happens to be:

  - *If the WCT turns out to be VT*- Procainamide may either convert the rhythm- or at least slow down the rate of the VT.
  - *If the WCT turns out to be an SVT*- the "Quinidine-like" action of Procainamide may either convert the rhythm- and/or prevent recurrence (by suppressing PACs/PJCs that typically precipitate these tachyarrhythmias).
  - *If the WCT turns out to be WPW*- Procainamide is the drug of choice for treatment of a WCT due to rapid A Fib in a patient with WPW. The reason Procainamide is effective for this indication is that it *slows* anterograde conduction down the accessory pathway. In contrast, Digoxin, Verapamil, and Diltiazem are all *contraindicated* for treatment of rapid A Fib with WPW because these drugs *accelerate* conduction in the forward direction down the accessory pathway.

> **Bottom Line-** *Lidocaine* is clearly the drug of choice for *initial* treatment of a WCT that is thought to be VT. *Adenosine* offers the advantage of effectiveness for treatment of PSVT- and diagnostic utility for determining the specific etiology of other types of SVT. *Procainamide* is a little bit more difficult to use- but may help in treatment *regardless* of what the cause of the WCT happens to be.

- ***Other Measures***. As was the case for VT, consideration might be given to the use of additional measures if the patient with sustained WCT fails to respond to Lidocaine/Adenosine/Procainamide. These may include:

  - *Search for a potentially correctable cause of the rhythm.*
  - *Use of* ***Magnesium***- which may be helpful in the treatment of *both* VT and certain SVTs (especially when serum magnesium levels are likely to be low).
  - *Use of* ***Bretylium***- which has become a 3rd-line agent for the treatment of sustained ventricular arrhythmias- but which may still be useful in selected cases.
  - *Use of* ***Synchronized Cardioversion***. As was the case for VT, synchronized cardioversion should be considered if medical therapy (as outlined above) fails- and/or if at *any* time in the process the patient shows signs of hemodynamic compromise.

Section 1D: *Bradyarrhythmias (including PEA/Asystole)*

The bradyarrhythmias encompass a wide variety of rhythm disturbances that range from the most often innocent *sinus bradycardia-* to the almost invariably lethal pulseless rhythms of *asystole* and *PEA.* Prognosis and recommendations for management depend on the particular rhythm itself, the associated clinical setting, and the patient's hemodynamic status. Although ECG manifestations of the various bradyarrhythmias are admittedly quite different- many of the principles used in evaluation and treatment of these patients are the same. We therefore combine discussion of PEA rhythms, asystole, and the other bradycardias into this final section of Chapter 1.

Initial Approach: *KEY Clinical Questions*

As was the case for evaluating the patient with tachycardia- three *KEY Clinical Questions* should be addressed in the earliest part of our clinical approach. These questions are:

i) Is there a pulse?
ii) Is the rhythm hemodynamically significant?
iii) What is the rhythm? (and/or- *What is our need to know?*)

Application of this *Initial Approach* is best illustrated by considering the tracing shown below (Figure 1D-1). *How would you interpret this rhythm?*

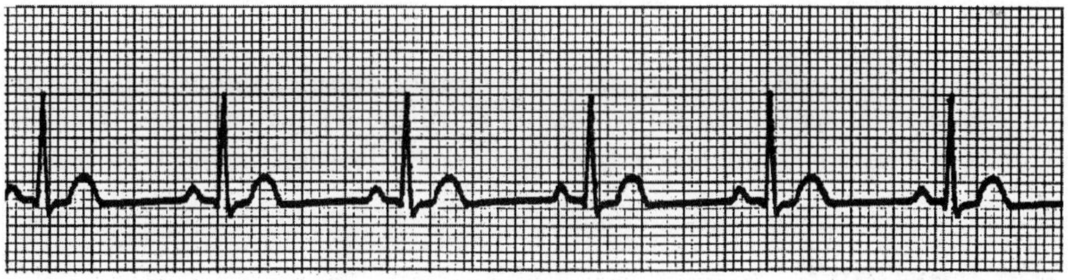

Figure 1D-1- ECG strip showing a sinus mechanism rhythm at a rate of 70 beats/minute.

Electrocardiographically- the ECG strip shown in Figure 1D-1 illustrates ***NSR*** (***N****ormal* ***S****inus* ***R****hythm*) at a rate of 70 beats/minute. The rhythm is regular, the QRS complex is narrow- and each QRS is preceded by a P wave with a constant and normal PR interval.

The point to emphasize is that clinical interpretation of the rhythm in Figure 1D-1 will *not* necessarily be NSR. Instead, clinical interpretation of this rhythm may vary- depending on answers to the *KEY Clinical Questions* that are listed above. Consider the following clinical scenarios. Note how interpretation of the rhythm in Figure 1D-1 will differ in each case:

- *If a pulse is present and BP is normal*- then the rhythm in Figure 1D-1 should be interpreted as it appears- as ***Normal Sinus Rhythm*** at a rate of 70 beats/minute No specific treatment is needed in this situation, other than routine supportive measures (i.e., observation, oxygen, establishment of IV access, etc.).

- *If a pulse is present- but the patient is hypotensive-* then specific treatment may be in order. Interventions aimed at improving hemodynamic status (i.e., fluid infusion, use of a pressor agent, etc.) should be considered.

  Although technically, the rhythm in Figure 1D-1 clearly does *not* qualify as *"bradycardia"* (since the heart rate is *more* than 60 beats/minute)- AHA Guidelines make the point that this rhythm *would* qualify as ***relative* bradycardia** if the clinical setting was that of a patient in shock with marked hypotension. In this situation, a normal hemodynamic response to the drop in blood pressure would be to *increase* heart rate (in an attempt to compensate for the hypotension). A heart rate of only 70 beats/minute (as shown in Figure 1D-1) should be interpreted as *inappropriately* slow (i.e., as *"relative"* bradycardia) for this clinical situation.

- *If no pulse is present-* then the rhythm in Figure 1D-1 should be interpreted as ***PEA*** (or ***EMD***). Clinical implications and recommendations for treatment will be very different than they are when a pulse is present (*See below*).

Is the Rhythm Hemodynamically Significant?

If a pulse *IS* present in association with bradycardia (and/or *relative* bradycardia)- then the next *KEY* issue to address is ***whether the bradycardia is hemodynamically significant.*** Specifically, one seeks to determine if the slow (or *relatively* slow) rhythm is causing the patient problems (i.e., producing *signs* or *symptoms* of concern)- as a *direct result* of the reduction in heart rate. For the purpose of this definition:

- ***Signs of Concern-*** include hypotension (i.e., systolic BP ≤80-90 mm Hg), shock, heart failure/pulmonary edema, and/or Acute MI.

- ***Symptoms of Concern-*** include chest pain, shortness of breath, and/or decreased mental status.

Pulseless rhythms will obviously be of hemodynamic significance. However, when a pulse *is* present- it will often be much more difficult to determine if a particular bradyarrhythmia is hemodynamically significant (and whether or not treatment is needed).

What is the Rhythm?

Our purpose in asking this third *KEY Clinical Question* is twofold: 1) To emphasize again the importance of assessing the patient for the presence of a pulse and for assessing hemodynamic status; and 2) To illustrate how the answer to this *KEY Question* may influence prognosis and treatment.

We have already shown how clinical interpretation of the same ECG rhythm strip may differ- depending on the patient's hemodynamic status at the time the tracing is recorded. Prognostic and therapeutic implications will also vary accordingly. For example, the prognosis is excellent (and no specific treatment is needed)- if the rhythm shown in Figure 1D-1 occurs in an asymptomatic patient who is hemodynamically stable (in which case the rhythm simply represents NSR). In contrast, prognosis is poor (and treatment is *urgently* needed)- if the *identical* tracing occurs in a patient without a pulse. This very same rhythm should now be interpreted as PEA (since it now occurs in association with a *pulseless* state).

An important point to make regarding this third *KEY Question* relates to ***our need to know*** *the* ***specific diagnosis*** *of the bradyarrhythmia.* As we have emphasized, it clearly *is* important to distinguish between NSR and PEA. Practically speaking, however- it matters little in the acute care setting if a particular bradycardia is the result of 3° AV block, idioventricular escape, Mobitz type I 2° AV block, or even marked sinus bradycardia- *as long as a pulse is present.* Initial clinical priorities (i.e., of attempting to speed up the heart rate with drugs and/or pacing) will probably *not* be much different- *regardless* of what the true rhythm happens to be.

Bottom Line- Initial priorities for assessing and treating the bradycardic (or *relatively* bradycardic) patient with a pulse will usually be the same- *regardless* of what the specific type of bradycardia happens to be. These priorities are:

i) To determine the patient's hemodynamic status.
ii) To initiate treatment based on this determination.

Practically speaking- we often do *not* have a "need to know" the specific diagnosis of the type of bradycardia in the emergency care setting.

With this introduction- we now move into the specific types of bradyarrhythmias- and present the corresponding algorithms for treatment.

Pulseless Electrical Activity

The term ***PEA*** (*Pulseless Electrical Activity*) has been added to AHA Guidelines in an attempt to *unify* an otherwise complex group of cardiac rhythms. Similarities among the entities included in this group are that they all share a common list of potential etiologies- and that they generally respond to the same treatment protocol. It should be noted that this newer term encompasses many rhythms that had previously been designated as ***EMD*** (*ElectroMechanical Dissociation*).

Clinically, the meaning of the term PEA is suggested by its name. Thus, the term is used to describe a group of diverse electrocardiographic rhythms that *by definition* manifest evidence of *Electrical Activity* (since they all produce an ECG rhythm)- but which are unified by the clinical finding of *Pulselessness.* According to this definition, PEA rhythms must therefore be *nonperfusing-* or at most no more than *minimally* perfusing (since they are by definition associated with the pulseless state).

Note- Recent echocardiographic studies demonstrate the surprising finding that many patients previously diagnosed on clinical grounds as having PEA rhythms actually have evidence of at least *some* meaningful ventricular contraction- albeit *not* enough to produce a blood pressure detectable by the usual methods of palpation or sphygmomanometer (AHA Text- Pg 1-21). Rather than an "all-or-none" phenomenon- it therefore appears that the clinical entity of PEA really encompasses a *spectrum* of disorders in which some mechanical function is actually present in many (if not most!) patients.

Many types of ECG rhythms have been associated with the clinical entity known as PEA. Most of these rhythms can be classified into one of the following groups:

- ***EMD Rhythms***- in which there is an *organized* ECG rhythm (usually with a *narrow* QRS complex)- but no pulse.
- ***Pseudo-EMD Rhythms***- in which the ECG rhythm is associated with at least some *meaningful* mechanical contraction (as might be evidenced by obtaining a pulse with doppler that is too faint to palpate clinically).
- ***Idioventricular*** or ***Ventricular Escape Rhythms***- in which the QRS complex of the escape rhythm is widened. Atrial activity is absent. There is no pulse. Included in this group are *post-defibrillation* idioventricular rhythms.
- ***Bradyasystolic Rhythms***- in which there is profound bradycardia, often with prolonged periods of asystole. There is no pulse.

An essential point to emphasize about PEA rhythms is that they are often associated with *specific* clinical states that *can* be reversed- *IF* these states can be *identified early* and *treated appropriately* (AHA Text- Pg 1-21).

> **Note-** The ECG appearance of a PEA rhythm may provide insight as to the relative likelihood that the condition can be reversed. In general, prognosis tends to be better if the ECG rhythm manifests *organized* atrial activity (in the form of P waves that conduct), a rate that is *not* excessively slow, and *narrow* QRS complexes- provided (of course) that the *underlying* cause of the PEA rhythm can be identified and corrected.
>
> In contrast- PEA is much more likely to be a *preterminal* rhythm when organized atrial activity is absent, the QRS complex is wide, and/or bradycardia persists despite medical treatment.

Treatment Algorithm for PEA Rhythms

AHA recommendations for treatment of the ***PEA rhythms*** are summarized in the algorithm we present in Figure 1D-2. Management priorities are best understood by awareness of the fact that they reflect two *KEY* clinical points:

i) That by definition- PEA is a *nonperfusing* (or at least *not* adequately perfusing) rhythm.

ii) That PEA is almost always a *secondary* disorder (that occurs as a result of *some other* underlying condition).

Figure 1D-2- *Treatment Algorithm for PEA*

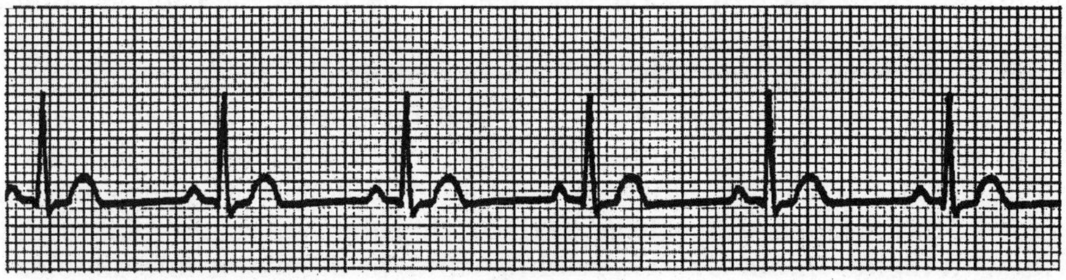

- *The above ECG rhythm in a patient without a pulse* = ***PEA*** !

KEY Treatment Options:

- *Begin/Continue* ***CPR*** :

  - Early performance of CPR is essential (since by definition PEA is a *non-perfusing* or *poorly* perfusing rhythm).
  - ***Supportive Actions*** (Intubate/Establish IV access, etc.).
  - Assess blood flow and other clinical parameters (i.e., use of ***doppler***, *End-Tidal* CO_2, *arterial line-* as possible).

- **Epinephrine:**
  - Begin with an **SDE** dose (i.e., **1.0 mg** by IV bolus).
  - May *either* repeat SDE (every 3-5 minutes- if/as needed)-
    - or *increase* the dose (i.e., to **HDE**) if there has been no response.

- *Search for the* ***Cause*** *of PEA* :

  - Consider the most common causes (*Table 1D-1 on page 96*):
    - i) Inadequate ventilation?
    - ii) Inadequate circulation?
    - iii) Metabolic disorder?

  - Once detected- try to correct the underlying/precipitating cause.
  - Consider empiric ***Volume Infusion*** (since hypovolemia is probably the most common *potentially correctable* cause of PEA).

- *Consider Other Options*:

  - ***Atropine***- likely to be helpful *only* if the PEA rhythm is associated with *absolute* or *relative* bradycardia. Give **1 mg** IV; may repeat every 3-5 minutes (if/as needed)- up to a *total* dose of 0.04 mg/kg (= **3 mg**).

  - ***Pacing***- likely to be helpful *only* if PEA is due to *temporarily* disturbed conduction (as may occur in some cases of drug overdose).

Perform CPR/Supportive Actions

Because PEA is a *non-perfusing* rhythm (or at most a *minimally* perfusing rhythm)- the *initial* priority in management must logically be to ***begin*** **CPR** (and/or to ***continue*** **CPR** if it has already been started). CPR will need to be performed for as long as the patient remains pulseless.

Other ***Supportive Actions*** should be accomplished at this time (i.e., intubation, establishment of IV access). In view of the fact that meaningful contractile activity *does* occur in a surprising number of patients with PEA- consideration may be given to one or more means of assessing the presence of *subclinical* blood flow. This may include use of ***End-Tidal*** **(ET) CO_2 monitoring**- and/or **doppler** determination of blood pressure. Patients with higher initial ET CO_2 readings and/or demonstrable doppler pressures may have a somewhat less severe form of PEA- and may respond better to intensive treatment. Clinically, awareness of this information may prove useful *prognostically* (when deciding how far to pursue the resuscitation effort)- as well as *therapeutically* (in determining the most appropriate dose of Epinephrine to use- as we discuss below).

Use of Epinephrine

The medical treatment of choice for PEA is ***Epinephrine.*** The reason for recommending this drug for treatment of this condition is that it favors perfusion to the heart and brain. It is therefore the most effective pharmacologic way to optimize blood flow to these vital organs. However, because PEA is most often a *secondary* condition- administration of Epinephrine *by itself* will usually not resolve the problem (unless the *precipitating* cause of the disorder can be identified and corrected).

The following points should be kept in mind regarding the use (and dosing) of Epinephrine in the treatment of PEA:

- PEA may occasionally be a *primary* disorder. That is, instead of an underlying precipitating cause- the principal problem may be a direct result of *inadequate coronary perfusion.* In this situation, the preferential *shunting* effect of Epinephrine (which favors blood flow to the coronary and cerebral circulation)- together with its potent *chronotropic* and *inotropic* effect (which increases contractility) may prove to be life-saving therapy.

- Epinephrine may be administered either *intravenously* ***(IV)*** or *endotracheally* ***(ET)***- depending on whichever route of access is established first. Although IV administration of drug is preferable- one should clearly *not* hesitate to use the ET route if this is the only access available for drug delivery. AHA Guidelines advise use of a larger dose (i.e., **2-2.5 mg**) when Epinephrine is given by the ***ET route.***

- If adequate IV access is available- the *initial* recommended dose of ***Epinephrine*** for treatment of PEA is **1.0 mg IV** (or 10 ml of a 1:10,000 soln.). This amount of drug is referred to as an ***SDE*** dose (i.e., *Standard-Dose Epinephrine*).

- The effect of an IV bolus of Epinephrine peaks in about 2-3 minutes. As a result, the drug should probably be repeated *at least* every 3-5 minutes- for as long as the PEA rhythm persists.

- During cardiac arrest- AHA Guidelines allow for *flexibility* in Epinephrine dosing if the patient fails to respond to the initial SDE dose (AHA Text- Pg 1-16). One may therefore *either* repeat the 1 mg SDE dose in 3-5 minutes (and continue thereafter as needed with 1 mg doses)- ***or*** *choose between several* ***H****igh-****D****ose* **alternative** *regimens.* These include:

  i) Administration of **2-5 mg** IV boluses (which AHA Guidelines describe as *"intermediate"* dose Epinephrine)

  - OR -

  ii) *Escalating* **1- 3- 5 mg** IV boluses

  - OR -

  iii) Dosing at **0.1 mg/kg** as an IV bolus.

> Flexibility in Epinephrine dosing is best illustrated by the AHA statement that- *"Use of higher doses of Epinephrine (**HDE**) can NEITHER be recommended NOR discouraged"* (AHA Text- Pg 7-4). Thus, after the initial SDE dose is given- the amount of Epinephrine for subsequent dosing is at the discretion of the treating clinician(s).

- Lower doses of Epinephrine (i.e., SDE) may be more likely to work for the subgroup of patients with less severe forms of PEA. As noted earlier, such patients probably have at least some meaningful contractile actvity- and may therefore respond better to intensive therapy. Clinical features that may help to identify such individuals include detection of a pulse by doppler, a higher initial ET CO_2 reading, and/or ECG findings of an organized rhythm with conducting P waves and narrow QRS complexes.

  In contrast, SDE dosing would seem to be less likely to work when there is no contractile activity (as is likely when no pulse is detected by doppler, the initial ET CO_2 reading is low, and a wide QRS complex rhythm is present that is slow and lacks P waves). Higher doses of Epinephrine should probably be considered at an earlier point for such individuals (if they are felt to be salvageable)- and even then, the chances for long-term survival are dismal.

Search for the Cause (and Cure) of PEA

As we have already emphasized- success in the treatment of PEA will most often depend on identifying and correcting the underlying (precipitating) cause of the disorder. The role of the emergency care provider in determining this cause can be greatly facilitated by keeping in mind the three major categories of potential etiologies:

i) PEA rhythms due to ***Inadequate Ventilation.***

ii) PEA rhythms due to ***Inadequate Circulation.***

iii) PEA rhythms due to a ***Metabolic Disorder.***

Specific entities in each of these categories are listed in Table 1D-1. Practically speaking, if PEA results from rupture of an aortic aneurysm or massive pulmonary embolism- there will be little one can do to save the patient. In such situations, development of PEA is most often a *preterminal* event. On the other hand, a number of *potentially reversible* causes of PEA exist that *can* be effectively treated- *IF* they are identified in time.

Table 1D-1: *Conditions Most Likely to Cause a PEA Rhythm*

Inadequate Ventilation

- Intubation of right mainstem bronchus- or *other cause* of hypoxemia
- Tension pneumothorax (*trauma, asthma, patient on ventilator*)
- Bilateral pneumothorax (*trauma*)

Inadequate Circulation

- Pericardial effusion with tamponade (*trauma, pericarditis, uremia, too vigorous CPR*)
- Myocardial rupture or rupture of aortic aneurysm
- Massive pulmonary embolism
- **Hypovolemia** due to:
  - Acute blood loss (*trauma, GI bleeding*)
  - Dehydration
  - Septic shock
  - Cardiogenic shock (*Acute MI, myocardial contusion*)
  - Anaphylactic shock
  - Neurogenic shock (*cervical spine fracture*)

Metabolic Disorders

- Electrolyte disturbance (*severe hyperkalemia, hypokalemia, hypomagnesemia*)
- Persistent severe acidosis (*diabetic ketoacidosis, lactic acidosis*)
- Overdose of cardiac depressant drugs (*tricyclic antidepressants*)
- Hypothermia

Clinically, attention should focus on specific aspects of the history and physical examination that may suggest one or more of the causes of PEA that are listed in Table 1D-1. Use of selected laboratory tests (either obtained from review of the patient's chart and/or ordered STAT) may provide additional clues to the underlying cause. (*Note how similar Table 1D-1 is to Table 1A-2 that was introduced on page 15 during discussion of the **D**ifferential **D**iagnosis in the* ***Secondary Survey***).

One of the most common sources of a PEA rhythm stems from a problem with ventilation. As a result, the first thing to check for on physical examination is the ***adequacy of respiration***. Absence of breath sounds on the *left* side of the chest suggests intubation of the *right* mainstem bronchus. Simply withdrawing the endotracheal tube a small distance may restore bilateral breath sounds. If this maneuver is not successful (and/or breath sounds are absent on the right in association with tracheal deviation)- the possibility of *tension* pneumothorax should be considered. One's index of suspicion for the presence of tension pneumothorax might be further increased in certain clinical settings (i.e., if there was a history of significant trauma, or in patients with asthma or chronic obstructive pulmonary disease- especially if they have been on a ventilator). In such cases, if time does not allow for the luxury of radiographic confirmation- a *diagnostic* (and *potentially therapeutic!*) tap with a large-bore needle (or Heimlich valve) may be indicated.

> **Note-** The point of insertion for ***emergency decompression*** of *suspected* ***tension*** **pneumothorax** is in the second or third intercostal space. Pass the large bore (16 or 18 gauge) needle *over the top* of the rib (to avoid the intercostal vessels that run along the lower border of each rib)- and insert the needle in the *midclavicular line* (to avoid the internal mammary artery that lies medially). Air under tension produces a hissing sound- and *dramatic improvement* in the patient's hemodynamic condition should *immediately* follow.

If inadequate ventilation is *not* the problem- attention should next be directed at evaluating the status of the patient's circulation. Specifically, the ***adequacy of intravascular volume*** should be assessed. Clinically, this may be done by attempting to answer the following questions:

- Was the patient *dehydrated* prior to the arrest?
- Is the patient in *cardiogenic shock* (i.e., from massive acute infarction)?
- Was the patient at risk for *pulmonary embolus* ?
- Was there a known *aortic aneurysm* ?
- Could the patient have been in *septic shock* ?

> ***KEY-*** Practically speaking, ***hypovolemia*** is probably the most common (and one of the more easily treatable) causes of PEA. With this in mind, even *without* any obvious reason for hypovolemia- *empiric* **volume infusion** (in the form of a ≈500-1,000 ml fluid challenge) should be strongly considered at this point.

A number of other *potentially reversible* causes of PEA should be considered. These include pericardial effusion with ***cardiac tamponade*** (from trauma, pericarditis, uremia, or as a complication of CPR)- *metabolic* disorders such as ***persistent acidosis*** (i.e., diabetic ketoacidosis, lactic acidosis) or severe ***electrolyte disturbance*** (i.e., hyperkalemia, hypokalemia, or hypomagnesemia)- ***drug overdose*** (from myocardial depressant drugs)- and ***hypothermia*** (which can be *subtle-* and ever so easy to overlook if the patient's temperature is never taken). Laboratory evaluation (i.e., with ABGs and STAT serum electrolytes) will assess some of these possibilities. The history may suggest others.

> <u>**Note-**</u> If ***cardiac tamponade*** is at all suggested, either by history (i.e., known uremia or pericarditis)- by the course of resuscitation (i.e., suspicion of fractured ribs from too vigorous CPR)- and/or by physical examination (presence of jugular venous distention or muffled heart sounds)- then *pericardiocentesis* should be attempted. *Withdrawing as little as 50 ml of fluid under these circumstances may be lifesaving.*
>
> ***Emergency pericardiocentesis*** is best performed through a subxiphoid approach- with insertion of the needle at a 20° to 30° angle with respect to the frontal plane. The needle should be directed toward the tip of the left shoulder. Aspiration is continuously applied. Entry into the pericardium usually produces a distinct "giving" sensation that should be followed by the appearance of *nonclotting* blood in the syringe. If the blood clots, it most likely has been removed from the right ventricle.

Finally, special consideration should be given to PEA that occurs in association with ***trauma***- which should prompt the emergency care provider to actively consider an alternative set of causes. In this situation, the *mechanism* of injury may be enlightening. For example- learning that a victim's automobile was demolished in a high-speed freeway accident in which the patient's chest deformed the steering wheel *before* his head crashed through the windshield- should suggest *at least* four possible etiologies for PEA. These include:

i) *Acute blood loss* (with internal hemorrhage from abdominal injury, pelvic fracture, etc.)
ii) *Cardiogenic shock* from myocardial contusion (the result of the steering wheel injury)
iii) *Neurogenic shock* from cervical spine injury
iv) Pericardial tamponade, bilateral pneumothorax, or tension pneumothorax from *trauma* to the chest wall.

<u>Other Treatment Options: *Atropine and Pacing*</u>

Because bradycardia is *not* the principal problem with PEA- treatment with Atropine and/or pacing will usually *not* restore perfusion. Use of these modalities should probably be reserved for the following situations:

i) When the rate of the PEA rhythm is *slow* (i.e., either absolute or relative bradycardia)- in which case both ***Atropine*** and ***pacing*** may be tried.

ii) With certain types of drug overdose, in which a healthy myocardium exists, but conduction is temporarily impaired by ingestion of one or more myocardial depressant drugs. In this case, implementation of cardiac pacing until the effect of the drug(s) wears off may be a lifesaving intervention.

Treatment Algorithm for Asystole

AHA recommendations for treatment of ***Asystole*** are summarized in the algorithm we present in Figure 1D-3. Unfortunately, prognosis of the patient who is found in this rhythm is never good. Nevertheless, a well defined treatment protocol has been described- and on occasion, may result in successful resuscitation.

An important point to emphasize is that ultimate outcome is not necessarily as bleak when asystole occurs *in* the hospital setting- as when this rhythm is seen as the primary mechanism of cardiac arrest that occurs in the field (i.e., *outside* of the hospital). Asystole that occurs outside of the hospital setting is most often a *preterminal* rhythm that results from deterioration of V Fib in patients with prolonged cardiac arrest. Resuscitation of such patients may sometimes restore a pulse temporarily- but meaningful long-term survival (i.e., with intact neurologic function) is rare.

In contrast, asystole that develops *within* the hospital setting may reflect a somewhat different process- and may be the *direct result* of a sudden massive discharge of *parasympathetic* activity. In such cases, the rhythm may sometimes be surprisingly responsive to Atropine. This phenomenon (of sudden massive parasympathetic discharge) is most likely to be seen with certain operative procedures (i.e., endoscopy or cardiac catheterization), induction of anesthesia, toxic drug reactions, vasovagal episodes, and/or with AV block from acute *inferior* infarction.

An additional reason for the less uniformly dismal prognosis of asystole in the hospital setting is that the time elapsed from the onset of this rhythm until discovery of the patient by trained personnel tends to be much less than when asystole occurs outside of the hospital. As a result, irreversible pathophysiologic changes may not yet have set in. Such patients are therefore more likely to respond to the treatment measures described below.

> **Bottom Line**- The long-term prognosis for patients with asystole is never good. The best chance for meaningful survival (with intact neurologic function) will be for those patients in whom the rhythm is promptly recognized- and for whom treatment is *immediately* started.

Is the Rhythm *truly* Asystole?

The diagnosis of asystole is made from the electrocardiographic finding of a flat line recording in *all* monitoring leads- that occurs in a patient who is *pulseless.* It is important to remember that conditions *other than* asystole may also produce a flat line recording. The differential diagnosis of a ***FLAT line recording*** should therefore include the following (AHA Text- Pg 1-14):

- ***Fine V Fib***- that may occasionally ***"masquerade"*** as asystole.
- ***Loose electrode leads*** (or leads *not* connected to the monitor).
- ***No power*** (for whatever technical reason).
- ***Signal gain turned down*** (to a point so low that it fails to produce a rhythm on the monitor).

The reason why fine V Fib may sometimes "masquerade" as asystole relates to the fact that when the lead being monitored is *perpendicular* to the predominent vector of the fibrillation rhythm, an *isoelectric* complex (in this case, a *flat* line) will be seen. Practically speaking, this phenomenon is *not* a common occurrence.

Figure 1D-3- *Treatment Algorithm for Asystole*

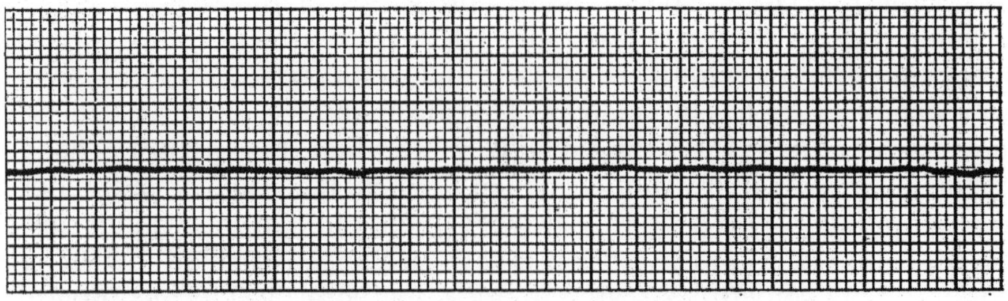

Is the Rhythm Truly Asystole?
- Pulseless and unresponsive pt?
- Monitoring leads correctly hooked up?
- Flat line recording in *more* than 1 lead?

- *Begin/Continue* **CPR** :
  - ***Supportive Actions*** (Intubate/Establish IV access, etc.).
- *Search for a possible* ***Cause(s)*** *of Asystole*
  - Potential causes (and many of the treatments) of asystole are similar to those of PEA (*Tables 1A-2 and 1D-1 on pages 15 and 96*).

KEY Treatment Options:

- *Consider Immediate use of* ***TransCutaneous Pacing (TCP)***
  - To be effective, TCP *must* be started *early* !
  - *IF available*- TCP should therefore be applied *immediately* in the treatment of asystole (either *before* or *simultaneously* with the use of drugs!).
- **Epinephrine:**
  - Begin with an **SDE** dose (i.e., **1.0 mg** by IV bolus).
  - May *either* repeat SDE (every 3-5 minutes- if/as needed)-
    - or *increase* the dose (i.e., to **HDE**) if there has been no response.
- **Atropine:**
  - Give **1 mg** IV; May repeat every 3-5 minutes- *if/as needed* (up to a *total* dose of 0.04 mg/kg ≈**3 mg**).
- *Consider Other Options*:
  - ***Aminophylline***- 250 mg IV over 1-2 minutes; may repeat. (Although use of this drug is *not* yet approved by AHA Guidelines- it *might* be considered if all else fails.)
  - ***Sodium Bicarbonate***- indications for use in asystole are generally quite limited (i.e., to *hyperkalemia*- severe *preexisting* and/or *bicarbonate-responsive acidosis*- and *tricyclic overdose*).
  - Termination of efforts . . . .

In the past, recognition of asystole was indication for delivery of an unsynchronized countershock- on the grounds that the rhythm "might possibly be V Fib" (masquerading as asystole)- and in the belief that shocking asystole "can't make the rhythm worse". *This practice is no longer justified* (AHA Text- Pg 1-23). Shocking asystole *can* make the rhythm worse- by "stunning" the heart and producing more damage to an already impaired conduction system that may reduce even further the chance for return of spontaneous activity (AHA Text- Pg 4-7).

- Practically speaking- operator (and/or technical) errors are a much more common cause of ***"false asystole"*** than isoelectric V Fib masquerading as this rhythm.
- The issue of whether or not electrical activity is present can be quickly resolved- simply by *rotating* quick look paddles by 90° (or for the monitored patient, by viewing the rhythm in *more* than a single monitoring lead).

> **Bottom Line**- Recognition of a flat line recording in a single monitoring lead does *not* justify routine defibrillation. Instead it should prompt clinical reevaluation of the patient (to ensure the *true* absence of a pulse)- check of additional leads (to verify *complete* lack of electrical activity)- and reassessment of patient and monitor lead hook-up (to rule out the possibility of technical errors).

CPR/Supportive Actions/Search for a Cause

Obviously there is no perfusion with asystole. As a result- ***CPR*** must be performed for as long as this rhythm persists. Other ***Supportive Actions*** (i.e., intubation, establishment of IV access, etc.) should be accomplished at the earliest opportunity.

As was the case for PEA- consideration should always be given to the possibility of an underlying cause predisposing to development of the rhythm. Potential causes of asystole are similar to those that are likely to precipitate PEA (*See Tables 1A-2 and 1D-1*). When such factors are responsible for the rhythm- success in treatment will depend on identifying and correcting this underlying cause.

> **Note**- Patients with bradyasystolic arrest that occurs in association with ***special circumstances*** (i.e., *hypothermia- electrocution- drug overdose- drowning- sudden failure of a permanent pacemaker*) represent a special group, for whom prognosis may even be favorable- IF the patient is promptly attended to. This is because underlying the rhythm disorder, the myocardium of such individuals may be relatively normal. As a result- *greater persistence in resuscitative efforts is usually appropriate* (in the hope of providing *supportive care* while precipitating factors are identified and treated).

Use of Pacing for Asystole

In general, pacemaker therapy is only effective in the treatment of bradycardia and asystole when myocardial function has been preserved. As a result, it is unlikely to be helpful in the treatment of asystole when this rhythm occurs as a preterminal event after prolonged (and unsuccessful) attempts at resuscitation. In acknowledgement of the almost uniformly dismal prognosis of such patients- AHA Guidelines emphasize that pacing is now an *optional* procedure that need *not* always be tried in such situations (AHA Text- Pg 1-23).

- Pacemaker therapy is most likely to be successful in the treatment of bradyasystolic cardiac arrest if attempted *early* in the process (i.e., *before* irreversibility has set in). As a result, if it is to be used- ***TCP*** (*__T__rans-__C__utaneous __P__acing*) should be applied as soon as the device is available- which may be *before* (and/or *simultaneously* with) the use of drugs (AHA Text- Pg 1-24).

- Pacemaker therapy is no longer recommended as routine treatment for patients with bradyasystolic cardiac arrest. Special attention should be given to the decision of whether to even attempt pacing in patients with out-of-hospital cardiac arrest who have not responded to other measures- especially when the period of arrest has been prolonged. The sombering reality is that long-term prognosis for most of these patients is dismal- *regardless* of what interventions are undertaken. AHA Guidelines suggest that pacing actually becomes relatively *contraindicated* when delay before initiation of treatment with this modality exceeds 20 minutes- since the chance for successful resuscitation with intact neurologic function is virtually nil in this situation (AHA Text- Pg 5-2).

Use of Epinephrine

The initial drug of choice for the treatment of asystole is ***Epinephrine***. Because the vasoconstrictor effect of Epinephrine in the arrested heart makes it the *KEY* pharmacologic agent for favoring blood flow to the coronary and cerebral circulation- the drug should be used *liberally* in the treatment of asystole.

- AHA Guidelines recommend *beginning* with an ***SDE*** dose of Epinephrine (i.e., **1 mg IV**). This dose may be repeated every 3-5 minutes for as long as the patient remains in asystole.

- Consideration should be given to increasing the dose of Epinephrine if the patient fails to respond to one or more doses of SDE. Practically speaking- you *can't* really overdose on Epinephrine when treating asystole (i.e., *"You can't be deader than dead"*). Escalation of the dose (i.e., to ***HDE***) is therefore appropriate- for *potentially salvageable* patients who are felt to have a reasonable chance for restoration of intact neurologic function. AHA Guidelines leave the decision of whether or not to escalate the dose of Epinephrine entirely at the discretion of the treating clinician (AHA Text- Pg 7-4).

Use of Atropine

As noted above- asystole may occasionally be caused by a sudden massive discharge of *parasympathetic* activity. As a result, treatment with *Atropine* should always be tried.

- The *initial* recommended dose of Atropine for treatment of asystole is **1.0 mg IV**. This dose may be repeated every 3-5 minutes if there is no response (up to a *total* dose of 0.04 mg/kg- or ≈**3 mg** for an *average-sized* adult).
- AHA Guidelines allow for use of Atropine at even more frequent intervals than every 3-5 minutes in the treatment of bradyasystolic cardiac arrest. Thus, the drug can be given at *1-minute* intervals in this situation (AHA Text- Pg 1-30).
- Practically speaking- the chance that Atropine will work in asystole is relatively small. This is particularly true when the drug is used in the treatment of prolonged out-of-hospital cardiac arrest.

When All Else Fails: *Use of Aminophylline?*

Although *not* included in AHA Guidelines, a drug to consider when all else fails (i.e., for what would *otherwise* be *lethal* bradyasystolic arrest) is ***Aminophylline***. Data on use of this agent for treatment of asystole are limited- but promising. The theory proposed to account for the beneficial effect of Aminophylline in this situation relates to potential mediation of severe ischemia and bradycardia/asystole by release of *endogenous adenosine* (in the body's attempt to vasodilate and restore myocardial oxygen supply). As a result, endogenous adenosine may accumulate- leading to further exacerbation of ischemia (by a "coronary steal" phenomenon) and/or contributing to (or causing) more profound bradycardia/asystole. The mechanism by which Aminophylline works may therefore result from the known *antagonistic* effect that this drug exerts on adenosine.

- If you decide to use Aminophylline- the dose we suggest is **250 mg IV**, to be given over 1-2 minutes. This dose may be repeated if there is no response.

> **Bottom Line**- Clearly, additional studies are needed. Nevertheless, it is difficult to imagine how administration of Aminophylline could worsen the prognosis of refractory asystolic cardiac arrest. *Consideration might therefore be given to empiric use of this drug for this otherwise almost certainly lethal condition.*

Use of Sodium Bicarbonate for Asystole

Indications for use of ***Sodium Bicarbonate*** in the treatment of asystole are limited. They include *hyperkalemia*- severe *preexisting* and/or *bicarbonate-responsive acidosis* (that is thought to have contributed to or precipitated the arrest)- and *tricyclic overdose*. Empiric use of Sodium Bicarbonate is no longer recommended in cardiac arrest.

Consider Termination of Efforts

AHA Guidelines intentionally *avoid* citing a time limit beyond which resuscitation will never be successful. Instead, they emphasize how "*special situations call for common sense and clinical judgement*" (AHA Text- Pg 1-25). Practically speaking, the prognosis of patients with out-of-hospital bradyasystolic arrest is exceedingly poor- especially if the patient fails to respond to initial attempts at resuscitation. In such situations- "asystole most often represents a *confirmation of death*- rather than a rhythm to be treated". *Resuscitation efforts may therefore be stopped*- after intubation, IV access, basic CPR, and a trial of Atropine/Epinephrine. A trial of pacing is *not* necessarily indicated for all patients.

Treatment Algorithm for Bradycardia

AHA recommendations for treatment of ***Bradycardia*** are summarized in the algorithm we present in Figure 1D-4. For the purpose of this algorithm- the term ***Bradycardia*** is used to encompass the diverse group of cardiac rhythms that are unified by the finding of a *slow* ventricular rate (i.e., of *less* than **60 beats/minute**). The principal entities included within this group are the following:

- ***Sinus bradycardia*** (which often occurs in conjunction with ***sinus arrhythmia***).
- ***A Fib*** with a ***slow*** **ventricular response**.
- The various forms of **AV block**.
- ***Escape rhythms*** (including ***junctional*** **escape** and ***slow*** **idioventricular rhythm**).

> **Note-** An additional category that should be considered in this group is ***"relative" bradycardia***- so defined as encompassing those rhythms for which the heart rate is *inappropriately slow* for the clinical situation at hand- *despite* the fact that the rate may be faster than 60 beats/minute. This might be the case for the example of sinus rhythm shown in the beginning of this section (Figure 1D-1 on page 89). Despite the fact that the rate of this rhythm is 70 beats/minute- this rate would be *inappropriately slow* if the patient was in shock with marked hypotension.
>
> **Bottom Line-** Description of heart rate as either *"appropriate"* for the clinical situation- or *"too slow"*- is usually more helpful from a clinical perspective than strictly defining a rhythm as bradycardic or not based on the actual rate. Practically speaking- clinical evaluation and treatment considerations will be similar- *regardless* of whether a bradycardia is *"relative"* or absolute.

Initial Approach: *KEY Clinical Questions*

As emphasized at the beginning of this section- three *KEY Clincal Questions* should be addressed in the earliest part of our clinical approach. These questions are:

i) Is there a pulse?
ii) Is the rhythm hemodynamically significant?
iii) What is the rhythm? (and/or- *What is our need to know?*)

Application of this *Initial Question Approach* is best illustrated by considering the rhythm that appears at the top of Figure 1D-4. We are told (in the legend *below* the Figure) that the patient has a pulse. If no pulse was present in association with this tracing- then the rhythm (*by definition!*) would be PEA- and the evaluative approach and management decisions would be those that are recommended in Figure 1D-2 (on page 93). Priorities are very different when the rhythm is PEA- in that the primary needs are to reestablish perfusion and identify and correct the underlying cause of the disorder, rather than simply increasing the rate.

Figure 1D-4- *Treatment Algorithm for Bradycardia*

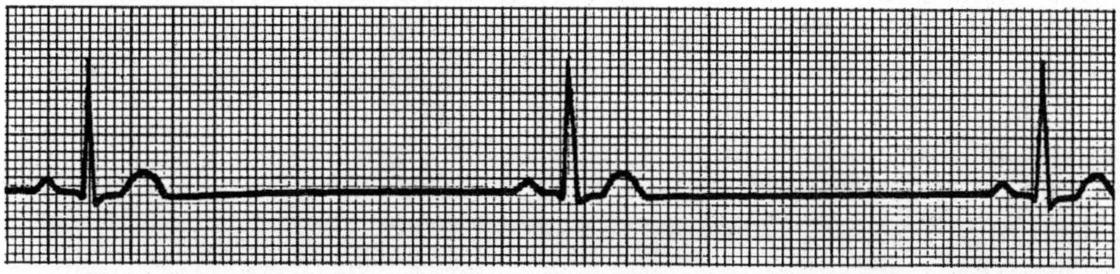

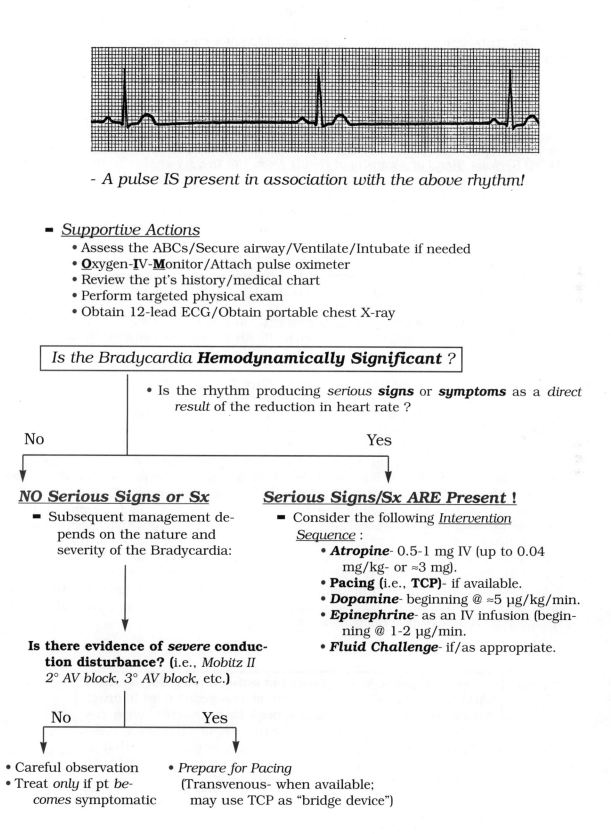

- A pulse IS present in association with the above rhythm!

- *Supportive Actions*
  - Assess the ABCs/Secure airway/Ventilate/Intubate if needed
  - **O**xygen-**I**V-**M**onitor/Attach pulse oximeter
  - Review the pt's history/medical chart
  - Perform targeted physical exam
  - Obtain 12-lead ECG/Obtain portable chest X-ray

Is the Bradycardia **Hemodynamically Significant** *?*

- Is the rhythm producing *serious* ***signs*** or ***symptoms*** as a *direct result* of the reduction in heart rate ?

No → ***NO Serious Signs or Sx***

- Subsequent management depends on the nature and severity of the Bradycardia:

Is there evidence of *severe* conduction disturbance? (i.e., *Mobitz II 2° AV block, 3° AV block*, etc.)

No →
- Careful observation
- Treat *only* if pt *becomes* symptomatic

Yes →
- *Prepare for Pacing* (Transvenous- when available; may use TCP as "bridge device")

Yes → ***Serious Signs/Sx ARE Present !***

- Consider the following *Intervention Sequence* :
  - ***Atropine***- 0.5-1 mg IV (up to 0.04 mg/kg- or ≈3 mg).
  - **Pacing** (i.e., **TCP**)- if available.
  - ***Dopamine***- beginning @ ≈5 μg/kg/min.
  - ***Epinephrine***- as an IV infusion (beginning @ 1-2 μg/min.
  - ***Fluid Challenge***- if/as appropriate.

Is the Rhythm Hemodynamically Significant?

Once told that a pulse is present- ***Supportive Actions*** should now be accomplished (as feasible, given the clinical situation). These actions include ensuring an adequate airway and ventilation, achieving IV access, attaching monitoring leads to the patient (if not already done), performing a *targeted* physical exam, gleaning information from the medical chart, and obtaining appropriate laboratory tests and x-rays. While these actions are being accomplished, attention can now be directed at answering the second *KEY* Clinical Question: ***Is the rhythm hemodynamically significant*** ? Specifically, one seeks to determine if the bradyarrhythmia is causing the patient problems as a *direct result* of the reduction in heart rate. There are two possibilities:

1) ***NO Serious Signs or Symptoms result from the Bradycardia.*** In this case, subsequent management will depend on the nature and severity of the bradycardia. In general- no immediate intervention (other than careful observation) should be needed (since the patient is *not* symptomatic). Preparation may need to be made for pacing (and/or for pacing *back-up*- known as ***"anticipatory pacing readiness"***)- depending on whether or not there is evidence of *severe* conduction disturbance (*See Figure 1D-4*). The advantage of using ***TCP*** (*TransCutaneous Pacing*) in this situation is that the device may be placed on the patient in *standby* mode (i.e., applied to the patient- but with pacing *not* turned on).

2) ***Serious Signs or Symptoms ARE present.*** In this case, immediate intervention *is* needed (since the patient *is* symptomatic!). AHA Guidelines suggest the intervention sequence that we show in Figure 1D-4 and describe below.

What is the Specific Rhythm? (*What is Our Need to Know?*)

Our purpose in adding a second part to this final *KEY Question* (i.e., ***What is our need to know?***)- is to emphasize how specific diagnosis of the type of bradycardia is much *less* important in the *acute* setting than the patient's hemodynamic condition.

For example- consider again the rhythm that appears at the top of Figure 1D-4. Despite the fact that the mechanism of this rhythm is sinus, the rate is exceedingly slow (i.e., *less* than 30 beats/minute). As a result- pacemaker therapy will probably still be needed if the onset of this rhythm was sudden and the patient fails to respond (with an increase in heart rate) to medical therapy. Much more important than whether a slow rhythm is the result of 2° or 3° AV block- or simply profound sinus bradycardia (as is the case here)- will be the patient's clinical condition and hemodynamic status (i.e., effective heart rate, blood pressure, mental status, presence of symptoms). Practically speaking- a patient with serious signs or symptoms from severe bradycardia will *initially* be treated the same (i.e., with Atropine, pacing, Dopamine, and/or Epinephrine)- *regardless* of what the specific type of bradycardia happens to be.

> **Bottom Line**- *Always* ***treat the patient- NOT the monitor!*** (AHA Text- Pg 1-30). Treatment of bradycardia (with drugs and/or pacing) will sometimes need to be started when the patient is symptomatic *without* being sure of what the specific diagnosis of the rhythm is. AHA Guidelines emphasize that in reality- diagnosis of the rhythm should proceed *simultaneously* with initiation of therapy (AHA Text- Pg 1-30).

From a clinical perspective- determination of the specific ECG diagnosis of the type of bradycardia becomes more important in the decision making process when the patient is hemodynamically stable. In this situation, determination of the need for pacemaker therapy will depend on the severity of the conduction disturbance. In general, pacing will be needed for patients with Mobitz II 2° AV block and/or 3° AV block with QRS widening.

> **<u>Note</u>**- The anatomic site of an acute infarction may provide insight to the expected clinical course and response to therapy for patients with new-onset conduction system disorders (AHA Text- Pg 1-32). Patients with **acute *anterior* infarction** who develop new-onset 2° AV block (which is typically of the Mobitz II type) or 3° AV block (which will typically manifest a *wide* QRS complex escape rhythm)- generally require transvenous pacing. This is because these conduction system disorders are usually *not* reversible. Atropine should *only* be used in such patients with extreme caution (if it is used at all). TCP may prove invaluable as a *"bridge"* device until transvenous pacing is available.
>
> In contrast, patients with **acute *inferior* infarction** typically manifest a *narrow* QRS complex escape rhythm- since the anatomic level of AV block is most often at the level of the AV node with this type of infarction. As a result, these patients generally respond well to Atropine (which opposes the vagotonic activity that most often causes the conduction defect). Fortunately, 2° AV block (most often Mobitz I) and 3° AV block that occur in association with acute *inferior* infarction are usually *transient* conduction disorders that are likely to *spontaneously* resolve in time). If symptoms are minimal or absent- *standby* use of TCP may be all that is needed in the interim.

Symptomatic Bradycardia: *Rationale for Intervention Sequence*

Many factors enter into the decision making process for the treatment of bradycardia. In the hope of optimizing the ***Intervention Sequence***- we emphasize the following points:

- The need for specific interventions in the treatment of bradycardia should be based on the *severity* of the clinical situation (AHA Text- Pg 1-30). AHA Guidelines emphasize that rather than slow and discrete stepwise progression through a well defined protocol- rapid decision making and *near simultaneous* implementation of *multiple* interventions may be needed (AHA Text- Pg 1-31). For example, the patient with severe symptomatic bradycardia may receive Atropine *at the same time* as preparation is made for cardiac pacing. Preparation may also be made at this time for IV infusion of Dopamine (and/or Epinephrine) in anticipation of the possibility that Atropine may be ineffective and application of TCP could be delayed.

- *<u>If Signs/Symptoms from Bradycardia are "Mild"</u>*- AHA Guidelines suggest selection of ***Atropine*** as the initial pharmacologic intervention "of choice" (AHA Text- Pg 1-30). The dose recommended in this situation is **0.5-1 mg IV**- which may be repeated every 3-5 minutes as needed (up to a *total* dose of 0.04 mg/kg- or ≈**3 mg**).

  - The lower dose of Atropine (i..e, **0.5 mg**) is preferable for *initial* treatment of the patient with less severe symptoms from the bradycardia. Consider increasing the dose (i.e., to **1.0 mg**) if the patient fails to respond to one or two 0.5 mg doses- and/or if the symptoms from bradycardia become more severe.

> **<u>Note</u>**- Use of Atropine is *not* benign. By blocking parasympathetic output, the drug may *unmask* previously contained enhanced sympathetic activity. This may lead to development of *tachycardia* and/or precipitation of potentially malignant ventricular arrhythmias (including VT and V Fib).
>
> **<u>Bottom Line</u>**- Atropine should *not* be used to treat the asymptomatic patient with bradycardia. Instead, use of the drug should be reserved for treatment of *symptomatic* bradycardia (i.e., bradycardia associated with chest pain or dyspnea)- and/or bradycardia accompanied by signs of *hemodynamic compromise* (i.e., hypotension, heart failure, ventricular ectopy, or altered mental status).

- Although one usually waits at least 3-5 minutes before repeating the dose of Atropine- the drug may be dosed more frequently (i.e., as often as every 1-3 minutes!) for selected patients with *marked* hemodynamic compromise from the slow rate (AHA Text- Pg 1-30).

- Atropine should be used with extreme caution (if at all) when the rhythm being treated is advanced AV block with ventricular escape (i.e., with a wide QRS complex). Theoretically, Atropine could even *worsen* hemodynamic status in such patients (if by increasing the atrial rate it reduced the number of impulses conducted to the ventricles). Pacing appears to be preferable for such patients- especially if the AV block occurs in association with acute *anterior* infarction (AHA Text- Pg 1-32).

- The denervated (transplanted) heart will *not* respond to Atropine. As a result, one should immediately intervene with either pacing and/or catecholamine infusion in such patients.

■ *<u>If Symptoms are "More Severe"</u>*- Consideration should be given to ***pacing*** as soon as this modality is available. AHA Guidelines emphasize that it *IS* appropriate to use ***TCP*** as the *initial* intervention in the treatment sequence- *<u>IF</u>* the bradycardia is severe and/or the clinical condition is unstable (AHA Text- Pg 1-31). Pacing is also *preferable* to Atropine when the rhythm being treated is advanced AV block with ventricular escape (for the reasons stated above).

- Pacing should *not* be delayed while attempting to achieve IV access (or while waiting for Atropine to take effect)- *especially if the patient is symptomatic* (AHA Text- Pg 1-29).

- Although admittedly, pacing is *not* very effective in the treatment of bradyasystolic cardiac arrest- it is generally much more effective (and may be *lifesaving*) when used to treat patients who *have* a pulse and who manifest symptomatic bradycardia. Because the primary problem in such patients is the slow rate- cardiac pacing would seem to be the *ideal* modality for responding to this situation.

- Keep in mind that it will *not* always be possible to implement external pacing (i.e., awake patients may not always tolerate the device; electrical capture with effective mechanical contraction may not always be obtained).

- *If Atropine is Ineffective and Pacing is Unavailable*- Consider the use of a pressor agent. With *less* severe symptoms- ***Dopamine*** is the agent that is generally preferred in this situation. AHA Guidelines suggest beginning at a dose of **5 μg/kg/minute**- and titrating the rate of infusion upward as needed according to the clinical response (AHA Text- Pg 1-31).

  If hemodynamic symptoms are more severe- AHA Guidelines suggest beginning directly with **IV infusion** of ***Epinephrine*** (instead of Dopamine). The initial rate recommended for IV infusion of Epinephrine is **1-2 μg/minute**- which can be rapidly titrated upward as needed according to the clinical response.

> **Note**- Epinephrine should *not* be given by IV bolus when using the drug as a *pressor* agent (i.e., to treat a patient who is *not* in cardiac arrest). Use of continuous IV infusion provides the advantage of *moment-to-moment* titration capability for altering the dose of drug given. Should an adverse effect occur, the IV infusion can *immediately* be turned down (or off). In contrast, if Epinpehrine is given by IV bolus and an adverse effect occurs- *"You can't take the bolus back."*

Additional Considerations/Pitfalls

In addition to standard recommendations for treatment of bradycardia that are listed above, a number of thoughts should be kept in mind:

i) Bradycardia will *not* always be the result of conduction system disease. Correction of other factors (i.e., *hypoxemia- hypovolemia- electrolyte disturbance*- etc.) may sometimes be all that is needed to "cure" the problem. This point emphasizes the importance of always considering the "**D**" component (i.e., *Differential Diagnosis*) of the ***Secondary Survey***- especially when confronted with an arrhythmia that does not respond to standard treatment measures.

ii) Patients with bradycardia and hypotension may be ***volume depleted***- either from volume loss (due to hemorrhage or dehydration), or as a result of inappropriate vasodilatation (from acute myocardial infarction, septic or neurogenic shock).

- Although most of the time, patients with hypotension will be *tachycardic*- this is *not* always the case. In particular, patients with acute *inferior* infarction frequently manifest excessive parasympathetic tone- which commonly leads to bradycardia and hypotension.

- Clinically, it will often be difficult to adequately assess volume status. As a result, it is important to always maintain a high index of suspicion for the possibility of hypovolemia. Placing such patients in Trendelenburg position, and cautious administration of a ***fluid challenge*** (with **150-500 ml** of normal saline) is the treatment of choice.

> **Note**- An extremely common problem in emergency cardiac care is ***hypotension***. It is important to realize that patients with hypotension may be tachycardic, bradycardic- or have a normal heart rate. Optimal management ideally entails identification and correction of the underlying cause of the hypotension. Although this goal often extends beyond immediate capabilities of the emegency care provider (who is faced with the problem of keeping alive a patient in extremis)- the point to emphasize is that ***empiric* volume infusion** should *always* be strongly considered as a *potential* therapeutic intervention for patients with hypotension of uncertain etiology- especially if they fail to respond to standard treatment measures.

iii) As we suggest in our section on asystole- administration of ***Aminophylline*** might also be *considered* as a treatment alternative for the patient with *severe* bradycardia who fails to respond to more standard measures (i.e., *Atropine*, *Epinephrine*, and *TCP*).

- If you decide to use Aminophylline- the dose we suggest is **250 mg IV**, to be given over a 1-2 minute period. This dose may be repeated if there is no response.

> **Note**- Use of Aminophylline is *not* yet included in AHA Guidelines. Standard measures should clearly be tried first. Nevertheless- if the patient remains symptomatic from severe bradycardia *despite* standard measures- consideration *might* be given to the use of this drug.

iv) Do *not* use **Lidocaine** as a prophylactic measure (to prevent V Fib) if the patient is in advanced AV block with ventricular escape beats (and/or a ventricular escape rhythm). In this situation- Lidocaine may abolish the *only* escape rhythm you have!

v) Use of **Isoproterenol** as a pressor agent has been strongly discouraged in recent years. This is because of the drug's potential to produce deleterious effects on the heart and circulation (including peripheral vasodilatation and an *increase* in myocardial oxygen consumption). If used at all (as it occasionally may be to provide *pure* chronotropic support)- the dose of Isoproterenol must be kept *low*- and extreme *caution* is urged! We emphasize that at the present time- *other* pressor agents (i.e., Dopamine, Epinephrine) *are clearly preferred* to the use of Isoproterenol (AHA Text-Pg 1-32).

vi) Clinical judgement is needed to determine whether ***CPR*** should be performed on the patient with bradycardia *in addition* to other therapeutic measures. The need to perform CPR clearly depends on the *severity* of hypotension and the degree of hemodynamic compromise. It is obviously *not* needed for treatment of mild bradycardia- or even for 2° or 3° AV block if the patient is alert and asymptomatic. On the other hand, continuation of CPR would be an essential component of therapy for an unresponsive patient in a slow ventricular escape rhythm with marked hypotension. *Whether to perform CPR in less clearcut situations is a matter of clinical judgement.*

CHAPTER 2

Essential Drugs and Treatment Modalities

Section 2A: *Drug Delivery/ General Principles*

The armamentarium of drugs and treatment modalities for cardiopulmonary resuscitation and emergency cardiac care is ever expanding. This situation could easily be overwhelming, especially for the ACLS provider who does not work with these drugs and modalities on a daily basis. In view of this and considering that the reader's need (and/or desire) to know about this material is likely to vary greatly- we have organized our presentation of the subject in as practical a format as possible. In this initial section, we briefly review several *KEY* concepts regarding ***Drug Delivery***- and then address a number of ***General Pharmacologic Principles*** (including the importance of the autonomic nervous system, the types and clinical implications of the various adrenergic receptors, determinants of cardiac performance, and considerations that go into selecting a pressor agent). Although this material may be basic and/or review for some readers- we have included it in the hope that it may lay the groundwork for understanding the description of the drugs and treatment modalities to follow.

For each drug that is covered, we include dispensing and dosing information, indications for current use, and *KEY* clinical concepts. Fortunately, the number of truly *essential* medications that one must be thoroughly familiar with in order to effectively manage a cardiac arrest is limited. These ***"KEY Drugs"*** (i.e., the ones you need to master to successfully complete the ACLS course)- are discussed in **Section B** of this chapter. In **Section C**, we present an easy-to-learn method for ***Simplified Calculation of IV Infusions*** for the commonly used medications in emergency cardiac care. This is followed in **Section D** by a brief discussion of the ***KEY Treatment Modalities*** (i.e., defibrillation, cardioversion, pacing).

The new guidelines have facilitated our task by *deemphasizing* or eliminating a number of agents that were previously recommended for use. These include Sodium Bicarbonate, Calcium Chloride, and Isoproterenol. Although there are still some indications for use of these agents, these ***Deemphasized Drugs*** (discussed in **Section F**) are no longer viewed as *essential* in the management of cardiopulmonary arrest. Familiarity with them may therefore be looked on as *optional*, particularly for the reader with only a limited time to prepare for the ACLS course. Similarly, the ***Additional Drugs*** we discuss in **Section E** comprise material *"beyond the core"* of what one needs to know to successfully complete the ACLS course. It may be useful for those exposed to cardiology and acute care medicine on a regular basis, and helpful as a reference to those who are not. Finally, we briefly review drugs used in ***Pediatric Resuscitation*** in **Section G.**

Drug Delivery: IV Access

Along with management of the airway and defibrillation, establishing IV (intravenous) access for drug delivery is one of the major priorities of cardiopulmonary resuscitation. Many techniques exist for achieving this goal- each with its own relative merits and drawbacks.

Circulation of drugs in the arrested heart is most effectively accomplished when administered directly into a ***central* vein** (such as the ***internal jugular*** or ***subclavian vein***). Compared to drug delivery from a peripheral IV access route, medication administered through a central IV line clearly attains *higher* peak concentrations and reaches the central circulation in *less* time (AHA Text- Pg 6-6).

Use of a central vein for IV cannulation offers the additional advantage of having a fairly constant location with respect to easily identifiable anatomic landmarks. This usually allows rapid cannulation- even in a state of cardiovascular collapse (when peripheral veins may be exceedingly difficult to visualize). However, selection of a central vein as the site for IV access is not without potential problems. These include:

- The need for an operator skilled in the technique
- The need to stop CPR while cannulation is being performed
- Significant risk of pneumothorax, hemothorax

In the past, use of the *femoral* vein was advocated as a site for central venous access, since it avoided the latter two problems listed above. However, the femoral vein can no longer be recommended- as it is now known that blood flow *below* the diaphragm is significantly diminished during CPR in the arrested heart (AHA Text- Pg 6-7). Drugs administered through the femoral vein during cardiopulmonary resuscitation are therefore unlikely to reach the central circulation in adequate concentration- *unless* a long catheter is threaded up from this site to *above* the diaphragm. For practical purposes, then- central line placement during CPR should be *limited* to use of *either* the internal jugular *or* subclavian veins.

> AHA Guidelines emphasize that the *primary determinant* of whether (and *at what point*) in the code to insert a ***central* IV line** should be "the *experience* of the operator" (AHA Text- Pg 6-1). An experienced operator who is able to *rapidly* insert an ***internal jugular*** or ***subclavian*** IV line with a relatively low complication rate may choose to do so at the *earliest* possible moment during a code.

Practically speaking, the most commonly chosen site for intravenous access during cardiopulmonary resuscitation is a ***peripheral* IV line**. This is particularly true when operators skilled in the insertion of central lines are not on the scene. One should remember that the smaller the catheter and the more distal the site- the less likely there will be adequate drug delivery to the central circulation. Several practical suggestions are made to help optimize drug delivery by the peripheral IV route (AHA Text- Pg 1-10):

i) Select as *proximal* a site as possible. For example, the antecubital vein is clearly superior to a small vein on the dorsum of the wrist.
ii) Use a large bore IV needle- ideally 16 gauge (or larger) if at all possible.
iii) Follow each drug administration with a ***flush*** (i.e., 20-30 ml bolus) of **IV fluid** to facilitate drug delivery to the central circulation.
iv) Elevate the arm after each IV medication.

> Despite the superiority of central lines for drug delivery- AHA Guidelines still recommend cannulation of a ***peripheral* IV site** as the *'procedure of choice'* during CPR. Their rationale for this recommendation relates "to the *speed*, *ease*, and *safety* with which this procedure can usually be performed" (AHA Text- Pg 6-1).
>
> The recommended ***"1st target"*** for IV access should be the ***antecubital* vein** (AHA Text- Pg 1-10). Another large and easily accessible vein to consider (when visible) is the ***external jugular* vein**.
>
> Once IV access is achieved, AHA Guidelines now recommend use of ***Normal Saline*** (rather than D5W) as the IV fluid vehicle of choice (AHA Text- Pg 1-10). Normal saline is a more effective volume expander than D5W- and will *not* increase the serum glucose level (which could potentially have an adverse effect on neurologic outcome).

Endotracheal Drug Administration

On occasion, IV access may be difficult (if not impossible) to achieve. In this situation- administration of drug by the ***EndoTracheal (ET) route*** provides a suitable alternative for three of the most commonly used medications in cardiopulmonary resuscitation (i.e., Atropine, Lidocaine, Epinephrine). Although pharmacokinetic properties (of drug absorption and delivery) are not as favorable with ET administration as they are with the IV route- one should *not* hesitate to give drugs endotracheally when this is the only route available.

> Use of the mnemonic ***A - L - E*** (*Atropine- Lidocaine- Epinephrine*) facilitates recall of the 3 *KEY* drugs used in ACLS that are relatively well absorbed by the ***ET route.***

Several additional points should be emphasized reagarding administration of drugs by the ET route:

- To increase the likelihood of adequate drug devliery- a *higher* dose of medication is advised when using the ET route. AHA Guidelines recommend administration of **2** to **2.5 times** the normal dose of medication (AHA Text- Pg 1-10).

- The most commonly used technique for ET administration consists of drawing up the drug in a 10- to 20- ml syringe with an 18-gauge neede firmly attached to the end of the syringe- then *rapidly* injecting the drug (diluted to a volume of at least 10 ml) down the lumen of the ET tube- and immediately following this with 3-5 forceful insufflations of the ventilation bag. External chest compressions should be *stopped* momentarily while the drug is injected (since this may result in expulsion of the medication). Medication may also be expelled if the patient happens to cough during the procedure- in which case it may be necesary to readminister the dose of the drug.

  Alternatively, drug may be given endotracheally by threading a long (35-cm) through-the-needle intracatheter down the inside of the ET tube- and injecting the drug through the catheter.

- ***A**tropine- **L**idocaine- **E**pinephrine* are not the only medications that can be given by the ET route. ***N**arcan* and ***V**alium* may also be administered endotracheally (for the patient in cardiopulmonary arrest due to either narcotic overdose or seizures). Use of the mnemonic ***N*** - ***A*** - ***V*** - ***E*** - ***L*** - may help to recall these 5 medications.

In summary- use *whatever* drug access site is established first. Usually this will be a peripheral IV line (that hopefully will be with a large bore catheter placed in a proximal site such as the anticubital or external jugular vein). As soon as a skilled operator adept at central line placement arrives on the scene- insertion of a central venous catheter (into either the internal jugular or subclavian vein) may be attempted- especially if the patient is *not* responding to treatment. In the event that IV access is unavailable but the patient *is* intubated- medication should be given first by the ET route (as described above). If needed- this may then be followed by *readministration* of medication once effective IV access has been established.

The Autonomic Nervous System

The ***Autonomic Nervous System*** is the *involuntary* nervous system of the body. It is made up of a series of reflex arcs which regulate functions of the body that are *not* under conscious control. Such functions include modulation of heart rate, control of blood pressure, intestinal motility, bladder function, and release of glandular secretions. Because it innervates the viscera, the autonomic nervous system is sometimes referred to as the *visceral* nervous system. Fibers from the autonomic nervous system are distributed to smooth muscles in all parts of the body. In contrast, the central nervous system per se supplies areas of the body that are under conscious control (or everything except the viscera).

The autonomic nervous system is divided into two major branches: the ***Sympathetic Nervous System*** **(SNS)** and the ***Parasympathetic Nervous System*** **(PNS).** A series of intricate interconnections exists between the central nervous system, efferent nerve fibers of the SNS and the PNS, autonomic ganglia, and the various target tissues and organs innervated by the autonomic nervous system.

- *Preganglionic* fibers of the autonomic nervous system transmit nerve signals from the central nervous system to the autonomic ganglia. Preganglionic fibers of both the SNS and the PNS stimulate nerve cells in these ganglia by releasing ***acetylcholine***- and are therefore said to be ***cholinergic***.

- *Postganglionic* fibers of the autonomic nervous system emanate from the ganglia and go on to innervate their respective target organs. Postganglionic fibers of the SNS are ***adrenergic*** (with the exception of those nerves stimulating sweat glands and portions of skeletal muscle). They are so called because they mediate their effects on target organs by releasing ***norepinephrine***. In contrast, postganglionic fibers of the PNS are cholinergic. Like preganglionic fibers of both branches of the autonomic system, they mediate their effects by releasing acetylcholine.

Generalized activation of the **SNS** results in a ***"fight or flight"*** reaction. In addition to adrenergic stimulation and release of the neurotransmitter norepinephrine- the adrenal gland is stimulated to release endogenous epinephrine. Heart rate and blood pressure increase, the pupils dilate, the individual perspires, bronchodilation occurs, intestinal peristalsis and glandular secretion are inhibited, and the anal sphincter contracts.

In contrast, the **PNS** is the ***"repose and repair"*** system. Its activation results in *slowing* of the heart rate, a fall in blood pressure, and resumption of glandular secretion and peristalsis.

Clinical Applications of the PNS and SNS

The autonomic nervous system exerts an extremely important influence on cardiac function. As is the case for other internal organs of the body, the heart is *doubly* innervated by both sympathetic and parasympathetic nerve fibers. (In contrast, blood vessels have only sympathetic innervation.)

Impulses from the **PNS** are transmitted to the heart via the ***vagus nerve***. The vagus innervates the sinoatrial (SA) and atrioventricular (AV) nodes- and primarily exerts an ***inhibitory* effect** on the heart. Its stimulation therefore results in *slowing* of the heart rate and *delay* in atrioventricular (AV) conduction. As a result of optimal conditioning, young athletes often exhibit significant vagal tone at rest. They may therefore demonstrate a fairly marked sinus bradycardia and/or arrhythmia, first-degree AV block, and/or second degree AV block Mobitz type I as *normal phenomena*- that simply reflect the presence of *marked* vagotonia at rest. On the other hand, excessive vagal discharge may also be commonly noted in association with acute *inferior* myocardial infarction. In this latter setting, the accompanying bradycardia, hypotension, and AV conduction disturbances are clearly pathologic.

Adrenergic fibers of the **SNS** innervate the myocardium and primarily exert an ***excitatory* effect**. This results in acceleration of the heart rate (enhanced *chronotropy*) and increased contractility (positive *inotropic* effect). Adrenergic innervation is also present in the respiratory system and in vascular smooth muscle. Stimulation of these fibers may result in bronchodilatation or changes in vasomotor tone (vasoconstriction or vasodilatation- depending on the predominant type of adrenergic receptor activity).

Clinical applications of autonomic nervous system activity can best be illustrated by examining the mechanism of action of several commonly used cardioactive drugs. For example- ***Atropine*** is optimally effective when used to treat bradycardia (and accompanying hypotension) associated with acute *inferior* infarction if the drug is given within the first few hours after onset. This is because *parasympathetic* activation is greatest at this time. In contrast, patients with acute *anterior* infarction are much more likely to manifest evidence of *sympathetic* overactivity (i.e., hypertension, tachycardia, arrhythmias) during the early hours of infarction. This is one reason why ***IV beta-blockers*** are most effective when given *early* in the course to such patients.

Another medication that exerts its clinical effect through an action on the autonomic nervous system is ***Digoxin***. Patients with new-onset atrial fibrillation often present with a rapid ventricular response to this rhythm. Digoxin is one of the most commonly used drugs for controlling the rate. This *rate-slowing* effect of Digoxin is mediated by stimulation of the *vagal* nerve (i.e., activation of the PNS). However, some patients fail to respond even to high doses of IV Digoxin. This is particularly true for acutely ill patients who are severely stressed by their illness. As a result of their illness, such patients are likely to have extremely high *endogenous* catecholamine levels that maintain the tachycardia *despite* the Digoxin-induced increase in vagal tone. For this reason, rate-slowing drugs that work by a mechanism *other than* increasing vagal tone (i.e., Verapamil, Diltiazem, and/or use of an IV beta-blocker) are increasingly favored (over Digoxin) for acute treatment of rapid A Fib.

The last clinical application we mention relates to ***vagal* maneuvers** (i.e., carotid massage)- that are commonly used as a diagnostic/therapeutic measure in patients with supraventricular tachyarrhythmias. The increase in vagal tone produced by these maneuvers *slows* AV conduction- which hopefully will either convert the rhythm to sinus- or at least temporarily slow the rate enough to allow detection of previously hidden atrial activity.

Adrenergic Receptors of the Autonomic Nervous System

As noted above, adrenergic innervation is present in the heart, lungs, and in vascular smooth muscle. Adrenergic activation is mediated by ***ALPHA-*** and ***BETA-adrenergic*** **receptors** that are located on cellular surfaces. Each of these receptor types are further subdivided into two subtypes: alpha-1 and alpha-2- and beta-1 and beta-2, respectively.

- ***Beta-1*** *receptors*- are predominantly located in the myocardium. Adrenergic stimulation of these receptors is responsible for enhanced chronotropy and positive inotropy of the heart.

- ***Beta-2*** *receptors*- are predominantly located in respiratory and vascular smooth muscle. Stimulation of these receptors results in bronchodilatation and vasodilatation.

> As an aid to remembering what each beta-adrenergic receptor does, you may find it helpful to think of *"**one** heart, **two** lungs"* :
>
> - *beta-**1** receptors* act on the ***heart***
> - *beta-**2** receptors* act on the ***lungs***

Clinically, *beta agonists* (activators) are useful in the treatment of asthma because of the bronchodilation they produce. Non-selective beta agonists (such as Isoproterenol) stimulate *both* beta-1 and beta-2 receptors- and are therefore more likely to produce tachycardia (from beta-1 stimulation)- as well as bronchodilation (from beta-2 stimulation). For this reason, use of a more *selective* beta-2 agonist (i.e., Terbutaline, Albuterol) is preferable- as it produces less cardiac stimulation (and tachycardia) in association with bronchodilation.

Beta-blocking drugs produce the opposite pharmacologic effects as beta agonists. Thus, a potential adverse effect of a beta-blocker is that it may precipitate bronchospasm. Theoretically- *"selective"* beta-blocking drugs should be less likely to precipitate bronchospasm because they primarily affect beta-1 receptors. In contrast, "non-selective" beta-blockers inhibit *both* beta-1 and beta-2 receptors. Practically speaking, however- *"beta-selectivity"* appears to be lost at relatively low doses of these drugs, so that the advantages of beta-selectivity are more theoretical than clinical reality.

- ***Alpha-1*** *receptors*- are primarily *postsynaptic* in location. That is, they are found on the effector cell (i.e., vascular smooth muscle)- *after* the synapse between the nerve that is stimulated and the target organ.

- ***Alpha-2*** *receptors*- are presynaptic *and* post-synaptic in location (and *not* just presynaptic as was previously thought!).

Alpha-1 receptors respond preferentially to neurotransmitter catecholamines that are released by presynaptic nerve endings. Stimulation of alpha-1 receptors results in potent vasoconstriction.

Stimulation of alpha-2 receptors also results in vasoconstriction. In addition, alpha-2 receptors participate in a feedback loop (in conjunction with alpha-1 receptors)- that acts to prevent further release of neurotransmitter catecholamines. As opposed to post-synaptic alpha-1 receptors (that respond preferentially to the neurotransmitter norepinephrine)- alpha-2 receptors respond preferentially to *circulating* catecholamines.

> With respect to cardiac resuscitation- ***vasoconstriction*** is the ***alpha-adrenergic* receptor activity** with which we are most concerned (because this is the property that favors coronary and cerebral blood flow when CPR is performed in the arrested heart).
>
> For simplicity (and unless otherwise specified) we will use the general term *alpha-adrenergic stimulation* to refer to stimulation of *alpha-1* adrenergic receptors.

Technically, the differential responsiveness of alpha-1 and -2 receptors explains why Epinephrine (which stimulates *both* types of alpha receptors) is a more effective agent in the setting of cardiopulmonary resuscitation than pure alpha-1 stimulating drugs (such as Methoxamine and Phenylephrine). Low-flow states such as cardiac arrest result in a *down-regulation* of alpha-1 receptor activity and an *up-regulation* of alpha-2 receptor activity. This effect enhances responsiveness to vasoactive agents that stimulate alpha-2 receptors (such as Epinephrine and Norepinephrine).

In contrast, pure alpha-1 stimulating agents are far less likely to produce effective vasoconstriction in the setting of cardiac arrest- because of the *down-regulation* of these receptors in this situation. As a result- Methoxamine and Phenylephrine generally exert little effect on aortic diastolic pressure (and therefore do not significantly augment coronary perfusion during CPR).

In our subsequent discussion of vasoactive drugs, note will be made of their relative degree of alpha- and beta-adrenergic receptor activity. For example, ***Isoproterenol*** is a *pure* beta-adrenergic receptor stimulator. It therefore exerts a potent chronotropic and inotropic effect on the heart (beta-1 action), as well as causing bronchodilatation and peripheral vasodilatation (beta-2 effect).

In contrast to Isoproterenol- ***Epinephrine*** possesses *both* alpha- and beta-adrenergic activity. Its beta-1 effects produce enhanced chronotropy and inotropy in a similar manner as does Isoproterenol. Its vasoactive action, however, will be somewhat dose dependent. At low doses, the beta-2 effects of Epinephrine predominate- and the result is vasodilatation. With higher doses (as are used in the treatment of cardiac arrest)- the alpha-adrenergic (vasoconstrictor) effect of Epinephrine overrides the beta-2 (vasodilatory) action of the drug. It is this vasoconstrictor effect of Epinephrine that becomes so vitally important in maintaining coronary blood flow during cardiopulmonary resuscitation.

> Under normal circumstances, *circulating* catecholamines (principally endogenous Epinephrine- and to a lesser extent Norepinephrine)- exert little influence on cardiac function. Instead, cardiac tone and function are mediated by the autonomic nervous system.
>
> However, with chronic stress-inducing conditions (such as congestive heart failure)- myocardial catecholamine stores may become depleted. In such situations, *circulating* catecholamines probably assume a much more important role.

Administered medication with adrenergic stimulating properties may exert profound chronotropic and inotropic effects on the heart. In contrast, administration of a *beta-blocking* agent (such as Propranolol) may dramatically depress myocardial function in patients who become dependent on *circulating* catecholamines to stimulate cardiac contraction. Thus, ***beta-blocking* agents** may depress cardiac function (and worsen heart failure) in a number of ways:

1) heart rate reduction
2) blood pressure reduction
3) direct *negative* inotropic effect
4) catecholamine inhibition

As suggested above- the latter effect (catecholamine inhibition) may be particularly important in acutely ill patients who are *dependent* on catecholamine secretion as their principal mechanism of compensation.

On the other hand, the sympatholytic and negative chronotropic/inotropic effect of beta-blockers may prove invaluable as a *beneficial* therapeutic measure in the treatment of patients with acute *anterior* infarction (in which tachycardia, hypertension and excessive sympathetic tone combine to increase myocardial oxygen consumption and exacerbate ischemia).

Determinants of Cardiac Performance

The principal parameter for assessing cardiac performance is ***cardiac output* (CO)**. This is simply a measurement of the volume of blood pumped out by the heart each minute. It is equal to stroke volume (**SV**) times heart rate (**HR**) as expressed by the following equation:

CO = HR X **SV**

where **SV** (= ***stroke volume***) reflects the *average* amount of blood ejected from the heart with each contraction.

Heart rate is a reflection of the interaction between *sympathetic* and *parasympathetic* tone of the autonomic nervous system. It is important to remember that under *normal* conditions- the resting heart is under the influence of *both* of these divisions of the autonomic nervous system. Parasympathetic tone usually predominates. This is especially true for the case of the young well-trained athlete who (as mentioned earlier) frequently manifests sinus bradycardia as the result of marked vagotonia. A certain amount of resting *sympathetic* tone is *also* usually present in most individuals. This is evidenced by experiments that demonstrate an increase in heart rate following parasympathetic denervation that far exceeds the original resting heart rate.

Clinically, this concept becomes important when ***Atropine*** is administered for treatment of hemodynamically significant bradyarrhythmias. Especially when a large dose of the drug (such as 1 mg at a time) is given- blockade of parasympathetic discharge may *unmask* underlying sympathetic hyperactivity (that had previously been held in check)- resulting in potentially deleterious effects (including increased myocardial oxygen consumption and/or tachyarrhythmias).

The second determinant of cardiac output in the above equation is ***stroke volume***. The amount of blood ejected from the heart with each contraction depends on the interplay between three factors:

i) ***Preload***- the amount of passive "stretch" placed on myocardial fibers *prior* to the onset of contraction.
ii) ***Afterload***- the force (or resistance) against which the heart must pump.
iii) ***Contractility***- the force with which contraction takes place.

Clinically- ***preload*** is determined by the degree of left ventricular volume and pressure at the end of diastole. Under normal circumstances, the greater the LVEDP (i.e., left ventricular *end-diastolic* pressure)- the more the heart will be "stretched" (and the stronger it will contract). Physiologically, this relationship is reflected by the ***Frank-Starling* principle**. This concept explains why a failing heart requires a higher left ventricular filling pressure in order to perform the same amount of work as does a normal ventricle. Unless adequate myocardial "stretch" occurs- *the heart will simply not contract forcefully enough to adequately eject blood.* As a result, one frequently tries to achieve slightly higher than normal filling pressures in patients with acute myocardial infarction in an attempt to improve cardiac function. However, because excessive filling pressures may precipitate cardiac decompensation (as the heart will be unable to contract when there is too much "stretch")- hemodynamic monitoring (with a Swan-Ganz catheter) may be needed to assist in making manipulations when adjusting preload.

> Recently, much attention has been given to the use of ***ACE-Inhibitors*** in the post-infarction period. The mechanism by which ACE-Inhibitors are felt to work is similarly related to the Frank-Starling principle. Beginning *within hours* of acute infarction, a process known as ***remodeling*** starts- in which myocardial tissue around the zone of infarction dilates (and therefore *expands* the left ventricular cavity). Remodeling continues over the ensuing weeks to months following infarction- ultimately resulting in the left ventricle assuming a more *spherical* configuration. The process of remodeling probably reflects the body's attempt to invoke the Frank-Starling principle to maximize *stretch* (which is clearly greater in this larger, more *spherical* left ventricular configuration). The objective of increasing "stretch" in this manner is to help *maintain* cardiac contractility. Unfortunately with time- too much "stretch" may occur, resulting in *decompensation* (and ultimate development of heart failure). Enthusiasm for the use of ACE-Inhibitors following acute infarction stems from the hope that this class of drugs may attenuate the process of remodeling- and therefore lessen the likelihood of ultimate heart failure.

Another manner by which cardiac output with acute infarction may be improved is to reduce ***afterload***. Blood pressure control becomes vitally important in this situation. What would normally constitute only mild-to-moderate elevation in blood pressure (i.e., a blood pressure of 150-160 mm Hg systolic and 90-100 mm Hg diastolic)- might *severely* overload an infarcting ventricle and precipitate overt cardiac decompensation. An agent such as ***IV Nitroglycerin*** would seem to be ideally suited for use in this clinical situation- since it improves cardiac function *both* by decreasing preload, *as well as* by reducing afterload in a patient in whom LVEDP is too high.

Clinically- a very fine balance must be sought so as to optimize cardiac function *without* adversely affecting hemodynamics. Producing too potent an inotropic effect might disproportionately increase myocardial oxygen consumption and become deleterious. This is the reason that agents which increase ***contractility*** (such as Isoproterenol) are usually *avoided* in acute infarction. On the other hand, drugs that produce too great an increase in peripheral vascular resistance (increasing afterload) may place too great a strain on the heart (and also result in a reduction of cardiac output). Thus, in order to select the *optimal* agent for a particular patient in a given situation- many factors must be kept in mind. Treatment needs to be *individualized* according to the hemodynamic response of that particular patient.

Selection of a Pressor Agent

The cardiovascular drugs used in emergency cardiac care all affect one or more of the determinants of myocardial performance that we have just discussed. For example:

- Adrenergic receptor agents with ***beta-1*** *stimulating* properties (i.e., Isoproterenol, Epinephrine, Dopamine, Dobutamine)- all increase heart rate and myocardial contractility.
- Adrenergic receptor agents with ***beta-2*** *stimulating* properties (i.e., Isoproterenol, *low-dose* Epinephrine)- produce vasodilation.
- Adrenergic receptor agents with ***alpha****-stimulating* properties (i.e., moderate-to-high doses of Epinephrine and Dopamine, Norepinephrine)- produce vasoconstriction.

> Collectively the drugs that we list above are frequently referred to as ***"pressor" agents***. However, in light of the fact that Isoproterenol and Dobutamine produce little vasoconstriction per se- this is probably *not* the most appropriate term. Instead it may be far better to think of these agents with regard to whether they provide ***chronotropic*** and/or ***inotropic*** *support* (i.e., act to improve cardiac output by increasing the rate and/or force of contraction)- or ***pressor*** *support* (i.e., act by increasing peripheral vascular resistance and blood pressure).

Drugs such as ***Dopamine*** may affect *all* of the above parameters- depending on the dose that is given. At low-to-moderate infusion rates, Dopamine increases cardiac output by its predominant beta-adrenergic effect, often with little change in blood pressure. At higher infusion rates- the vasoconstrictor (alpha-adrenergic) effect of the drug predominates and the pressor effect takes over. At this *higher* dose range- *Dopamine acts very much like Epinephrine or Norepinephrine.*

Which drug is selected for a particular situation depends principally on the needs of that situation. In the case of *cardiac arrest*- this means that the primary concern is to *restart* the heart and maintain adequate coronary and cerebral flow until a spontaneously perfusing rhythm takes over (Table 2A-1). The drug of choice in this situation is ***Epinephrine***. Its alpha-adrenergic action favors coronary flow (by raising aortic diastolic blood pressure) and cerebral flow (by shunting blood from the external to the internal carotid artery)- while its beta-adrenergic effect stimulates contractility. High dose *Dopamine* will probably provide similar success as Epinephrine during cardiac arrest.

In contrast to the beneficial effect of Epinephrine (and high dose Dopamine) during cardiac arrest- ***Isoproterenol*** is *contraindicated* in this clinical situation. This is because *despite* the potent chronotropic and inotropic activity of Isoproterenol, the *pure* beta-adrenergic stimulation it produces results in vasodilatation. This leads to a *lowering* of peripheral vascular resistance and aortic diastolic pressure- with a corresponding *reduction* in coronary blood flow to the arrested heart.

Table 2A-1: ***Selection of a Pressor Agent in the Arrested Heart- and the Period Immediately Thereafter***

	In the Arrested Heart (i.e., V Fib, asystole)	**Once the Heart Has Been Restarted**
Needs of Therapy	- To restart the heart - To maintain coronary and cerebral perfusion	- To improve cardiac output and peripheral perfusion
Drug of Choice	- **Epinephrine** by bolus or infusion. Increase to higher doses of Epinephrine as needed.	- **Dopamine** infusion (at low-to-moderate doses)
Alternative Agent(s)	- **Dopamine** infusion (at moderate-to-high doses)	- **Epinephrine** by **IV infusion** (for a slow idioventricular rhythm with a low blood pressure) - Possibly Isoproterenol (if *only* chronotropic support is needed and blood pressure is adequate)
Drugs that are Contraindicated	- **Isoproterenol** (since the vasodilation it produces will reduce coronary perfusion pressure)	- **Epinephrine** by **IV bolus** (since it is difficult to judge how much drug is needed- and once an IV bolus is given, *"you can't take the bolus back"*)

As indicated in Table 2A-1, once the heart has been restarted (and a *perfusing* rhythm is restored)- *priorities change.* Achievement of a high aortic diastolic pressure is no longer essential for maintaining coronary flow. Instead, the goal of therapy *after* restarting the heart becomes improvement of cardiac output and peripheral perfusion:

- Once the heart has been restarted- ***Dopamine*** (at low-to-moderate infusion rates) is probably the drug of choice.

- ***Epineprhine*** *by* ***IV bolus*** is a relatively *contraindicated* drug for a patient *with* a spontaneous pulse. This is because of the difficulty in determining the *appropriate* dose when Epinephrine is administered by this route to a patient with a pulse. If too much of the drug is inadvertently given- there unfortunately is *no way* to take the IV bolus back.

- In contrast- administration of ***Epinephrine*** *by* ***IV infusion*** is an effective way to give the drug to a patient with a pulse (as might be indicated for treatment of a slow idioventricular rhythm with associated hypotension). The moment-to-moment *titratability* of an IV infusion allows careful regulation of the dose administered (which can easily be adjusted according to the patient's hemodynamic response).

> Caution is advised when using Epinephrine infusion to treat a patient with only minimal hypotension. This is because the drug may be *deleterious* if the increase in afterload that it produces overrides the improvement in cardiac output. For this reason, the agent of choice for pressor support when treatment is needed but hypotension is relatively mild is Dopamine.

- ***Isoproterenol*** may be effective for treatment of hemodynamically significant bradyarrhythmias- if *chronotropic support* is the primary need (i.e., if the heart rate is slow but the blood pressure is adequate). However, if hypotension accompanies the bradycardia (as is usually the case)- use of Isoproterenol is likely to *exacerbate* the situation by producing further vasodilatation.

Section 2B: *Key Drugs in ACLS*

Epinephrine

How Dispensed:

- As a **1:10,000 Soln.** of Epi (1 mg per 10 ml syringe- i.e., **0.1 mg/ml)**- for **SDE**
- As a **1:1,000 Soln.** of Epi (30 mg per 30 ml vial- i.e., **1.0 mg/ml)**- for **HDE**

Indications → V Fib/Pulseless VT, asystole, EMD/PEA.

- Use of Epinephrine (by IV infusion) may also be considered for treatment of hemodynamically significant bradyarrhythmias that have *not* responded to Atropine.

Mechanism:

Epinephrine is an endogenous catecholamine that exerts both *alpha-* and *beta-adrenergic* properties. Although the latter effect increases the force and rate of myocardial contraction (inotropic and chronotropic actions)- the *alpha-adrenergic* (= vasoconstrictor) effect of Epinephrine is *far more* important in the setting of cardiac arrest. This is because this vasoconstrictor effect:

i) favors blood flow to the coronary circulation (by increasing aortic *diastolic* pressure- which enhances the flow gradient to the coronary arteries).

ii) preferentially *shunts* blood to the *internal* carotid artery (and therefore enhances *cerebral* blood flow).

Under the best of circumstances, cardiac output produced by basic life support during cardiac arrest is no more than 20% to 30% of cardiac output during spontanous circulation. Without the use of medication, however, only a fraction of this output is delivered to the heart and brain. Epinephrine is probably the most effective drug available for optimizing blood flow to these vital organs.

Insight into the relative role of alpha- and beta-adrenergic activity for maintaining coronary perfusion during CPR can be gained by reflecting on previous practice. In the past, pure beta-adrenergic agents such as *Isoproterenol* were routinely recommended for treatment of cardiac arrest- in the hope that potent chronotropic and inotropic stimulation might facilitate *ROSC* (*Restoration Of Spontaneous Circulation*). Unfortunately, *pure* beta-adrenergic stimulation also produces peripheral *vasodilatation*- an effect that is counterproductive because it *reduces* peripheral vascular resistance and aortic end-diastolic pressure. It is precisely for this reason that Isoproterenol is no longer indicated during cardiac arrest. The reduction in aortic diastolic pressure that Isoproterenol produces leads to a corresponding reduction in coronary perfusion pressure- and generally *counteracts* any beneficial effect that might be obtained from positive chronotropic and inotropic actions of the drug.

In contrast to the vasodilatory effect of Isoproterenol- the vasoconstrictor (i.e., *alpha-adrenergic*) effect of Epineprhine acts to *increase* aortic diastolic pressure. This is why Epinephrine *enhances* the gradient for coronary blood flow during CPR. Still unresolved, however, is the *dose* of Epinephrine needed to produce *optimal* coronary perfusion in the non-beating heart.

Terminology:

Before reviewing current dosing recommendations for Epinephrine, it is important to be comfortable with the following two definitions:

- ***SDE*** = ***S**tandard-**D**ose **E**pinephrine* = **1.0 mg** by **IV bolus**. This is the dose of Epinephrine that has been traditionally recommended for the treatment of cardiac arrest in adults.

- ***HDE*** = ***H**igh-**D**ose **E**pinephrine* = administration of any IV dose of Epinephrine that is *greater* than the SDE dose.

Dose & Route of Administration:

Based on available clinical data- there appears to be little reason to alter the *initial* IV dose of Epinephrine from that which was recommended for use in the past (AHA Text- Pg 7-4). *Recommendations are less certain for subsequent dosing.* Therefore, when treating a patient in cardiac arrest for whom effective IV access has been established- the following approach is suggested (AHA Text- Pg 1-16):

- ***Initial* IV Dose**- Begin with the ***SDE*** dose = **1.0 mg** of Epinephrine by IV bolus (= 10 ml of a 1:10,000 soln.).

- ***Subsequent* IV Dosing** - Repeat the IV bolus of Epinephrine in 3 to 5 minutes. Continue to give Epinephrine *every* **3-5 minutes** thereafter (as needed)- for as long as the patient *remains* in cardiac arrest.

  After the *initial* **SDE** (= 1 mg) IV dose, one may *either* continue with 1 mg IV doses- *OR*- chose between several ***HDE* alternatives** :

  i) Administration of **2-5 mg** IV boluses (which AHA Guidelines describe as *"intermediate"* dose Epinephrine)

  \- *OR* -

  ii) *Escalating* **1- 3- 5 mg** IV boluses

  \- *OR* -

  iii) Dosing at **0.1 mg/kg** as an IV bolus.

In addition to IV bolus administration- Epinephrine may also be given by the ET route- *and/or* by continuous IV infusion. Dosing and clinical considerations for these forms of administration are noted below:

- **ET Administration** - is an effective route for delivery of Epinephrine. However, absorption of the drug is somewhat *slower* and *less* complete by this route than it is for IV administration. As a result:

  - IV administration is preferable during cardiac arrest- *IF* (as soon as) effective IV access has been established.

  - If IV access is unavailable- do *not* hesitate to use the ET route. To ensure adequate dosing, a larger amount of drug will need to be given by the ET route. Dosing recommendations are to instill 2-2.5 times the IV dose (i.e., **2-2.5 mg** of 1:10,000 soln.) down the ET tube- and then to follow with several forceful insufflations of the Ambu bag.

- **<u>IV Infusion of Epinephrine</u>**- is another effective alternative method for drug delivery. A decided advantage of this form of administration is the extremely wide range of dosing it allows. For example, IV infusion of Epinephrine for treatment of a bradycardic patient who is *not* in cardiac arrest is usually begun at a rate of between 1-2 μg/minute. The rate of infusion can then be titrated upward (as needed) according to the patient's clinical response. By way of comparison, a dose on the order of 100 times greater (i.e., 100-200 μg/minute) is generally recommended as the *starting* rate for *"higher-dose"* IV infusion of Epinephrine (which is comparable to the dose that is usually used for treatment of cardiac arrest).

  A second important advantage of administering Epinephrine by continuous IV infusion is the capability of *moment-to-moment* titration in the dose of drug given. This feature enhances safety by allowing the clinician to *immediately* turn down (or off) the IV infusion as soon as an adverse effect occurs. In contrast, if Epinephrine is given by IV bolus and an adverse effect occurs- *"You can't take the bolus back."*

  Despite these beneficial features- most emergency care providers prefer to administer Epinephrine by IV bolus instead of by IV infusion when treating a patient in cardiac arrest (i.e., with ventricular fibrillation or asystole). Moment-to-moment dose titration is far less important in this clinical situation (since the patient is *pulseless* and likely to need significantly *larger* doses of drug). From a purely practical standpoint- giving Epinephrine by IV bolus is both quicker and simpler than having to set up and administer an IV infusion. On the other hand- use of a *lower* (and more carefully regulated) dose of drug is clearly preferable when treating a patient with severe bradycardia (and/or hypotension)- but who is *not* cardiac arrest.

IV infusion of Epinephrine may be administered at *low* dose (for treatment of the patient *with* a pulse)- or in more concentrated form that we designate *higher* dose (for the patient who *is* in cardiac arrest). For ease of recall, we suggest the following preparations:

- ***<u>Lower Dose</u>*** **<u>Epinephrine Infusion</u>**- Mix 1 mg of a 1:10,000 soln. of Epinephrine in 250 ml of D5W- and *begin* the infusion @ 15-30 drops/minute (=**1-2 μg/minute**). Titrate the rate of infusion upward as needed.

- ***<u>Higher Dose</u>*** **<u>Epinephrine Infusion</u>**- Mix 50 mg of a 1:1,000 soln. of Epinephrine in 250 ml of D5W- and *begin* the infusion @ 30-60 drops/minute (=**100-200 μg/minute**). Titrate the rate of infusion upward as needed.

It should be emphasized that the *total* amount of Epinephrine delivered in a unit of time by *lower dose* IV infusion will be small compared to the dose that is typically given by IV bolus. For example- IV infusion of between 1-10 μg/minute (which is the range usually recommended when using Epinephrine as a *pressor* agent) will only deliver between 0.06-0.6 mg of drug in an *hour*.

By way of comparison- IV infusion of Epinephrine at the above cited *higher dose* rate of **200 μg/min** will deliver 1,000 μg = **1 mg** of Epinephrine every **5 minutes** (= 200 X 5 = 1,000 μg)- *which is comparable to the amount of drug contained in the recommended SDE dose by IV bolus* !

In Summary- Use of ***Lower Dose*** **Epinephrine Infusion** is appropriate for treatment of the patient with severe bradycardia (and/or hypotension) who is *not* in cardiac arrest. When using the drug as a *pressor agent* in this manner, the infusion is usually begun at a rate of **1-2 µg/minute**- and then titrated upward as needed according to the clinical response. Moment-to-moment titration of dose and the ability to immediately turn off the infusion if adverse effects occur are important features when treating the patient who is *not* in cardiac arrest. The recommended range of infusion is between 1-10 µg/minute.

In contrast- *either* **IV bolus** therapy *or* IV infusion of Epinephrine may be used when treating the patient in cardiac arrest. If using IV infusion in this situation- ***Higher Dose*** **Epinephrine Infusion** is recommended (usually *beginning* at **100-200 µg/minute**- and titrating the dose upward as needed).

Regarding the "Optimal" Dose of Epinephrine:

Epinephrine is clearly the *most* important drug used in the treatment of cardiac arrest. Unfortunately- *the optimal dose of Epinephrine remains unknown.* Results from several recent prospective, randomized clinical trials (on more than 2,000 human subjects with out-of-hospital cardiac arrest)- suggest that use of HDE in patients with refractory ventricular fibrillation may *increase* the rate of ROSC. However, these same studies *fail* to show a statistically significant improvement in long-term survival with the use of HDE when compared to SDE (AHA Text- Pg 7-3). Whether such studies sufficiently investigate *all* possible subsets of patients who could *potentially benefit* from the use of higher doses of drug (HDE) is uncertain. Nevertheless, several important conclusions can be derived from results of these clinical trials:

i) Survival rates for patients in cardiac arrest are low- *regardless* of the dose of Epinephrine used.
ii) Most patients who do survive cardiac arrest- do so as a result of *defibrillation* (and *not* as a result of receiving Epinephrine) !
iii) Administration of Epinephrine to patients in cardiac arrest does *not* appear to be harmful- even if large doses of drug (i.e., HDE) are given.

In view of these results- AHA Guidelines currently recommend use of **SDE** for the *initial* dose of drug. Thereafter the Guidelines clearly allow for *flexibility* in Epinephrine dosing by stating-*"Use of higher doses of Epinephrine (**HDE**) can NEITHER be recommended NOR discouraged"* (AHA Text- Pg 7-4).

Cautions:

As suggested above- use of HDE in the treatment of patients with refractory out-of-hospital cardiac arrest may *increase* the likelihood of ROSC. Unfortunately, patients who are salvaged by this approach are also more likely to suffer permanent neurologic sequelae- primarily because of the longer time until discovery and treatment for many of these patients. Practically speaking- the chance for long-term survival (with *meaningful* neurologic recovery) is exceedingly small- IF patients with out-of-hospital cardiac arrest fail to respond to countershock in the field. This raises the ethical dilemma of whether HDE should be tried if patients fail to respond to SDE- and if so, how to decide which patients should receive this form of treatment.

Bottom Line- Judgement is clearly needed on the part of the emergency care provider in deciding whether or not to use **HDE**- and if so, under what circumstances. Factors that might enter into making this decision include:

- time until discovery of the patient- initiation of CPR- and delivery of countershock. The longer the interval between the onset of arrest and the initiation of treatment- the less the chance for meaningful survival with intact neurologic status.
- the patient's premorbid condition.
- the mechanism (i.e., initial rhythm) of the arrest (be this V Fib, asystole, PEA- or other bradyarrhythmia). In general, higher doses of Epinephrine are more likely to be needed when the initial rhythm is asystole or very fine V Fib.
- beliefs and personal preferences of the treating clinician.

Special Points:

- Other pressor agents (i.e., higher dose infusion of *Dopamine* or *Norepinephrine*) may exert similar beneficial effects as Epinephrine in the setting of cardiac arrest. However, experience with Epinephrine is far greater- so this drug clearly remains the standard.
- The effect of an IV bolus of Epinephrine peaks in 2-3 minutes. As a result, AHA Guidelines now allow for repetition of each bolus of drug as often as every 3 minutes- if needed- as long as the patient remains in cardiac arrest.
- Epinephrine should *not* be given by IV bolus if using the drug as a *pressor* agent (i.e., to treat a patient who is *not* in cardiac arrest). This is because if adverse effects occur- *"you can't take a bolus back."*
- If using Epinephrine by IV infusion- remember to turn down the rate of infusion at the *earliest* opportunity- as soon as the desired hemodynamic response is acheived (and/or to consider switching to a Dopamine infusion if a pressor agent is still needed).
- Take comfort in the fact that *either* continued use of SDE (1 mg IV boluses) *throughout* the code- *or* escalation to HDE dosing (if the patient fails to respond to initial SDE)- are *both* perfectly reasonable alternatives. Use of HDE dosing might be most appropriate when the patient is felt to be salvageable, and a reasonable chance still exists that irreversible brain damage has *not* yet occurred.
- *Intracardiac Epinephrine* is no longer recommended (*unless* performing open cardiac massage). This is because of uncertain benefit from administration of the drug by this route during closed chest cardiac massage- and the *very high* risk of coronary artery laceration (with induction of *intractable* ventricular fibrillation).

Lidocaine

How Dispensed:

- **IV Bolus-** 100 mg per 10 ml syringe.
- **IV Infusion-** *Pre-mixed* bags of 1g/250 ml and 2g/500 ml (as *pre-filled* syringes for IV infusion are *no longer* available).

Indications:

- Drug of choice for *Refractory V Fib* and acute treatment of ventricular arrhythmias (i.e., *frequent PVCs, VT*)- when such treatment is indicated. Use of Lidocaine is also appropriate for the treatment of *WIDE-complex* tachycardias of *uncertain* etiology (which statistically are most likely to be VT).

> **Note**- AHA Guidelines list **Lidocaine** as the *first **Antifibrillatory Agent*** to use in the treatment of Refractory V Fib. Reasons for this recommendation are that emergency personnel are generally more familiar (and comfortable) with the use of this drug- and that it is *faster-acting* (and probably *safer*) than the 2nd and 3rd-line agents (*Bretylium* and *Procainamide*) in the setting of cardiac arrest (AHA Text- Pg 1-19).

Mechanism:

The antiarrhythmic effect of Lidocaine is attributed to its ability to decrease automaticity in ventricular myocardium- as well as to alter conduction velocity in reentrant pathways of ischemic tissue. The drug also appears to raise fibrillation threshold (which means that spontaneous V Fib is *less* likely to occur- and less likely to *recur* after successful defibrillation). Although difficult to prove in controlled studies- there is evidence suggesting that *combined* use of Lidocaine and Bretylium may produce a *synergistic* beneficial effect on fibrillation threshold (AHA Text- 7-7).

Dose & Route of Administration:

- **IV Bolus** (*Treatment of* ***PVCs/VT***)- Give **1.0- 1.5 mg/kg** (most often ≈50-100 mg) as an *initial* IV bolus. Repeat boluses of ≈50-75 mg (i.e., ≈0.5-0.75 mg/kg) may be given every 5-10 minutes up to a total dose of 3 mg/kg (≈225 mg).

> - **IV Infusion**- Mix 1g in 250 ml of D5W, and *begin* drip @ 30 drops/minute (= **2 mg/minute**).
>
> - Usual *range* of infusion = 0.5- 4 mg/minute (although most patients are adequately treated at a rate of between 1-2 mg/minute).

- **<u>IV Bolus</u>** (*Treatment of* ***V Fib***)- Give **1.0- 1.5 mg/kg** (≈50-150 mg) as an *initial* IV bolus. May repeat in 3-5 minutes- although a *single* IV dose (of **1.5 mg/kg**- or ≈100-150 mg) is acceptable in cardiac arrest. (*IV infusion is NOT necessarily needed while the patient remains in V Fib!*)

- **<u>ET Administration</u>**- Use 2 to 2.5 times the IV dose (≈100-150 mg) when giving the drug by the ET route. Be aware that endotracheal absorption of Lidocaine and delivery of drug to the central circulation during cardiac arrest is *not* nearly as reliable as when the drug is given by the IV route.

Cautions in Use: For most patients, an IV infusion rate of ≈**2 mg/minute** will provide adequate serum antiarrhythmic levels of the drug. However, a *lower* infusion rate (i.e., of **0.5-1.0 mg/min**) should probably be used (if possible) in certain subsets of patients who are at particularly high risk of developing Lidocaine toxicity. Such patients include the elderly- patients with heart failure, liver disease or shock- and those who have been on Lidocaine infusion for more than 24 hours. Additional caveats to keep in mind regarding the use of Lidocaine are that:

- ***Not every PVC need be eliminated for Lidocaine to exert a protective effect.*** Maintenance of a therapeutic serum level of Lidocaine may be all that is needed to protect against development of VT/V Fib- *even if "break through" PVCs are still occurring.* It is usually best *not* to try to eliminate all PVCs in such patients.

- ***One need NOT necessarily increase the infusion rate of Lidocaine each time that a bolus is given*** ! This is especially true during the period of initial IV loading with Lidocaine (when steady state levels of drug have *not* yet been reached!). Higher infusion rates (i.e., of 3-4 mg/min) will usually *not* be needed in most patients- *and may predispose to development of toxicity.*

- ***Lidocaine should NOT be used to treat chronic*** (*i.e., long-standing*) ***PVCs in asymptomatic patients*** !!! Treatment of chronic PVCs has *never* been shown to improve survival.

Adverse Effects/Lidocaine Toxicity:

In general, Lidocaine is an extremely well tolerated antiarrhythmic agent. Development of toxicity is relatively uncommon when the drug is dosed appropriately (*See above*). When adverse effects do occur (from excessive blood levels of Lidocaine)- they usually involve the central nervous system. Manifestations of toxicity most commonly include perioral paresthesias, feelings of dissociation, dizziness, drowsiness, euphoria, mild agitation, dysarthria, hearing impairment, disorientation and confusion. At higher blood levels there may be muscle twitching- which may ultimately lead to seizures and/or respiratory arrest.

Lidocaine has the potential to produce (and/or aggravate) conduction disturbances in susceptible patients. Fortunately, therapeutic doses of the drug *can* be used safely in most patients- even when minor conduction disturbances are present. However- *caution is advised* when giving the drug to patients with preexisting bundle branch block and/or 2° or 3° AV block. Although not common- marked bradycardia and even *asystole* have been precipitated by use of the drug in such patients.

A final, less well known adverse effect of Lidocaine is that the drug may occasionally *accelerate* the ventricular response of some patients with supraventricular tachyarrhythmias. As a result- we caution against *indiscriminate* use of the drug in patients with WCT of unknown etiology- since the chance exists that Lidocaine may aggravate the condition (i.e., *accelerate* the ventricular response) if the rhythm turns out to be supraventricular. We emphasize that use of Lidocaine *is* appropriate for treatment of a WCT when there is reasonable suspicion that the rhythm is VT (as it will be *most* of the time).

Use of Lidocaine: Prophylaxis vs Treatment:

We emphasize the importance of distinguishing between Lidocaine prophylaxis and treatment.

- ***Lidocaine Prophylaxis***- entails use of the drug in an attempt to *prevent* the occurrence of a life-threatening arrhythmia. Two principal settings for Lidocaine prophylaxis have been described:

  i) As ***primary* prophylaxis** in the setting of **Acute MI**- in which Lidocaine is administered to patients with only rare PVCs (*or no PVCs at all*) in the hope of *preventing* development of VT/V Fib. Although routine administration of prophylactic Lidocaine was common practice in the past- use of the drug for this indication is *no longer recommended* (AHA Text- Pg 7-7). The reason for discouraging use of prophylactic Lidocaine for patients with Acute MI (or suspected Acute MI) is that the drug has *not* been shown to improve survival in this setting- and its use is *not* without risk.

  ii) As ***secondary* prophylaxis** in the setting of ***cardiac arrest***- in which Lidocaine is given as a prophylactic measure in an attempt to *prevent recurrence* of V Fib in patients who have beeen converted *out* of this rhythm. AHA Guidelines strongly recommend initiation of a *prophylactic* Lidocaine infusion for this purpose *as soon as* a patient is converted out of V Fib (AHA Text- Pg 7-7).

- ***Lidocaine Treatment***- differs from prophylactic use in that the drug is given to *actively treat* (i.e., suppress) *new-onset* and frequent PVCs (including couplets/VT) in patients with either acute ischemic heart disease and/or Acute MI. AHA Guidelines recommend Lidocaine as the drug of choice for acute treatment of potentially life-threatening ventricular arrhythmias that occur in the setting of emergency cardiac care and/or ACLS situations.

It should be emphasized that indications (and enthousiasm) for treating ventricular arrhythmias are *not* nearly as liberal as they had been in the past. Long-standing PVCs- even if frequent- are no longer viewed as an acceptable indication for treatment- *unless* they are associated with exceedingly severe symptoms (that truly upset the patient's lifestyle).

On the other hand- treatment with Lidocaine *is* still appropriate (and advised)- when ventricular ectopy is *new* in onset and associated with *acute* ischemia and/or a cardiac arrest situation- especially when new-onset PVCs are *frequent* and *repetitive* forms (i.e., couplets, salvos) are present.

Special Points:

- Always initiate Lidocaine administration with an IV bolus of the drug. Failure to do so will greatly *delay* achieving therapeutic blood levels- because a period *at least* several hours is required to reach steady state if only IV infusion is used.
- Keep in mind that in the *spontaneously beating heart*- the half-life of Lidocaine is short (i.e., ≈10 minutes). As a result- IV infusion of the drug *must* be started *within* 5-10 minutes of giving an IV bolus (or the effect of the bolus will be dissipated).
- The pharmacokinetics of Lidocaine differ in the *arrested heart.* This is because clearance of the drug is *markedly reduced* in this situation. As a result- it will *not* be essential to begin an IV infusion soon after a bolus is given. AHA Guidelines therefore allow for use of a *single* (1.5 mg/kg) IV bolus dose in V Fib. Once the patient is converted out of V Fib- a second IV bolus should then be given *prior* to starting the IV infusion.

> **Note**- AHA Guidelines recommend *only* giving Lidocaine by IV bolus during cardiac arrest. We differ with this recommendation- and instead prefer to routinely begin an IV infusion *whenever* we initiate use of this drug. Our rationale for doing so is that the relatively *small amount* of Lidocaine administered during a code (at a rate of 2 mg/minute) should *not* pose a significant risk of developing drug toxicity. Our concern is that it may be all too easy to *forget* to start the Lidocaine IV infusion after the patient *is* converted out of V Fib- if you did not already do so at the time of the initial bolus.
>
> The point to emphasize is that if you chose *not* to begin the Lidocaine maintenance infusion at the time you administer the loading bolus- it is *imperative* to remember to do so *as soon as* the patient is converted out of V Fib. Failure to begin a Lidocaine infusion after conversion to sinus rhythm would substantially increase the risk of V Fib recurrence.

- Practically speaking- if one dose of Lidocaine fails to work for the patient in *refractory* V Fib, it is relatively unlikely that additional boluses will fare much better. As a result- we favor consideration of *alternative* antifibrillatory measures (i.e., use of Bretylium, Magnesium, etc.) if the initial 1.5 mg/kg Lidocaine bolus is ineffective.
- Despite its shortcomings, Lidocaine is an extremely effective antiarrhythmic agent- and the acute *treatment of choice* for ventricular arrhythmias that occur in the emergency setting (when such arrhythmias need to be treated).

Bretylium Tosylate

How Dispensed → 500 mg per 10 ml ampule.

Indications:

- Drug of *2nd choice* for refractory V Fib (after Lidocaine); *3rd-line* agent for acute treatment of PVCs/VT.

> **Note**- Bretylium has been used less in recent years. This is probably the result of several factors:
>
> i) Bretylium has *not* been shown to be superior to Lidocaine in the treatment of V Fib.
>
> ii) Lidocaine appears less likely to produce adverse hemodynamic effects during CPR.
>
> iii) Most clinicians are more familiar (and comfortable) with the use of Lidocaine (AHA Text- Pg 7-10).
>
> Despite these factors- it should be emphasized that Bretylium is an effective *antifibrillatory* agent that should be considered in the treatment of V Fib after one (*or at most two*) boluses of Lidocaine have been tried.

Mechanism/Adverse Effects:

The *initial* mechanism of action of Bretylium is ***adrenergic stimulation***- followed by ***adrenergic blockade***. As a result of its mechanism:

- PVCs and BP may actually *increase* at first after Bretylium is given (due to the initial *adrenergic stimulation* effect of the drug). For this reason, caution is urged when using Bretylium to treat PVCs/VT- especially when these arrhythmias occur in association with Dig toxicity.

- Hypotension is common (and a limiting factor) with IV maintenance infusions of the drug (as a result of the *adrenergic blockade* that follows the adrenergic stimulation). Nausea and vomiting are other common side effects noted in patients who are conscious- especially if the rate of IV infusion is rapid. *Infusing the drug at a slower rate may resolve these problems.*

Dose & Route of Administration:

- **IV Bolus (*for Refractory V Fib*)**- Give an initial IV bolus of ≈5 mg/kg (*or* a single **500 mg** IV bolus = **1 amp** of the drug). Defibrillate the patient approximately one minute later. If V Fib persists- a **2nd dose** (of 10 mg/kg *or* ≈1-2 amps) may be given approximately 5 minutes after the first dose. This 10 mg/kg dose may then be repeated *twice* at 5-30 minute intervals (until a total loading dose of 30-35 mg/kg has been given).

- Dosing of Bretylium in the setting of V Fib is by nature somewhat empiric. In the interest of simplicity- we therefore favor administration of one complete ampule (= 500 mg) for the initial IV bolus (rather than strict calculation on a body weight basis).

- Be sure to circulate the drug with CPR (for ≈1-2 minutes) after each administration of Bretylium- and then *defibrillate* again.

- The effect of an IV bolus of Bretylium lasts for about 2-6 hours. There is therefore time to decide whether or not to follow up IV bolus administration with a continuous IV infusion of the drug.

- IV infusion of Bretylium is likely to be most helpful in the management of those patients with refractory cardiac arrest who *only* converted out of V Fib *after* Bretylium was given.

▪ **IV Infusion-** Mix 1g in 250 ml of D5W, and *begin* drip @ 15-30 drops/min (=1-2 mg/minute).

- Usual *range* of infusion = 1-2 mg/minute.

▪ **IV Loading Infusion (*for VT*)-** Dilute **500 mg** (≈1 amp) in 50 ml of D5W, and infuse over a10 minute period (i.e., giving a dose of ≈5-10 mg/kg). May repeat IV loading of another 5-10 mg/kg (i.e., ≈500 mg) in 10-30 minutes (again infused over another 10 minute period).

Special Points:

▪ Remember that the onset of action of Bretylium may be *delayed* for a few minutes when treating V Fib. It may sometimes be *delayed* for a substantially *longer* period of time (of up to 10-20 minutes!) when treating VT. As a result- *it is important not to abandon resuscitative efforts until the drug has had an adequate chance to work!*

▪ Although Bretylium is extremely effective as an *antifibrillatory* agent- use of the drug has been deemphasized for the treatment of ventricular arrhythmias including VT. Currently the drug is viewed as *no more* than a 3rd-line agent for these indications- primarily because of a relatively high incidence of hypotension and its potential for initially exacerbating the arrhythmia being treated.

Procainamide

How Dispensed → **IV bolus-** 100 mg/ml (10 ml vials).

IV infusion- 1 g per 2 ml vial.

Indications:

- Drug of 2nd choice (after Lidocaine) for acute treatment of ventricular arrhythmias (i.e., *frequent PVCs, VT*).
- Treatment of A Fib/Flutter (similar antiarrhythmic effect as Quinidine that may help to convert these arrhythmias to normal sinus rhythm).
- Rapid A Fib with WPW (Wolff-Parkinson-White Syndrome).
- *WIDE-complex* Tachycardia (WCT) of *uncertain* etiology.
- Refractory V Fib- *maybe . . . .* (See below).

Mechanism/Clinical Effects:

Procainamide is a type IA antiarrhythmic agent with electrophysiologic and clinical properties that are similar to those of Quinidine. As a result, it decreases conduction velocity and automaticity- and is therefore effective in the treatment of *both* atrial and ventricular arrhythmias.

In the setting of cardiac arrest, Procainamide is the second drug of choice (after Lidocaine) for the treatment of frequent and complex PVCs (including sustained VT). As a single agent, the drug may even be more effective than Lidocaine for treating sustained VT in certain non-ischemic settings. At times it may be used together with Lidocaine to produce a *synergistic* antiarrhythmic effect. An additional advantage of using Procainamide in the treatment of sustained VT is that even if the drug fails to convert the rhythm- it will often *slow* the rate of the ventricular tachycardia. Thus, VT at a rate of 140 beats/minute may be much better tolerated hemodynamically than if the rate was 180 beats/minute.

Procainamide is a drug of choice for the medical treatment of atrial fibrillation or flutter. Like Quinidine, it may help to convert these arrhythmias to sinus rhythm. It is also effective in suppressing PACs/PJCs that may precipitate recurrence of these arrhythmias. A special feature of Procainamide is its abiility to prolong the anterograde refractory period of the accessory pathway in patients with WPW. This action makes the drug a treatment of choice for patients with WPW who present with very rapid A Fib. In contrast to Procainamide, drugs such as Digoxin, Verapamil and Diltiazem all *facilitate* conduction over the accessory pathway- and are therefore likely to precipitate V Fib if inadvertently given to a patient with A Fib and WPW.

As a result of these diverse clinical effects- Procainamide appears to be an excellent agent to consider in the *empiric* treatment of a **WCT** of ***uncertain* etiology:**

- *If the WCT turns out to be VT*- Procainamide may either convert the rhythm- or at least slow down the rate of the VT.

- *If the WCT turns out to be an SVT*- the "Quinidine-like" action of Procainamide may convert the rhythm (by affecting conduction properties down one or both reentrant pathways)- and/or prevent PSVT recurrence (by suppressing PACs/PJCs that typically precipitate this tachyarrhythmia).

- *If the WCT turns out to be WPW*- Procainamide is the drug of choice for treatment of a WCT due to rapid A Fib in a patient with WPW. The reason Procainamide is effective for this indication is that it *slows* anterograde conduction down the accessory pathway. In contrast, Digoxin, Verapamil, and Diltiazem are all *contraindicated* for treatment of rapid A Fib with WPW because these drugs *accelerate* conduction in the forward direction down the accessory pathway.

Dose & Route of Administration:

- **IV Loading**- Administer Procainamide in increments of **100 mg IV**- given *slowly* over a 5 minute period (i.e., at ≈20 mg/minute)- *until* one or more of the following ***End Points*** are reached:

  i) The arrhythmia is suppressed
  ii) Hypotension occurs
  iii) The QRS complex widens by ≥50% over its baseline value
  iv) A total loading dose of **17 mg/kg** has been given. (This comes out to ≈1,000 mg for the *average-sized* adult.)

  Slowing the rate of IV infusion may minimize the chance of developing hypotension.

- ***Alternative* IV Loading Regimen**- Mix ≈500-1,000 mg of drug in 100 ml of D5W- and infuse this over 30-60 minutes (keeping in mind the *end points* of infusion that are noted above).

> - **IV Infusion**- Mix 1g in 250 ml of D5W, and *begin* drip @ 30 drops/minute (=2 mg/minute).
>   - Use of an IV Infusion may be considered to *maintain* the effect of Procainamide following IV loading.
>   - Usual *range* of infusion = 1-4 mg/min.

Special Points:

- AHA Guidelines currently list Procainamide as the 3rd drug to use (after Lidocaine and Adenosine) in the protocol for treatment of WCT of *uncertain* etiology. While fully acknowledging the potential drawbacks of using Procainamide in an acute care situation (i.e., risk of hypotension, QRS and QT widening- and the longer time needed to achieve therapeutic levels)- we feel the merits of this drug may favor its *earlier* consideration- especially when VT is thought to be present (since Adenosine is *unlikely* to be helpful in this situation).

- Although AHA Guidelines allow for use of IV Procainamide as an *antifibrillatory agent* in the treatment of *refractory* V Fib- they emphasize that *both* Lidocaine and Bretylium should be used *before* Procainamide in this situation. AHA Guidelines also acknowledge the unfortunate reality of "poor likelihood of success" with this treatment- especially in view of the prolonged time required to administer effective doses of Procainamide (AHA Text- Pg 1-20; Pg 7-8).

- An additional advantage of using IV Procainamide is the availability of an oral form of the drug for long-term maintenance therapy.

- Procainamide is *contraindicated* for treatment of Torsade de Pointes (i.e., for VT associated with QT interval prolongation).

Magnesium Sulfate

How Dispensed → 5 g/10 ml (i.e., as a 50% solution).

Indications:

- *Torsade de Pointes*- Magnesium is the medical treatment of choice!
- *Refractory VT/V Fib*- Mechanism is unclear, but *empiric* administration of Magnesium *may* be helpful (and should be considered)-*especially* if standard measures have been tried and failed!

> **Note-** AHA Guidelines list routine use of Magnesium in the treatment of refractory VT/V Fib as a **Class IIb** indication (acceptable- *possibly helpful*). It is listed as a **Class IIa** indication (*probably helpful*)- if serum magnesium levels are known (or *suspected*) to be low (AHA Text- Pg 1-20).

- *Acute MI* (as an antiarrhythmic treatment/prophylactic measure)- Use in this setting is clearly controversial! Magnesium is most likely to be beneficial if given *early* (i.e., within the first few hours of infarction)- especially if given to patients for whom thrombolytic therapy is *not* used. While acceptance of this treatment is more widespread when serum magnesium levels are *known* to be low- Magnesium appears to be beneficial in some patients even when serum levels are normal.
- *Possibly* in the treatment of *other* cardiac arrhythmias (i.e., PVCs, MAT, PSVT, A Fib or Flutter).

Mechanism:

The mechanism by which Magnesium works remains uncertain. In all probability- a *combination* of factors is operative. These include restoration of myocardial cell membrane stability, correction of electrolyte abnormalities (with adequate magnesium stores also being essential to ensure correction of hypokalemia), prolongation of the effective refractory period of the AV node (and of individual myocardial cells), and/or a *"cardioprotective effect"* that results from Magnesium's ability to limit infarct size, decrease platelet aggregation, reduce peripheral vascular resistance, and produce coronary vasodilatation.

Dose & Route of Administration:

Dosing of Magnesium is empiric. We suggest the following dosing considerations:

- For ***Life-Threatening Arrhythmias***- Give **1-2 g IV** of Magnesium Sulfate (= 2-4 ml of a 50% soln.)- by **IV push** for VFib (or IV over 1-2 minutes for VT or Torsade de Pointes). May repeat this dose in 5-10 minutes if no response. AHA Guidelines indicate that higher doses of Magnesium (i.e., of up to 5-10 grams!) have been used with success in the treatment of patients with Torsade de Pointes (AHA Text- Pg 7-14).
- For ***LESS Urgent Treatment Situations*** (i.e., treatment of other arrhythmias and/or Acute MI in patients who are magnesium deficient)- Consider *more gradual IV infusion* (i.e., of ≈1-2 g of Magnesium Sulfate over ≥20 minutes)- or simply adding the drug to the patient's IV fluids and infusing it over a period of hours (i.e., at a rate of between ≈0.5-1 g/hour for up to 24 hrs).

Special Points:

Guidelines for the use and dosing of Magnesium Sulfate in the acute care setting are *not* well defined. While need for the drug is clear in patients who develop problematic cardiac arrhythmias in association with low serum magnesium levels- the emergency care provider will often *not* have this information readily available at the time of a code or other emergency situation. This leaves the clinician with a dilemma: *What to do at the bedside (or in the field) when confronted with a patient in a potentially life-threatening arrhythmia- and the serum magnesium level is unknown?* Consideration of the following clinical points may help you determine your answer.

- Serum magnesium levels do *not* necessarily tell you if the patient needs Magnesium. Serum levels merely reflect *extracellular* magnesium. However, because the overwhelming majority of body magnesium stores are contained *within* the intracellular compartment- the serum level may sometimes be normal despite significant *intracellular* (and therefore *intramyocardial*) magnesium depletion.
- Certain clinical conditions are commonly associated with ***intracellular magnesium depletion***- *regardless* of whether or not the serum magnesium level falls within the normal range. These conditions include:
    - *Other electrolyte abnormalities* (especially hypokalemia, hyponatremia, hypocalcemia, or hypophosphatemia)
    - *Acute myocardial infarction* and *cardiac arrest*
    - *Digitalis* or *diuretic therapy*
    - History of *alcohol abuse*
    - *Renal impairment*
- A *comparable* beneficial antiarrhythmic effect is often achieved with administration of Magnesium to patients with normal serum levels as is seen when the drug is administered to patients with documented hypomagnesemia.
- Administration of Magnesium to patients with cardiac arrhythmias and/or Acute MI is usually *not* associated with significant adverse efffects- even when large doses of the drug are given. For example- in the LIMIT-2 Trial (which involved *more* than 2,000 patients)- 2 g of Magnesium Sulfate were given IV over the first 5 minutes- and followed by a total of 16 g IV that were infused over the next 24 hours. Despite these high doses- adverse effects were minimal (and essentially limited to slight

flushing, transient bradycardia, and mild hypotension). Adverse effects that do occur usually resolve simply by *slowing* the rate of IV infusion.

> **Note-** AHA Guidelines suggest ready availability of Calcium Chloride as a "safeguard" when administering Magnesium in the rare event that marked hypotension or asystole is produced (AHA Guidelines- Pg 7-14).

- There may be little to lose (and a *lot* to gain)- from *empiric* use of Magnesium in potentially life-threatening situations- especially if standard measures have already been tried and failed.

Atropine

How Dispensed→ 1 mg per 10 ml syringe.

Indications:

- Bradyarrhythmias that are *hemodynamically* significant. This may also include patients with ***"relative bradycardia"***- for whom the heart rate is faster than 60 beats/minute but still *inappropriately slow* for the clinical situation.

> A clinical example of *relative* bradycardia would be a heart rate of "only" 70 beats/minute that occurs in a patient with hypovolemia and marked hypotension. Treatment with Atropine (and/or pacing) may be appropriate for *selected* patients with *relative* bradycardia- if the rhythm is hemodynamically significant.

- PEA rhythms (when the heart rate is inappropriately slow).
- Asystole.

Mechanism/Adverse Effects:

Atropine is a *parasympathetic-blocking* (i.e., *vagolytic*) agent that is used in the treatment of bradyarrhythmias. However- the drug is *not* without adverse effects. In addition to its vagolytic action on the AV node- Atropine also enhances the rate of discharge from the SA node. As a result, the drug may precipitate atrial tachyarrhythmias. Moreover, by blocking parasympathetic output- Atropine may *unmask* underlying enhanced *sympathetic* activity that had previously been contained. This may lead to development of ventricular arrhythmias (including VT and even V Fib)- as well as increased myocardial oxygen consumption and development of angina.

> Because of these potentially deleterious effects- use of Atropine is now recommended *only* for the treatment of bradycardia that is felt to be ***"hemodynamically significant"***- and/or for treatment of frequent ventricular ectopy in which development of PVCs is felt to be *directly* attributed to the reduction in heart rate (AHA Text- Pg 7-4).

Another effect of Atropine in adddition to its vagolytic action is to improve conduction through the AV node. This helps to explain the beneficial effect of Atropine in the treatment of 2° and 3° AV block during the *early hours* of acute *inferior* infarction (at a time when these conduction defects are most likely to reflect excessive vagal tone). Atropine should *not* be expected to work as well if the drug is given *after* the first 6 to 8 hours of inferior infarction (or with anterior infarction)- because excessive parasympathetic tone is less likely to be the cause of the bradycardia.

- The clinical effects of Atropine may sometimes act as a *double-edged* sword. That is- the fact that the drug enhances the rate of sinus node discharge may actually *counteract* its beneficial action on AV nodal conduction. For example- in the setting of acute *inferior* infarction, the AV node may be able to conduct every sinus impulse to the ventricles when the heart rate is 50 beats/minute. However, *acceleration* of the heart rate (i.e., to 80 beats/minute- such as may occur following Atropine administration)- could result in a rate that is simply too rapid for an *ischemic* AV node to continue to conduct with a 1:1 AV ratio. If at this faster rate the AV node was only able to conduct every *other* sinus impulse- then for an atrial rate of 80, the ventricular response might *only* be 40 beats/minute (2:1 AV conduction). In this theoretical example- *administration of Atropine would actually have made the patient's condition worse* (i.e., by *decreasing* the overall ventricular response from 50 to 40 beats/minute).

- This phenomenon (in which administration of Atropine paradoxically *reduces* the overall ventricular response)- is particularly likely to occur in a patient with 2° AV block of the Mobitz II type. This is because Atropine is unlikely to improve AV nodal conduction of this rhythm disturbance.

> **In Summary**- Atropine is most likely to be effective for treatment of hemodynamically significant bradyarrhythmias that result from excessive *parasympathetic* tone (i.e., 2° AV block of the Mobitz I type, or 3° AV block with a *narrow* QRS complex escape rhythm)- especially when these conduction disturbances occur during the *early* hours of acute *inferior* infarction.

Atropine has also been recommended for treatment of asystole. The rationale for use in this setting stems from the finding that certain individuals demonstrate at least some parasympathetic innervation of the ventricles.

- The prognosis for asystole is *never* good. However, we emphasize the point that the outlook for asystole is not quite as poor when it occurs *inside* the hospital as when it occurs *outside* the hospital. Asystole in this latter setting is most often a *preter-*

minal event that results after *prolonged* cardiopulmonary arrest (and that follows deterioration of V Fib). On a cellular level- this type of asystole is usually associated with tissue hypoxia, acidosis, and cellular disruption. The response to treatment is typically dismal.

- In contrast- asystole that occurs *within* the hospital setting can sometimes be due to massive parasympathetic discharge. This is most likely when asystole occurs in association with an operative or diagnostic procedure, induction of anesthesia, toxic drug reactions, vasovagal episodes- and/or in association with heart block from acute inferior infarction. The time from the onset of asystole until discovery by trained personnel will usually also be significantly less in the hospital than when the condition occurs on the outside. As a result- asystole that occurs in a hospital setting may sometimes respond surprisingly well for a "prelethal" arrhythmia to Atropine therapy.

Dose & Route of Administration:

- **IV Bolus** (*for patients who are* ***NOT*** *in* ***Cardiac Arrest***)- Give **0.5-1.0 mg IV** initially. May repeat this IV bolus every 3-5 minutes- *if/as needed* (up to a total dose of 2-3 mg).

  - Consider use of the lower dose (i.e., **0.5 mg**) of Atropine when treating the patient with less severe symptoms (i.e., "mild" bradycardia with minimal signs of hemodynamic compromise)- at least for the initial dose. On the other hand, the larger dose (i.e., **1 mg**) may be preferable for the patient with more marked bradycardia and more severe hypotension- *and/or* if one or two 0.5 mg doses fail to produce the desired clinical response.

- **IV Bolus** (*for patients who* ***ARE*** *in* ***Bradyasystolic Arrest***)- Give **1.0 mg IV** at a time. May repeat this dose every 3-5 minutes- *if/as needed* (up to a total dose of **0.04 mg/kg**- which comes out to ≈**3 mg** for an *average-sized* adult).

- **ET Administration**- Use 2 to 2.5 times the IV dose (≈1-2 mg) when giving the drug by the ET route. Be aware that endotracheal absorption of Atropine during cardiac arrest is *not* as reliable as when the drug is given by the IV route.

Special Points:

- *Atropine is NOT a benign drug* !!! Because the drug blocks parasympathetic output- it may *unmask* previously undetected and underlying sympathetic activity (and thus precipitate ventricular tachyarrhythmias!). As a result- use of Atropine should be reserved for treatment of patients who *truly* have *hemodynamically significant* bradyarrhythmias.

- Although 2 mg will usually be the *full atropinization dose* for most patients- occasionally up to **0.04 mg/kg** (i.e., *up to* ≈**3 mg**) may be needed to obtain maximal effect. In general, use of a maximal dose of Atropine (i.e., ≈3 mg) should be *reserved* for treatment of patients with bradyasystolic cardiac arrest (AHA Text- Pg 7-5).

- AHA Guidelines allow for more frequent dosing of Atropine (*as often as every 1-3 minutes!*) for patients with *marked* hemodynamic compromise from bradycardia (AHA Text- Pg 1-30).

- Cardiovascular effects of Atropine last an estimated 2 to 4 hours. Other systemic effects (including pupillary dilation) tend to persist much longer. Practically speaking- despite producing a small (but definite) amount of pupillary dilatation, Atropine administration in conventional doses during cardiopulmonary resuscitation will usually *not* abolish pupil reactivity to light. Thus, the presence of fixed and dilated pupils in a patient who has failed to respond to resuscitation efforts is most likely to reflect severe neurologic (hypoxic-ischemic) injury- and should *not* be attributed to Atropine administration.

- Although recommended for treatment of PEA- Atropine is *unlikely* to be beneficial for this condition *unless* the associated rhythm is a bradycardia (or at least a "relative bradycardia").

- Atropine is most likely to work when used to treat bradycardia in the early hours of acute *inferior* infarction (when increased *parasympathetic* tone is most likely to be the mechanism of the slow heart rate).

- AHA Guidelines acknowledge that use (and the efficacy) of Atropine is *controversial* for treatment of patients with Acute MI and 2° or 3° AV block with QRS widening. *Despite "inconsistent recommendations" by experts-* AHA Guidelines continue to recommend Atropine as *"the initial pharmacologic intervention of choice for symptomatic bradycardia"* (AHA Text- Pg 1-30)- albeit they strongly advise *caution* if the drug is used when the QRS complex is *wide*- especially in the setting of acute *anterior* infarction. Pacing may be preferable to Atropine in this situation.

- Denervated transplanted hearts do *not* respond to Atropine. As a result, one should immediately intervene with either pacing and/or use of catecholamines in such patients.

Dopamine

How Dispensed → 200 mg per 5 ml ampule (or 400 mg per 10 ml); also comes in *premixed* bags (of 200 or 400 mg in 250 ml- and 400 mg in 500 ml).

Indications:

- Hemodynamically significant bradyarrhythmias that have *not* responded to Atropine (when cardiac pacing is unavailable); medical treatment of cardiogenic shock.

Dose & Route of Administration:

- **IV Infusion**- Mix 1 amp (200 mg) in 250 ml of D5W, and *begin* drip @ 15-30 drops/minute (≈2-5 μg/kg/minute). Titrate to clinical response.
  - AHA Guidelines recommend *starting* at 5 μg/kg/minute for treatment of *symptomatic bradycardia* (AHA Text- Pg 1-31).
  - Remember that there is patient-to-patient *variability* in the dose-dependent effects of Dopamine (See next page). *Careful titration is clearly needed in each patient.*

Mechanism/Infusion Characteristics:

Dopamine is a chemical precursor of Norepinephrine with ***dopaminergic, alpha-*** and ***beta-**adrenergic* receptor stimulating properties. Which of these pharmacologic actions predominates generally depends on the *rate of infusion* of the drug:

- ***At LOW infusion rates*** (i.e., 1-2 µg/kg/minute- and perhaps up to 5 µg/kg/minute)- dilates renal and mesenteric blood vessels (so urine output may increase)- but heart rate and blood pressure will usually *not* be affected (i.e., predominant *dopaminergic* effect).

- ***At MODERATE infusion rates*** (i.e., 2-10 µg/kg/minute)- increases cardiac output- usually with only a modest effect on peripheral vascular resistance and blood pressure (i.e., *beta-adrenergic* effect prevails).

- ***At HIGH infusion rates*** (i.e., >10 µg/kg/minute)- results in intense peripheral vasoconstriction (as *alpha-adrenergic* effect takes over)- producing a significant increase in peripheral vascular resistance and blood pressure.

Special Points:

Dopamine is a favored (and perhaps the most commonly used) *pressor* agent for treatment of hypotensive states that are not the result of hypovolemia. At moderate doses the drug may be effective for treatment of hemodynamically significant bradyarrhythmias that have *not* responded to Atropine (during the period *until* pacemaker therapy can be initiated). The drug may also be used at higher doses (i.e., >10-20 µg/kg/minute) to improve coronary perfusion in the arrested heart- although Epinephrine (by bolus or infusion) is usually preferred for this purpose.

A large part of the appeal of Dopamine appears to lie in its *flexibility*- which allows this one drug to be used not only for management of cardiac arrest, but also for blood pressure support and maintenance of vital organ perfusion during the immediate post-resuscitation period.

- The *dopaminergic* (i.e., renal vasodilatory) effect of *low-dose* Dopamine is an extremely attractive feature of the drug- especially for management of hypotensive patients with oliguria. As an extension of this principle- *combined* pressor treatment is sometimes tried in which a potent vasoconstrictor (such as Norepinephrine) is used to increase blood pressure *together with* low-dose Dopamine (for its dopaminergic effect)- in an attempt to maintain adequate renal perfusion and urine output.

- Other combinations of pressor agents and/or vasodilator drugs are sometimes tried. For example- Dopamine may be combined with Dobutamine in the hope of integrating the positive inotropic effect of this latter drug- with the vasoconstrictor pressor effect of Dopamine. Alternatively- *vasodilating* agents (such as IV Nitroglycerin or Nitroprusside) are sometimes combined with Dopamine- in the hope of minimizing the potentially deleterious increase in afterload produced by Dopamine, while still maintaining adequate blood pressure for systemic perfusion (AHA Text- Pg 8-4).

> Clearly- *combined* use of pressor agents in the manner described above is an *advanced* subject that extends *beyond* ACLS core material. Patients for whom this is tried almost invariably require ongoing invasive hemodynamic monitoring in an ICU setting.

- As a rule- the *dopaminergic* effect of Dopamine tends to be lost as the rate of infusion is increased (i.e., usually at levels of more than 2 to 5 µg/kg/minute).
- Moderate to high infusion rates of Dopamine tend to produce an effect that resembles Epinephrine (and may be used to maintain coronary perfusion in the arrested heart). As the infusion rate is increased even further (i.e., to 15-20 µg/kg/minute)- the drug becomes more and more like Norepinephrine (i.e., a pure vasoconstrictor).

Note- Although the *relative* degree of dopaminergic, alpha- and beta-adrenergic receptor activity can usually be anticipated for *most* patients from the rate of infusion- *individual differences in responsiveness do occur* (AHA Text- Pg 8-3). For example, the dopaminergic effect of the drug may be replaced by a potent beta-adrenergic response in some patients at infusion rates as low as 1-2 µg/kg/minute. In other patients- the potent alpha-adrenergic effect may already be in place at infusion rates of 5 µg/kg/minute. *Dose titration of Dopamine infusion must be highly individualized-* and carefully adjusted according to *each* patient's response.

- As with *all* pressor agents- remember that Dopamine may precipitate ventricular ectopy and/or tachyarrhythmias. If this occurs- be ready to *reduce* the rate of infusion (and/or *stop* the drip entirely).

Oxygen

Indications:

- *Suspected hypoxemia* of any cause (including cardiopulmonary arrest, acute ischemic chest pain, Acute MI, etc.).

Mechanism

Ambient air contains 20-21% oxygen. Expired air (as is delivered when administering mouth-to-mouth or mouth-to-mask resuscitation) contains no more than 16-17% oxygen. This concentration of oxygen is *not* enough to adequately oxygenate the victim of cardiopulmonary arrest- a condition that produces severe oxygen desaturation abnormalities. Use of supplemental oxygen ensures adequate arterial oxygen content and greatly improves tissue oxygenation.

Dose & Route of Administration:

- **Nasal Canula**- 24-40% oxygen can be delivered with flow rates of 6 L/minute.
- **Face Mask/Pocket Mask**- Up to 50% oxygen can be delivered with flow rates of 10 L/minute.

- **Venturi Mask**- offers a decided advantage over the nasal canula and face mask in that *fixed* oxygen rates (of 24%, 28%, 35%, and 40%) may be delivered. This is an especially helpful feature for patients with COPD (chronic obstructive pulmonary disease) and a history of CO_2 retention.

- ***Non-Rebreathing* Oxygen Mask**- Superior device for delivering high oxygen concentrations (of up to 90%).

Special Points:

Oxygen is one of the truly *essential* drugs in cardiopulmonary resuscitation and emergency cardiac care. It is the treatment of choice for *suspected* hypoxemia of *any* cause (including cardiopulmonary arrest, acute ischemic chest pain, and Acute MI). Supplemental oxygen should *never* be withheld for fear of causing CO_2 retention in an emergency situation. Instead, comfort should be taken in the fact that because such patients are *continually* monitored- respiratory suppression (if it occurs) will *not* be unnoticed:

- AHA Guidelines recommend administration of **100% oxygen** during the period of cardiopulmonary resuscitation (AHA Text- Pg 7-2).

- Supplemental oxygen is indicated in an emergency situation- *even* for patients with COPD. Practically speaking- respiratory drive will *seldom* be depressed enough in such patients to require ventilatory support in the emergency situation (AHA Text- Pg 7-2).

- Oxygen toxicity may become a problem with *continual* delivery of high oxygen concentration (F_{IO2} ≥50%)- when it is given for a *prolonged* period of time (i.e, *more* than 3 days). It is *not* a problem with short term delivery of 100% oxygen during the period of cardiopulmonary resuscitation.

Morphine Sulfate

How Dispensed → 5, 10, or 15 mg per ampule.

Indications:

- Acute ischemic chest pain (as well as the anxiety that so often accompanies it); pulmonary edema.

Mechanism:

Morphine works in a number of different ways. In addition to its extremely potent analgesic effect, it also allays anxiety in patients with acute chest pain or air hunger from pulmonary edema. Hemodynamically- the drug markedly increases venous capacitance. This significantly reduces preload (by decreasing venous return) and relieves symptoms of pulmonary congestion. Morphine also induces mild arterial vasodilatation- which improves cardiac performance by lowering afterload. Finally, the drug *indirectly* reduces the level of circulating catecholamines (and the tendency toward arrhythmias) by its analgesic and antianxiety effect.

Dose & Route of Administration:

- **IV Bolus**- Give in small (i.e., **1-3 mg**) *incremental* **IV doses**. Higher doses (i.e., of 3-5 mg) may be used if the drug is tolerated and symptoms are severe. May repeat IV dosing every 5-30 minutes (as needed).

Adverse Effects:

When carefully dosed in small incremental amounts, Morphine sulfate is usually well tolerated in most patients. Adverse effects that may occur include occasional bradycardia and hypotension- both of which often resolve when the drug is stopped (and respond well to placing the patient in Trendelenburg position and administration of Atropine or IV fluid if treatment is needed). Other adverse effects include oversedation, nausea, and respiratory depression. Fortunately, the latter effect may be quickly reversed with 0.4-0.8 mg IV **Naloxone (Narcan)**.

Special Points:

Morphine Sulfate is a drug that has withstood the test of time. Even today it remains an excellent agent for treatment of acute ischemic chest pain and pulmonary edema.

- *Don't forget about Morphine Sulfate.* Although acute ischemic chest pain is probably best *initially* treated with Nitroglycerin- incremental dosing with Morphine may be an extremely helpful adjunct when symptoms are severe and persistent. Efforts should *always* be made to relieve acute ischemic chest pain as soon as possible- and Morphine remains an excellent drug for accomplishing this goal.

- In conjunction with IV Furosemide- Morphine remains a treatment of choice for acute pulmonary edema. As noted, beneficial effects of the drug in the treatment of this condition include marked reduction in preload, a mild decrease in afterload, and attenuation of the anxiety and air hunger inherent with pulmonary edema.

Verapamil

How Dispensed → 5 mg per ml ampule.

Indications:

- PSVT- more than a 90% success rate in converting this rhythm to sinus.
- Atrial Fib/Flutter- effectively slows ventricular response.
- MAT- medical treatment of choice when rate control is needed.

> **Note**- Clinical indications for using Verapamil are the *same* as for Diltiazem. The mechanism of action, cautions and adverse effects that we list here are also similar for these two drugs.

Mechanism/Clinical Effects:

Verapamil exerts its primary physiologic effect on AV nodal tissue. The drug *slows* conduction and prolongs the effective refractory period *within* the AV node. As a result, conduction properties are altered in one or both arms of the *reentrant* pathway in patients with PSVT. This action serves to *interrupt* the reentrant cycle- which terminates the arrhythmia.

Verapamil is also a very useful agent for acute treatment of atrial fibrillation and flutter. Although conversion to sinus rhythm occurs *less* than a third of the time- the AV nodal depressant effect of the drug reliably slows the ventricular response to both of these tachyarrhythmias.

Verapamil is a drug of choice for the treatment of MAT in those patients for whom rate control is needed (i.e., for patients who remain symptomatic despite improved oxygenation and correction of electrolyte disturbances). In addition to its rate slowing effect on the AV node- Verapamil works to correct MAT by exerting a direct depressant effect on atrial automaticity (that reduces the number of ectopic atrial impulses).

Dose & Route of Administration:

- **IV Dosing**- Begin with an initial dose of **2.5-5 mg** (to be given IV over a 1-2 minute period). Give the drug *slower* (i.e., over 3-4 minutes) in the elderly or to those with borderline blood pressure. Peak effects from an IV bolus of Verapamil are usually seen within 5 minutes.

  The dose of IV Verapamil may be repeated one or more times after 15-30 minutes (if/as needed)- up to a *total* dose of ≈30 mg. If the initial 2.5-5 mg dose is well tolerated- then a larger dose (i.e., of 5-10 mg) may be given for subsequent IV boluses.

- **Oral Dosing**- The usual oral dose range for Verapamil is between 120-320 mg daily (maximum dose up to 480 mg daily). This amount of drug is typically divided into three equal doses- or given less often if sustained release preparations are used.

Pre-Treatment with Calcium Chloride:

Use of calcium *pre-treatment* is a helpful technique for *minimizing* the hypotensive response of Verapamil- *without* diminishing its antiarrhythmic effect (AHA Text- Pg 1-37). A dose of between 500 to 1,000 mg of ***Calcium Chloride*** (i.e, 5 to 10 ml of a 10-ml ampule of 10% Calcium Chloride) is infused IV over 5 to 10 minutes. Too rapid infusion may produce a generalized sensation of heat in the patient. Conversion of the rhythm or slowing of the ventricular response occasionally results from calcium infusion alone- even *before* Verapamil is administered. This probably reflects the blood pressure raising effect of calcium infusion (and resultant stimulation of carotid baroreceptors).

Consideration of *pre-treatment* calcium infusion would seem to be most suitable for those patients with supraventricular tachyarrhythmias whose pre-treatment hemodynamic status is borderline (i.e., systolic blood pressure <90 to 100 mm Hg). In patients with SVT who are given Verapamil *without* such pre-treatment- one should *not* forget about possible *post-treatment* use. That is, should hypotension occur following Verapamil administration- IV infusion of Calcium Chloride may help in restoring the blood pressure to normal.

Cautions/Contraindications:

Verapamil and Diltiazem are *both* extremely effective antiarrhythmic agents for the treatment of supraventricular tachyarrhythmias. However, optimal use of these drugs requires full appreciation of the clinical situations for which they are intended- and full awareness of the *cautions* and *contraindications* to their use:

- ***Do NOT use Verapamil/Diltiazem to treat*** :
  - *WIDE-complex* tachycardia (WCT) of *uncertain* etiology.
  - rapid A Fib in a patient with WPW.
  - sinus tachycardia.

- ***Do NOT give IV Verapamil/Diltiazem if*** :
  - you have administered an IV beta-blocker to the patient within the *preceding* 30 minutes.

- ***Use Verapamil/Diltiazem ONLY with special caution*** :
  - in patients with sick sinus syndrome- especially if the patient is also receiving Digoxin.
  - in patients with heart failure.
  - in patients whose blood pressure is low or borderline in association with the tachycardia.

Practically speaking- Verapamil and Diltiazem do *not* have any role in the acute treatment of ventricular arrhythmias. This point *cannot* be emphasized too strongly! These drugs should therefore *never* be given indiscriminately as a diagnostic and/or therapeutic trial to patients with a regular WCT of *uncertain* etiology. This is because if the WCT turns out to be VT- use of these calcium channel blocking agents will be likely to precipitate deterioration of the rhythm to V Fib.

Despite the efficacy of Verapamil for treatment of rapid A Fib in the usual patient- the drug should *not* be used to treat this arrhythmia if WPW is present. This is because Verapamil (or Diltiazem) may *accelerate* anterograde (i.e., forward) conduction down the accessory pathway in such cases- an effect that may precipitate deterioration of the rhythm to V Fib.

Verapamil/Diltiazem should *not* be used for the purpose of slowing the heart rate of a patient in sinus tachycardia. This is because the rapid heart rate in such patients is likely to be *compensatory* (and therefore necessary to maintain cardiac output). Instead, treatment of sinus tachycardia should *always* be directed at identifying and treating the *underlying* cause of the sinus tachycardia.

Neither IV Verapamil *nor* IV Diltiazem should be given within 30 minutes of administering an IV beta-blocker. The reason for avoiding combined IV use of these drugs is that the resultant *additive* effect may produce profound bradycardia- *and even asystole.* Deciding in advance- *either* to use an IV beta-blocker- *or* calcium channel blocker (but *not* both!) for the treatment of any given arrhythmia- is the best way to avoid this potentially problematic situation.

In addition to these *contraindications*- we draw attention to a number of clinical situations for which IV Verapamil/Diltiazem *may* be used- but for which *caution* (and special monitoring) is strongly suggested. Anticipation of these situations is forthcoming from awareness of the adverse cardiovascular effects that may be seen with use of these drugs. The most important of these are hypotension, exacerbation of heart failure, and aggravation of bradycardia and/or conduction system defects. Consider the case of a patient with heart failure and rapid A Fib. Clearly, this patient may benefit from the rate-slowing effects of Verapamil/Diltiazem. However, caution is needed because of the potential negative inotropic effects of these drugs. Fortunately, the improvement in cardiac output that results from slowing the rate of rapid A Fib (and therefore increasing diastolic filling) will usually outweigh any decrease in cardiac contractility. However, on occasion- cardiac decompensation may occur.

Similarly, patients with PSVT and a borderline or slightly decreased blood pressure will usually be able to tolerate IV administration of Verapamil/Diltiazem- if these drugs are given *slowly* with *careful* monitoring. As noted earlier, consideration may be given to the use of *pre-treatment* Calcium Chloride in this situation (with hope of *minimizing* the hypotensive response to this treatment). Blood pressure typically normalizes as soon as the patient is converted to sinus rhythm. The point to emphasize is that IV Verapamil/Diltiazem *can* be used- but that *caution* and awareness of potential complications is essential (as is *anticipation* of how to respond in the event of an adverse reaction).

The last clinical situation we mention relates to the patient *suspected* of having sick sinus syndrome (SSS). Patients with this condition often present with *alternating* slow and fast rhythms (hence, the alternate name of *"Tachy-Brady" syndrome*). Bradyarrhythmias typically include sinus arrhythmia and bradycardia (that may be marked), any of the forms of SA node block, sinus pauses and sinus arrest, and slow AV nodal escape rhythms. The most common tachyarrhythmias are rapid A Fib and PSVT. Caution is urged when contemplating treatment of tachyarrhythmias in a patient who *may* have SSS since IV use of Verapamil/Diltiazem may at the same time *exacerbate* the bradyarrhythmias. This is particularly true if such patients are also receiving Digoxin. Clinically, SSS should be suspected in elderly patients- especially if they present with a history of syncope or frequent falling espisodes. If IV Verapamil/Diltiazem is selected to treat rapid A Fib in such individuals- a *lower* dose of drug should be given at a *slower* rate than for other patients.

Special Points:

Although caution is urged when combining use of rate-slowing drugs in patients who may have SSS- we emphasize that such combinations will *usually* be safe and effective if such patients do *not* have underlying conduction system disease:

- A pearl to consider in treatment is that *combining* small doses of IV Digoxin with IV Verapamil (or IV Diltiazem) will often produce a *synergistic* rate-slowing effect in the management of rapid A Fib/Flutter- that ultimately allows lower doses of each agent to be used.

- Combination therapy (i.e., use of Digoxin *and* one of these calcium channel blockers)- may also be effective in providing long-term rate control for patients with chronic A Fib. Surprisingly, oral maintenance therapy with *either* Verapamil or Diltiazem as a *single* agent is more effective for long-term rate control of A Fib than maintenance Digoxin.

- Despite awareness of all precautions described above- potentially serious adverse effects may still occur from acute administration of *either* IV Verapamil or IV Diltiazem. Manifestations of acute ***Calcium Channel Blocker Toxicity*** include profound bradycardia, hypotension- and *even* asystole. AHA Guidelines recommend the following treatment approach to this problem (AHA Text- Pg 10-23):

  i) If not done already- immediately *stop* administration of IV Verapamil/Diltiazem.
  ii) Treat hypotension with fluid administration- rapidly giving 500-1,000 ml of ***Normal Saline.***

iii) If there is no response to Saline- give ***Calcium Chloride*** (500-1,000 mg)- which may be repeated one or more times (up to a maximal dose of 2-4 g).
iv) Give ***Epinephrine*** (by IV bolus or IV infusion- depending on the rhythm). Keep in mind that in *refractory* cases- Epinephrine may *sensitize* the vasculature to the action of calcium. Therefore, be sure to *repeat* the Calcium Chloride dose *after* giving Epinephrine if the patient still has not responded.
v) Consider the use of ***Glucagon*** (in a dose of 1 to 5 mg IV).
vi) Consider *pacing.*
vii) Consider the use of *other* pressor agents *in addition* to Epinephrine (i.e, Dopamine, Norepinephrine).

Adenosine

How Dispensed → 6 mg are contained in a 2 ml vial.

Indications:

- PSVT and other *reentry* tachyarrhythmias (including PSVT associated with WPW). The key determinant of whether Adenosine will be effective is the presence of a *reentry* loop- in which at least a portion of the loop involves the AV node. AHA Guidelines now recognize Adenosine as the initial drug of choice for treatment of hemodynamically stable PSVT (AHA Text- Pg 1-37).

- As a ***diagnostic* maneuver** (i.e., "*chemical* Valsalva")- in patients with SVT of *uncertain* etiology. Adenosine will probably convert the rhythm if it turns out to be PSVT. Otherwise, it will probably at least produce *transient slowing* of the rhythm. This may enable atrial activity to be seen- and hopefully allow the correct diagnosis to be made. *Adenosine is probably the safest and most effective drug to use in evaluation and management of an SVT of uncertain etiology.*

- Treatment of PSVT in infants and children (as adverse effects are much less likely to occur with Adenosine than with Verapamil/Diltiazem in this age group).

- Treatment of PSVT during pregnancy (if acute treatment is needed)- since the *duration* of fetal exposure is minimized compared to other drugs (because of Adenosine's extremely short half-life).

Mechanism/Clinical Effects:

Adenosine is a naturally occurring endogenous nucleoside that is found in *all* cells of the body in the form of ATP. Its primary effect is to slow conduction through the AV node. It also depresses SA node automaticity, and alters repolarization characteristics of atrial tissue.

As noted above, Adenosine is most effective in terminating *reentry* tachyarrhythmias such as PSVT- especially when a portion of the reentry circuit involves the AV node. Alteration of conduction properties in at least one arm of the reentry loop- even if it is of only *momentary* duration- is usually all that is needed to interrupt the cycle and restore sinus rhythm. In contrast, the drug will *not* be useful in the treatment of A Fib or MAT- because these arrhythmias do *not* depend on the AV node for perpetuation of the rhythm.

The reduction in ventricular rate that Adenosine produces with these arrhythmias will last *only* as long as the duration of the drug.

For similar reasons- Adenosine will usually *not* convert A Flutter to sinus rhythm. However, by *transiently* increasing the degree of AV block- it may slow the ventricular response enough to allow recognition of flutter activity that may not have been evident at the more rapid rate (i.e., "chemical Valsalva").

Pharmacokinetics:

By far, the most intriguing clinical characteristics of Adenosine are its extremely *rapid* onset of action and *ultrashort* half-life (which is estimated to be *less than* 10 seconds!):

- Because of its rapid onset of action- *little time is needed to find out if the drug will work.* Therapeutic effects are typically seen *within* 10 to 40 seconds.
- If adverse effects do occur- they will usually be extremely *short-lived.*
- The *therapeutic* effect of Adenosine may also be short-lived. This is a definite drawback to the use of Adenosine (and may lead to *recurrence* of the arrhythmia if conditions that predisposed to the initial episode have not been corrected).

> Adenosine *can* be repeated if PSVT recurs. Clinically, strong consideration should be given to using (and/or adding) *another* drug with a *longer* duration of action (i.e., Verapamil, Diltiazem, or a beta-blocker)- in the event that recurrence is seen.

Dose & Route of Administration:

- **IV Bolus-** Begin with administration of **6 mg** by **IV push**. If there is no response after 1-2 minutes, give **12 mg** by IV push (which may be repeated a final time 1-2 minutes later)- for a ***total* dose** of 6 + 12 + 12 = **30 mg**. If there is still no response by this time- it is *unlikely* that Adenosine will work (and *alternative* therapy should be tried).

> **Note**- Adenosine is one of the few drugs that *must* be given ***"IV push"***- injecting the drug *as fast as possible* (i.e., over a period of 1-3 seconds!). Failure to do so may result in the drug breaking down while still in the IV tubing. Drug distribution and absorption may be further facilitated by *immediately* following each dose with a ***saline flush*** (of ≈20 ml of fluid).

Adverse Effects:

Adverse effects to the use of Adenosine are relatively common. Fortunately, they are usually not serious- and typically resolve spontaneously (most often *within* 1-2 minutes). Adverse effects that are most commonly seen include:

- Facial flushing (since the drug is a mild cutaneous vasodilator).

- Coughing/dyspnea (since the drug is a mild bronchoconstrictor). For this reason Adenosine should be avoided in patients with frank bronchospasm or asthma.

- Chest discomfort (that may similate angina).

- Marked *slowing* of the heart rate (including sinus pauses of up to several seconds in duration!). Special caution is therefore urged when contemplating use of Adenosine in the treatment of patients with underlying conduction system disease or sick sinus syndrome (because of the risk of producing excessive bradycardia and/or prolonged sinus pauses).

WCT of Uncertain Etiology: Empiric Use of Adenosine

AHA Guidelines have now incorporated use of Adenosine into the protocol for treatment of a ***W**IDE-**C**omplex **T**achycardia* (***WCT***) of *Uncertain Etiology* when Lidocaine fails to convert the rhythm (AHA Text- Pg 1-33). Their rationale for doing so is that Adenosine is *unlikely to be harmful* if the WCT turns out to be VT (because of its ultrashort duration of action)- and that the drug is likely to convert the rhythm if the WCT turns out to be PSVT (with QRS widening from aberrant conduction).

The points we emphasize is that Adenosine is *unlikely* to work if the WCT turns out to be VT- and that use of this drug is *not* completely benign. Therefore, if it is *known* (or strongly suspected) that a particular rhythm is VT- we feel Adenosine should *not* be given. Instead, we strongly favor use of Lidocaine, Procainamide, and/or cardioversion in this situation. On the other hand- Adenosine may be an *excellent* agent to try as a diagnostic/therapeutic measure for treatment of a regular WCT that is felt to *probably* be supraventricular in etiology.

Special Points:

- Alteration in the degree of underlying adrenergic or vagal tone may affect individual patient susceptibility to Adenosine- and account for at least some of the variation in the therapeutic dose range. Patients with a higher degree of underlying sympathetic tone are therefore more likely to require a higher dose of the drug.

- Higher doses of Adenosine are also likely to be needed for patients receiving Theophylline or consuming large quantities of caffeine. This is because Adenosine is *competitively* antagonized by methylxanthines.

- Lower than usual doses (i.e., 3 mg or less) of Adenosine should be used in patients receiving Dipyridamole (Persantine)- because this drug *inhibits* Adenosine transport and greatly potentiates its effect. Extra caution (and lower than usual doses) should also be used in patients receiving Carbamezepine (Tegretol)- because this drug may potentiate the degree of AV block produced by Adenosine.

Diltiazem

How Dispensed → 5 mg/ml (25 mg in a 5 ml vial *or* 50 mg in a 10 ml vial)

Indications:

- PSVT- more than 90% success rate in converting this rhythm to sinus.
- Atrial Fib/Flutter- effectively slows ventricular response.
- MAT- medical treatment of choice when rate control is needed.

> **Note**- Clinical indications for using Diltiazem are the *same* as for Verapamil. The mechanism of action, cautions and adverse effects are also quite similar for these two drugs.

Mechanism/Clinical Effects

See Verapamil (Page 146).

Dose & Route of Administration:

- **IV Dosing**- Begin with an *initial* **IV bolus** of 0.25 mg/kg (or ≈**20 mg** for an *average-sized* adult)- to be given over a 2 minute period. The *onset* of action from an IV bolus of Diltiazem is usually *within* 3 minutes- *peaking* by 7 minutes- and *lasting* for up to 1-3 hours.

  If the desired clinical response is *not* obtained within 15 minutes after administration of the first IV bolus- a **2nd IV bolus** (of 0.35 mg/kg- or ≈**25 mg** for an *average-sized* adult) may be given. Dosing for subsequent boluses should be individualized (depending on patient age, body weight, underlying disease, and response to the initial boluses).

> ***KEY***- Remember that the doses cited above are for an *average-sized* adult! Significantly *smaller doses* (i.e., of ≈10-15 mg) should be given to patients of lighter body weight- especially if they are older (and more likely to have underlying conduction system disease).

- **IV Infusion of Diltiazem**- Availability of an approved formulation for use as a *continuous* IV infusion is the major advantage that IV Diltiazem offers over IV Verapamil. This greatly facilitates dose titration- and allows *maintenance* of the antiarrhythmic effect achieved by IV bolus. We suggest the following preparation:

- **IV Infusion**- Mix 250 mg of Diltiazem in 250 ml of diluant (to make a *concentration* of 1,000 mg in 1,000 ml =**1 mg/ml**).

The recommended ***initial* infusion rate** for IV Diltiazem is **10 mg/hr** (= 10 mg/60 minutes)- to be started after the 1st or 2nd IV bolus. In order to infuse this amount of drug (i.e., 10 mg) over a 60 minute period- the rate of the IV infusion should be set to deliver **1 mg** of drug (= the contents of **1 ml**) every **6 minutes**.

Application of the following relationship allows conversion of the number of mg (or ml) administered- into an infusion rate expressed in *drops/minute* :

1 ml = **60 drops** for a ***microdrip***

Thus, in order to deliver 10 mg/hr- the ***initial rate*** of the IV infusion should be set to run at **10 drops/minute**.

The dose *range* for IV infusion of Diltiazem is relatively easy to remember. Practically speaking- most patients achieve adequate antiarrhythmic control at infusion rates *between* **5** to **15 mg/hr** (i.e., 5 to 15 drops/minute). Use of the lower rate should be considered for patients who appear to be sensitive to the effects of the drug. Infusion rates above 15 mg/hr are *not* recommended (AHA Text- Pg 7-12).

In general, Diltiazem infusion should *not* be continued for more than 24 hours. Hopefully by this time, the rhythm (usually A Fib) will either have converted to sinus- or *other* (preferably oral) antiarrhythmic drugs that were started will be taking effect.

- **Oral Dosing**- The usual oral dose range for Diltiazem is between 90-360 mg daily. This amount of drug is typically divided into three or four equal doses- or given less often if sustained release preparations are used.

Cautions/Contraindications:

The major *contraindications* to using IV Diltiazem are the same as the contraindications to using IV Verapamil. That is- *neither* drug should be used to treat a WCT of *uncertain* etiology, rapid A Fib in a patient with WPW, or sinus tachycardia. In addition- *neither* drug should be given within 30 minutes of administering an IV beta-blocker (because of the potential for precipitating marked bradycardia- or even asystole!).

Although *cautions* for using these two drugs are also similar- IV Diltiazem may offer some features that make it preferable to IV Verapamil in some situations. For example, IV Diltiazem appears to be somewhat *less* likely to produce hypotension and depression of left ventricular function than IV Verapamil (provided that *comparable* doses of each drug are used). Availability of an approved formulation for IV infusion of Diltiazem further contributes to its safety by allowing *moment-to-moment* titration capability. Finally, serum Digoxin levels seem to be affected to a much greater degree by concomitant use of Verapamil than they are by Diltiazem. With long-term use of Verapamil, the serum

Digoxin level may *increase* by as much as 50%. In contrast, use of Diltiazem tends to increase serum Digoxin levels by only a small (and usually clinically unimportant) amount.

Special Points:

- The clinical niche for IV Diltiazem is probably in the management of rapid A Fib. The drug is highly effective in *slowing* the ventricular response to this rhythm, with an onset of action *within* 3 minutes of administering an IV bolus. Availability of a *continuous* IV infusion is a decided advantage of Diltiazem over Verapamil and Digoxin- and obviates having to coninuously bolus the patient to control the rate.
- IV Diltiazem may offer an additional advantage over IV Verapamil in that its negative inotropic effect is less, and its use is associated with a lower incidence of systemic hypotension.

Comparison of IV Verapamil/Diltiazem to Adenosine

All 3 drugs- Verapamil, Diltiazem, and Adenosine- are equally effective in the treatment of PSVT- with greater than 90% success in converting this rhythm to sinus. Comparative features of these drugs are shown in the table below:

Table 2B-1: ***Clinical Comparison of IV Verapamil, Diltiazem, and Adenosine***

Adenosine	IV Verapamil/Diltiazem
- Works faster - Side effects tend to be short-lived - Therapeutic effect is also short-lived (which leads to a high recurrence rate!) - Only effective for PSVT (reentry tachyarrhythmias) - May help diagnostically (i.e., "chemical Valsalva") - Preferred for use in children and during pregnancy - Relatively expensive	- Lasts longer than Adenosine- and has oral formulation for continued (maintenance) therapy - Effective for PSVT and MAT; reli-ably slows the ventricular res-ponse of A Fib/Flutter - Should never be used if the QRS complex is wide and the diagnosis is uncertain - Avoid for A Fib in patients with WPW - Less expensive than Adenosine

Propranolol

How Dispensed → 1 mg/1 ml vial.

Indications:

Indications for the use of an IV beta-blocker in an acute care situation are relatively limited:

- *Refractory ventricular arrhythmias* (including VT/V Fib)- especially if acute ischemia, excesssive sympathetic discharge, digitalis toxicity, and/or cocaine overdose are suspected as contributing etiologic factors.

- *Supraventricular tachyarrhythmias*- as an alternative agent for patients who have not responded to IV Verapamil/Diltiazem, Adenosine, and/or Digoxin.

> **Note**- Clinical indications for using IV Propranolol are the *same* as for IV Esmolol (and for other IV beta-blockers). The mechanism of action, cautions and adverse effects are also fairly similar for all drugs in this class of agents (with slight differences attributed to the relative amount of beta-selectivity).

Mechanism/Clinical Effects

Propranolol is a *non-selective* beta-blocking agent with a *multifactorial* mechanism of action. The drug decreases automaticity, reduces the sinus rate of discharge, and prolongs AV conduction time. In addition, it blocks catecholamine stimulation, reduces myocardial contractility, and decreases oxygen consumption. Despite these beneficial actions, it appears that use of IV Propranolol in the acute care setting has greatly decreased in recent years. This is unfortunate because- *there are situations when this IV beta-blocking agent (or Esmolol) becomes the drug of choice for the treatment of life-threatening ventricular tachyarrhythmias* !

The most difficult part about making recommendations for using IV beta-blockers in the setting of cardiopulmonary arrest is knowing when to administer these drugs. Clearly there are times when all other antiarrhythmic agents will fail- and *only* IV beta-blockers may save the patient. Situations in which IV beta-blockers are most likely to be successful in the treatment of life-threatening ventricular arrhythmias are those in which *excessive sympathetic tone* is implicated as an important etiologic factor. This is most likely to be the case in patients who develop VT/V Fib in association with acute *anterior* infarction- especially when the arrhythmia was preceded by a period of sinus tachycardia and/or systolic hypertension. It may also occur when cardiac arrest is precipitated by *cocaine* or (*amphetamine*) overdose- or an extremely *stressful/anxiety-producing* event. Another situation in which IV beta-blockers are likely to be successful is in the treatment of patients who demonstrate a period of antecedent *ischemia* (as may be suggested by development of ST segment depression on monitoring prior to the arrest). Administration of *empiric* IV beta-blocker therapy would also be reasonable (if not advisable) for patients with *recurrent cardiac arrest*- especially if other antiarrhythmic agents have failed (and/or sinus tachycardia appears to precede each recurrence).

Dose & Route of Administration:

- **IV Dosing**- Give **0.5** to **1 mg**- by ***slow* IV** administration (i.e., *not to exceed 1 mg/minute!*). Allow several minutes for the drug to work. Repeat increments of 0.5 to 1 mg may be given up to a total dose of 3-5 mg.

Contraindications/Cautions

Propranolol (and other IV beta-blockers) are *contraindicated* in patients with acute bronchospasm, heart failure, and/or significant conduction system abnormality. If IV Verapamil/Diltiazem has been given- an IV beta-blocker should *not* be used for *at least* the next 30 minutes (because the combination of these agents may result in excessive bradycardia or even asystole).

Special Points:

- We are definitely *not* advocating IV Propranolol as a panacea treatment for all ventricular tachyarrhythmias that occur in the seting of cardiopulmonary arrest. Lidocaine clearly remains the treatment of choice for such arrhythmias- and Procainamide, Bretylium, and/or Magnesium are next in line. However, in *select* situations (such as those described above)- a *trial* of an IV beta-blocker may occasionally prove to be *lifesaving*- especially if other standard measures have failed.
- Because of ease of administration and familiarity with its use, ***Propranolol*** is the IV beta-blocker most commonly selected for treatment of patients in cardiac arrest. Alternatively- *other* IV beta-blockers could be used:

  - ***Atenolol***- 5 mg IV over 5 minutes; may repeat in 10 minutes.
  - ***Metoprolol***- 5 mg IV over 2-5 minutes; may repeat twice at 5 minute intervals (up to a total dose of 15 mg).
  - ***Esmolol***- *See Section 2E* (Page 193).

  In general, IV Atenolol and Metoprolol are the beta-blockers most commonly selected for IV administration to hemodynamically stable patients with acute myocardial infarction. Optimal cardioprotective effect is achieved by continued beta-blocker administration- switching over to the oral form of these durgs over the ensuing 12 to 48 hours (after initial stabilization of the infarct)- and continuing with long-term oral maintenance in the post-infarction period.

Section 2C: *Simplified Calculation of IV Infusions*

The Rule of 250 ml

For the uninitiated, calculation of IV infusions may appear as a formidable task requiring a minimum of a Masters degree in mathematics to attain proficiency. In most cases, calculation of IV infusions is carried out by those assigned to the care of intravenous (IV) lines that have already been established- namely, by nurses and paramedics. Physicians often go no further than a request for the following:

"Please mix up a drip of drug X- *and run the infusion as fast as we need to.* "

Practically speaking, the experienced nurse will usually have already anticipated the situation and be "ready and waiting" almost before the order is given. Occasionally, however, the team leader may find himself/herself working with code team members who are less familiar with the preparation of IV infusions. For this reason, *all* ACLS providers should at least be familiar with a method for formulating IV infusions of the most important drugs.

Another reason for learning how to prepare IV infusions is to successfully complete the ACLS Provider Course. Most ACLS Instructors will ask this information of the Code Leader during the MEGA CODE Station. Fortunately, the calculation of IV infusions for those drugs most commonly used in emergency cardiac care (and ACLS) *need not be difficult!* Application of a simplified and easily remembered rule greatly facilitates the process. The method we favor invokes the ***"Rule of 250 ml"***, and works as follows:

- Mix ***1 unit*** of *whatever* drug you are using in **250 ml** of D5W- and set the infusion to *begin* at a rate of between **15-30 drops/minute.**

Application of the *Rule of 250 ml* allows you to estimate an appropriate *initial* IV infusion rate for *most* of the essential drugs used in ACLS. Adjustments in dosing can then be made based on the patient's clinical response.

The *KEY* to application of the ***"Rule of 250 ml"*** lies with determining the amount of drug contained in *one* **"unit"** of drug. Because the contents of a vial or ampule often vary from one hospital to the next (and are sometimes pre-mixed in varying amounts by the pharmaceutical company)- it is essential to become familiar with the drug formulary used in your particular institution.

Our calculations in this section assume the following:

- *For the* ***Antiarrhythmic Drugs*** :
  - **1 g** of ***Lidocaine***
  - **1 g** of ***Procainamide***
  - **1 g** of ***Bretylium***
- *For the* ***Pressor Agents*** :
  - **1 mg** (1 vial) of ***Isoproterenol***
  - **1 mg** (1 amp) of ***Epinephrine*** (in a 1:10,000 soln.)- when using *lower* dose (SDE) IV infusion of Epinephrine
  - **200 mg** (1 amp) of ***Dopamine***

(All of the above) = *1 Unit of Drug*

Substitution into the ***Rule of 250 ml*** of the quantities listed above for **"one unit"** of drug (for any of the three *antiarrhythmic agents,* two *catecholamines,* or for *Dopamine*)- will automatically result in an appropriately prepared *initial* IV infusion rate. For example:

- For Preparing an IV Infusion for the *Antiarrhythmic Agents* :

Lidocaine- Mix **1 g** (= 1 unit) of *Lidocaine* in **250 ml** of D5W (or 2 g in 500 ml)- and set the infusion to run at **30 drops/minute** (= 2 mg/min).

Procainamide- Mix **1 g** (= 1 unit) of *Procainamide* in **250 ml** of D5W (or 2 g in 500 ml)- and set the infusion to run at **30 drops/minute** (= 2 mg/min).

Bretylium- Mix **1 g** (= 1 unit) of *Bretylium* in **250 ml** of D5W (or 2 g in 500 ml)- and set the infusion to run at **15 drops/minute** (= 1 mg/min).

The usual *initial* IV infusion rate for Lidocaine and Procainamide in the setting of cardiac arrest is 2 mg/minute (= 30 drops/minute). On the other hand, for Bretylium- it is more common to begin IV infusion at 1 mg/minute (= 15 drops/minute).

As emphasized in Section B, many factors (including age, body weight, hepatic function, presence of heart failure, etc.) influence the rate of Lidocaine clearance from the body. As a result, a *lower* rate (of 0.5-1.0 mg/minute) may be preferable for maintenance infusion of Lidocaine in patients at increased risk of developing toxicity (such as the elderly, lighter patients, and patients with heart failure).

- For Preparing an IV Infusion for the *Catecholamines* :

Isoproterenol- Mix **1 mg** (i.e., 1 vial = 1 unit) of *Isoproterenol* in **250 ml** of D5W- and set the infusion to run at **30 drops/minute** (= 2 µg/min).

Lower Dose **Epinephrine Infusion**- Mix **1 mg** (i.e., 1 ampule = 1 unit) of a *1:10,000 solution of Epinephrine* in **250 ml** of D5W- and set the infusion to run at between **15-30 drops/minute** (= 1-2 µg/min).

Indications for administration of Isoproterenol have been greatly curtailed in recent years. In general, use of the drug is now limited to providing *chronotropic* support for the bradycardic patient who is not hypotensive. The recommended initial IV infusion rate for this indication is 2 µg/minute. Although this may be increased- the rate of an Isoproterenol infusion should generally *not* exceed 10 µg/minute.

Recommendations for the rate of Epinephrine infusion vary to a much greater degree. Both the concentration of drug and the rate of IV infusion depend primarily on the indication for use. For example, when treating a patient with severe bradycardia or hypotension who is *not* in cardiac arrest- ***Lower Dose*** **Epinephrine Infusion** is advised- beginning at a rate of 1-2 µg/minute. The usual range of IV infusion for this purpose is between 1-10 µg/minute. In contrast- a much higher dose of Epinephrine is recommended when IV infusion is used for treating the patient in cardiac arrest (*See page 162*).

- For Preparing an IV Infusion for *Dopamine* :

Dopamine- Mix **200 mg** (i.e., 1 ampule = 1 unit) of *Dopamine* in **250 ml** of D5W- and set the infusion to run at between **15-30 drops/minute**.

Although preparation of a Dopamine IV infusion is somewhat complex- the *Rule of 250 ml* may *still* be used to *approximate* an appropriate *starting dose* for IV infusion of this drug! Setting the initial infusion rate at between 15-30 drops/minute should deliver in the range of **2-5 µg/kg/minute** for most patients. The lower rate (i.e., 15 drops/min) may be preferable as a starting dose for patients who weigh less- and/or when preferential flow to the renal vascular bed is a high priority (i.e., dopaminergic effect of the drug). As is the case for other pressor agents, the rate of the Dopamine infusion may then be progressively increased *as needed*- depending on the patient's clinical response.

Clinical Application of the Rule of 250 ml

Being able to apply of the *Rule of 250 ml* for the drugs we have listed should be more than sufficient for passing this aspect of the ACLS Provider Course. To do this, all one need remember is the Rule itself, and the quantity of drug contained in "1 unit" for each of the agents. *Derivation of the Rule of 250 ml takes the process one step further, and facilitates understanding the method of preparation.*

Consider the following illustrative problems:

Problem: *Make up a* ***Lidocaine*** *infusion.* How fast should the drip be set to infuse 2 mg of Lidocaine per minute?

Answer: Applying the *Rule of 250 ml* for any of the three *antiarrhythmic agents* (Lidocaine, Procainamide, or Bretylium) suggests that ***1 unit*** of drug (i.e., 1 g) be mixed in ***250 ml*** (or 2 g in 500 ml) of D5W. The following calculation illustrates how doing so results in a concentration of 4 mg of Lidocaine per ml:

$$\frac{\mathbf{1\ g}}{\mathbf{250\ ml}} \text{ or } \frac{2\text{ g}}{500\text{ ml}} = \frac{4\text{ g}}{1000\text{ ml}} = \frac{4000\text{ mg}}{1000\text{ ml}} = \frac{4\text{ mg}}{\text{m l}} = \frac{\mathbf{2mg}}{\mathbf{0.5\ ml}}$$

The problem posed above in this particular case is to determine how fast to set the infusion so as to deliver 2 mg of Lidocaine per minute. Since we calculated the *concentration* of drug to be **4 mg/ml**- this means that in order to deliver 2 mg of Lidocaine per minute, the drip would have to be set to infuse 0.5 ml/minute. That is:

$$\frac{4\text{ mg}}{\text{m l}} \div 2 = \frac{\mathbf{2\ mg}}{\mathbf{0.5\ ml}}$$

The last piece of information required for determining the rate of the infusion is awareness of the ***conversion factor*** between *ml* and *drops* when a microdrip is used:

> **1 ml = 60 drops** for a ***Microdrip***
>
> - This means that 0.5 ml/min = 30 drops/minute.

Thus, IV infusion with a microdrip set at a rate of **60 drops/minute** will deliver the amount of drug contained in **1 ml** of fluid. It follows that:

- IV infusion at a rate of **30 drops/minute** will deliver *half* this amount (i.e., the amount of drug contained in 1 ml ÷ 2) or:

> **30 drops/min** delivers **0.5 ml/min**

and

- IV infusion at a rate of **15 drops/minute** will deliver *one quarter* this amount (i.e., the amount of drug contained in 1 ml ÷ 4) or:

> **15 drops/min** delivers **0.25 ml/min**

In this particular case, setting the drip to infuse at a rate of 60 drops/minute will therefore deliver 4 mg of drug (since the concentration of Lidocaine is 4 mg/ml). Thus, *the drip should be set to run in at a rate of* ***30 drops/minute*** *to deliver half this amount (or* ***2 mg/minute****) of* ***Lidocaine****.*

> For **Lidocaine** then (at this same concentration), an IV infusion rate of:
>
> - **15** drops/minute delivers **1 mg/minute** of drug
> - **30** drops/minute delivers **2 mg/minute** of drug
> - **45** drops/minute delivers **3 mg/minute** of drug
> - **60** drops/minute delivers **4 mg/minute** of drug

We again emphasize that with the exception of Epinephrine (when *higher* dose infusion is used)- the *Rule of 250 ml* works well for estimating an appropriate *initial* infusion rate for *each* of the drugs we have listed (i.e., Lidocaine, Procainamide, Bretylium, Isoproterenol, and Dopamine).

> Note that most manipulations in the above calculations involve *unit conversions* (i.e., 1 ml = 60 drops for a microdrip; 1,000 mg = 1 g; 1,000 µg = 1 mg; etc.) Thus, the *KEY* for determining the correct drug concentration and initial infusion rate is to *carefully maintain equivalent units of measure throughout each calculation!*

Application of the *Rule of 250 ml* for calculating an appropriate initial infusion rate for *Isoproterenol* and *Dopamine* is demonstrated in the next two illustrative problems.

Problem: *Make up an* ***Isoproterenol*** *infusion.* How fast should the drip be set to achieve an initial infusion rate of 2 μg/minute?

Answer: Applying the *Rule of 250 ml* for the *catecholamines* (Isoproterenol or Epinephrine- when *lower* dose infusion is being used) suggests that **1 unit** of drug (i.e., 1 mg) be mixed in **250 ml** of D5W. The following calculation illustrates how doing so results in a *concentration* of 4 μg/ml:

1 mg	or	4 mg	=	4000 μg	=	4 μg	=	**2 μg**
250 ml		1000 ml		1000 ml		ml		**0.5 ml**

Since the problem posed above is to determine the infusion rate needed to deliver 2 μg/minute- the drip should again be set to infuse at a rate of **30 drops/minute** (i.e., at 0.5 ml/min). Infusion at this rate will deliver 2 μg per minute (since this is the amount of drug contained in each 0.5 ml of IV fluid).

Problem: *Make up a* ***Dopamine*** *infusion.* How fast should the drip be set to achieve an initial infusion rate of 5 μg/kg/minute for a patient who weighs 80 kg?

Answer: Applying the *Rule of 250 ml* for *Dopamine* suggests that **1 unit** of drug (i.e., 200 mg) be mixed in **250 ml** of D5W. The following calculation illustrates how doing so results in a concentration of 800 μg/ml:

200 mg	=	800 mg	=	800,000 μg	=	800 μg	=	**400 μg**
250 ml		1000 ml		1000 ml		ml		**0.5 ml**

An initial infusion rate of 5 μg/kg/minute entails delivery of **400 μg/minute** of Dopamine for a patient who weighs 80 kg (i.e., 5 X 80 = 400). Since 400 μg is the amount of drug contained in each 0.5 ml of IV fluid at the concentration calculated in this example- the drip should again be set to infuse at a rate of **30 drops/minute.**

As emphasized earlier in this section (and on page 142 in Section B under our discussion of Dopamine)- the vasoactive effects of this drug depend on the rate of infusion. In the setting of cardiac arrest, IV infusion of Dopamine is most often begun at a rate of between 2-5 μg/kg/minute (which comes out to about 15-30 drops/minute for most patients). The rate of infusion is then progressively increased until the desired clinical response is achieved. At higher infusion rates (i.e., ≥10-20 μg/kg/minute), alpha-adrenergic (vasoconstrictor) effects predominate, and the actions of the drug become similar to those of Norepinephrine. This usually occurs at infusion rates of *greater* than 60 drops/minute.

Epinephrine: *Higher Dose IV Infusion*

As we acknowledged in the beginning of Section B of this chapter, the optimal dose of Epinephrine for treatment of cardiac arrest remains unknown. Moreover, the dosing requirements for any given patient will vary, being influenced by many factors including the condition being treated (i.e., ventricular fibrillation, asystole, or PEA), the duration of the code until medication is administered, and patient specific variables (such as age, body weight, the presence of underlying medical conditions, and the patient's response to other treatment measures).

The one point about Epinephrine dosing that has become clear is that *significantly higher doses than were used in the past may be needed by some patients to achieve and maintain adequate coronary perfusion pressure for as long as CPR is in progress.* Whether the use of higher doses of drug will ultimately lead to improved long-term survival in certain subsets of patients with cardiac arrest is still uncertain.

Clinically- when IV infusion of Epinephrine is used to treat severe bradycardia (and/or hypotension) in a patient who is *not* in cardiac arrest- ***Lower Dose*** **Epinephrine Infusion** is recommended. AHA Guidelines suggest beginning the rate of infusion at **1-2 µg/minute**- and then increasing this up to **10 µg/minute** as needed according to the patient's clinical response (AHA Text- Pg 7-4).

Much higher doses of drug are recommended when treating the patient who *is* in cardiac arrest. AHA Guidelines allow for use of *either* IV bolus therapy- or ***Higher Dose*** **Epinephrine Infusion** in this situation. Because the recommended *initial* infusion rate for *higher dose* Epinephrine infusion is *at least* 100-fold *more* than the initial rate commonly selected for *lower dose* IV infusion- it would appear preferable to use a different formulation for administration of these two dosing regimens. Incorporation of two modifications into the *Rule of 250 ml* allows it to be used in an alternative form for calculation of *higher dose* Epinephrine infusion:

i) Instead of the 1:10,000 dilution of drug that is used for preparing *lower dose* Epinephrine infusion- consider using a **1:1,000 solution** of Epinephrine. *This alteration increases the concentration of drug by a factor of 10- and thus facilitates IV infusion by minimizing the amount of fluid that needs to be administered for any given quantity of drug.* Whereas 10 ml of a 1:10,000 solution of Epinephrine would have to be given to deliver 1 mg of drug, the same amount of Epinephrine (1 mg) can be given in 1 ml of a 1:1,000 solution.

ii) Use **50 mg** (instead of 1 mg) as the quantity of drug contained in **"1 unit"**. *This alteration increases the concentration of drug for higher dose Epinephrine infusion by a factor of 50- compared to the concentration of drug used for lower dose Epinephrine infusion.*

Thus, preparation of IV infusion of *Epinephrine* might proceed as follows:

- **For Preparation of *Lower Dose* Epinephrine Infusion:** Mix **1 unit** of drug (i.e., 1 mg = 1 ml of a 1:10,000 solution) in **250 ml** of D5W, and set the infusion to run at **15-30 drops/min** (to achieve an *initial* infusion rate of 1-2 µg/minute).

$$\mathbf{\frac{1\ mg}{250\ ml}} \text{ or } \frac{4\ mg}{1000\ ml} = \frac{4000\ \mu g}{1000\ ml} = \frac{4\ \mu g}{ml} = \mathbf{\frac{2\ \mu g}{0.5\ ml}}$$

Infusion at a rate of **30 drops/minute** (i.e., at 0.5 ml/min) will deliver 2 µg per minute (since this is the amount of drug contained in each 0.5 ml of IV fluid at this concentration). Infusion at *half* this rate (i.e., at **15 drops/minute**, or at 0.25 ml/minute) will therefore deliver 1 µg per minute. *Note that preparation of* ***Lower Dose Epinephrine Infusion*** *according to the Rule of 250 ml is virtually the same as preparation of an Isoproterenol infusion.*

- **For Preparation of *Higher Dose* Epinephrine Infusion:** Mix **1 unit** of drug (i.e., **50 mg** = 50 ml of a **1:1,000** solution) in **250 ml** of D5W. The following calculation illustrates how doing so results in a *concentration* of 200 µg/ml:

$$\frac{\mathbf{50\ mg}}{\mathbf{250\ ml}} = \frac{200\ \text{mg}}{1000\ \text{ml}} = \frac{200{,}000\ \mu\text{g}}{1000\ \text{ml}} = \frac{\mathbf{200\ \mu g}}{\mathbf{1\ ml}}$$

Setting the *initial* infusion rate to run at **30-60 drops/minute** will deliver 100-200 µg/minute. *This rate can then be increased as needed according to the patient's clinical response.*

IV Infusion of Nitroglycerin/Nitroprusside:

The *Rule of 250 ml* is practical, as well as being easy to learn and remember. *It works.* It also encompasses what you'll need to know regarding IV infusions in order to successfully complete the ACLS Provider Course. We now conclude this section with suggestions for calculating the IV infusion rates for two drugs that do *not* follow the *Rule of 250 ml.*

Sodium Nitroprusside and IV Nitroglycerin are two potent *vasodilating* agents that share a number of important indications in emergency cardiac care. These relate to the treatment of hypertensive urgency/emergency, and preload/afterload reduction for treatment of patients with heart failure. Of the two agents- ***IV Nitroprusside*** is clearly the more potent arterial vasodilator (afterload reducer). As a result, it is a drug of choice (and the *most* effective drug currently available) for treatment of hypertensive emergencies including hypertensive encephalopathy and the severe hypertension associated with intracranial hemorrhage, acute head injury, dissecting aneurysm, catecholamine crisis, and perioperative complications. Unfortunately, a drawback of the drug is its potential to produce *coronary "steal"*- with shunting of blood *away* from ischemic areas of myocardium.

While not as potent an arterial vasodilator as Nitroprusside- ***IV Nitroglycerin*** appears less likely to produce coronary steal. For this reason, it is the preferred agent for initial treatment of mild-to-moderate hypertension associated with acute ischemic heart disease/acute infarction. Because IV Nitroglycerin also exerts a potent vasodilating effect on the venous side (reducing preload), it is a favored agent for the acute treatment of heart failure.

Although *neither* Nitroprusside nor Nitroglycerin follow the *Rule of 250 ml* (because the initial infusion rate is *not* 15-30 drops/minute)- preparation of an IV infusion for either agent may still be facilitated by using the same parameters as were suggested for preparation of *higher dose* IV infusion of Epinephrine. Therefore:

- **To Prepare an IV Infusion of IV Nitroprusside or Nitroglycerin:** Mix **1 unit** of drug (= **50 mg**) in **250 ml** of D5W. As was the case for *higher dose* Epinephrine Infusion- this results in a *concentration* of 200 µg/ml:

50 mg / **250 ml**	=	200 mg / 1000 ml	=	200,000 µg / 1000 ml	=	**200 µg** / **1 ml**

IV infusion of *Nitroprusside* and *Nitroglycerin* is usually begun at a rate of **10 µg/minute**. The rate of infusion can then be carefully titrated upward as needed to obtain the desired clinical response.

Problem: At what rate should the drip be set (for *either* **Nitroprusside** or **Nitroglycerin**) to achieve an initial IV infusion rate of 10 µg/minute?

Answer: At the concentration of drug derived above (i.e., 200 µg/ml)- 1/20th of a ml would have to be infused each minute to deliver 10 µg of drug per minute (i.e., 200 ÷ 20 = 10 µg/minute). Since **60 drops = 1 ml** with a microdrip, 1/20th of 1 ml will be 3 drops (i.e., 60 ÷ 20 = 3). Therefore, *the drip should be set at **3 drops/minute** to achieve an initial infusion rate of **10 µg/minute.***

Problem: By how many drops per minute should a drip of either *Nitroprusside* or *Nitroglycerin* be increased- to infuse an *additional* 10 µg each minute?

Answer: Since we established above that a rate of 3 drops/minute infuses 10 µg/ minute- *the drip would have to be increased by **3 drops each minute** to infuse an additional 10 µg/minute.* Thus:

- to infuse **20** µg/min, set the drip to infuse at a rate of **6 drops/minute**
- to infuse **30** µg/min, set the drip to infuse at a rate of **9 drops/minute**
- to infuse **40** µg/min, set the drip to infuse at a rate of **12 drops/minute**, and so forth . . . .

Problem: What would be the *maximum* infusion rate recommended for Nitroprusside for a patient who weighs 80 kg?

Answer: The *maximum* recommended infusion rate for IV Nitroprusside is **8 µg/kg/minute**. This comes out to 640 µg/minute for an 80 kg patient (i.e, 80 X 8= 640 µg/minute).

At the concentration of drug derived above (i.e., 200 µg/ml)- the maximum recommended infusion rate would therefore be 3.2 ml/minute (640 ÷ 200). Since 60 drops = 1 ml with a microdrip, *the maximum recommended infusion rate of Nitrprusside for a patient who weighs 80 kg is 192 drops/minute (60 X 3.2).*

In summary- familiarity with the ***Rule of 250 ml*** facilitates recall of an easily applied method for calculating IV infusions for the drugs most commonly used in ACLS (ie., *Lidocaine, Procainamide, Bretylium, Isoproterenol, Dopamine,* and *Epinephrine at lower dose*). Incorporation of two modifications (i.e., use of a 1:1,000 solution of Epinephrine and use of 50 mg as the unit size) allows the *Rule of 250 ml* to also be used in an alternative form for calculation of IV infusion of Epinephrine at *higher* dose.

Section 2D: *Diagnostic/Therapeutic Modalities*

Vagal Maneuvers

Vagal maneuvers have been used in the evaluation and management of patients with cardiac arrhythmias for well over half a century. They remain today an extremely helpful diagnostic/therapeutic tool for tachyarrhythmias in which atrial activity is either absent or only intermittently present.

Vagal maneuvers work by slowing the heart rate and/or prolonging atrioventricular conduction time. They bring about these effects by producing an increase in *parasympathetic* tone that results in *transient slowing* of conduction through supraventricular and AV nodal tissues *while* the maneuver is being applied. This action may interrupt a *reentry* pathway that involves the AV node (as occurs with abrupt termination of PSVT)- or it may temporarily reduce the number of impulses passing through (and allow diagnosis of the arrhythmia).

Types of Vagal Maneuvers/Clinical Responses

Although carotid sinus massage (CSM) is the most commonly employed vagal maneuver- there are many others. These include coughing, nasogastric tube placement, gag reflex stimulation (i.e., by tongue blades, fingers, and oral ipecac), facial submersion in ice, eyeball pressure, squatting, use of MAST trousers, placement of the patient into Trendelenburg position, performing a Valsalva maneuver, breath-holding, and digital rectal massage. Because of complications and/or patient discomfort- use of some of these methods has become quite limited. For example, application of ocular (eyeball) pressure is no longer recommended because of the risk of retinal detachment. Induction of gagging and activation of the diving reflex (i.e., facial submersion in ice) are both extremely unpleasant for the patient. Gagging may produce vomiting with the associated risk of subsequent aspiration. Facial submersion in ice is still used in pediatrics, but is not really practical in an acutely ill adult. We therefore limit discussion in this section to application of those vagal maneuvers that are most likely to be used in clinical practice.

The potency of effect from application of the various vagal maneuvers will vary significantly- depending on operator technique, patient-related factors (which are often intangible), and the particular maneuver selected. In general, however- certain cardiac arrhythmias can be expected to produce certain characteristic clinical responses (Table 2D-1). Thus, vagal stimulation of a patient in ***sinus tachycardia*** will usually produce *gradual* heart rate slowing- with resumption of the tachycardia upon completion of the maneuver. "Telltale" P waves may become evident *during* the maneuver- allowing definitive diagnosis and direction of therapy toward alleviating the underlying cause of the sinus tachycardia. In contrast, with an AV nodal *reentry* tachycardia (such as ***PSVT***), application of a vagal maneuver will either *terminate* the tachyarrhythmia- or have *no effect* at all.

Table 2D-1: Clinical Responses to Vagal Maneuvers

Tachyarrhythmia	Characteristic Clinical Response
Sinus Tachycardia	Gradual slowing of the sinus tachycardia *during* the vagal maneuver (with resumption of the tachycardia *after* the maneuver).
PSVT	*Abrupt termination* of the tachyarrhythmia (with conversion to sinus rhythm)- - or - *No response at all.*
Atrial Flutter or Atrial Fibrillation	Increased degree of AV block (with *transient* slowing of the ventricular rate- that will hopefully allow diagnosis of the arrhythmia by enabling atrial activity to be seen).
Ventricular Tachycardia	*No response to the vagal maneuver.*
WCT (*Wide-Complex Tachycardia*) of *Uncertain* Etiology	No response if the WCT is ventricular tachycardia. If the WCT is PSVT, there may either be no response- - or - Abrupt termination of the rhythm.

Practically speaking- ***ventricular tachycardia*** does not respond to vagal maneuvers. In view of the fact that PSVT may also fail to respond- the *lack of response* to a vagal maneuver will *not* be helpful from a diagnostic standpoint if the rhythm in question is an undifferentiated ***wide-complex* tachycardia (WCT)**. On the other hand, if the cause of the WCT turns out to be PSVT (with QRS widening from *either* aberrant conduction or preexisting bundle branch block)- then use of a vagal maneuver may sometimes work, and abruptly convert the rhythm to sinus.

The remaining two rhythms are ***atrial fibrillation*** and ***atrial flutter***. Both respond similarly to vagal maneuvers- most often with a temporary *decrease* in atrioventricular conduction (and resultant reduction in heart rate). This transient *slowing* of the ventricular response while the vagal maneuver is being applied may allow atrial activity that was previously hidden to become evident- thereby facilitating diagnosis of the arrhythmia (Figure 2D-1). Resumption of the tachyarrhythmia will occur upon completion of the maneuver.

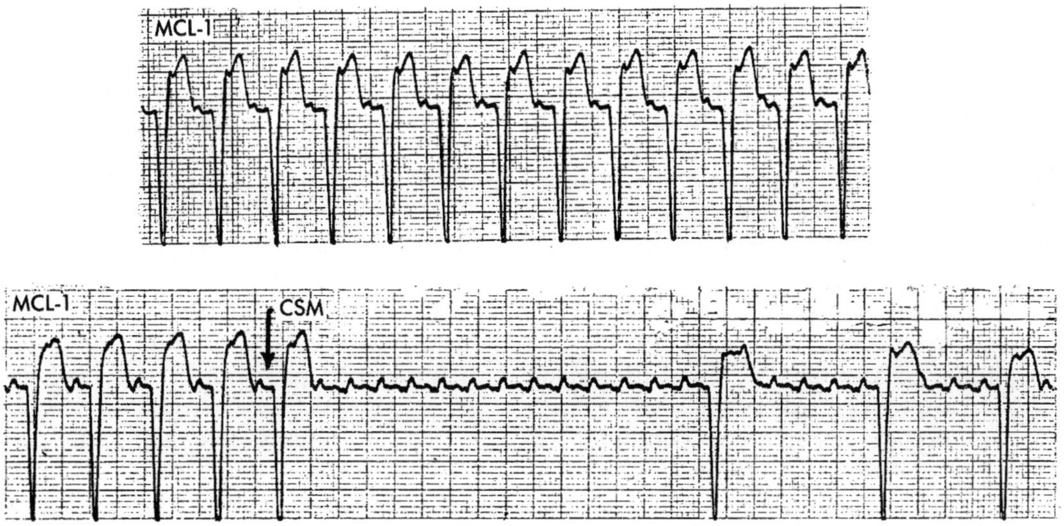

Figure 2D-1: Application of carotid sinus massage (CSM) at the point indicated by the arrow to an elderly man who had been in supraventricular tachycardia. As can be seen, CSM decreased (almost too well in this case) conduction through the AV node- revealing *flutter* waves (at a rate of just under 300 beats/minute) that had been obscured by the tachycardia.

It should be emphasized that vagal maneuvers may need to be repeated a number of times. In particular, patients with PSVT who fail to respond to *initial* application of a vagal maneuver- may still be successfully converted to sinus rhythm on *reapplication* of the vagal maneuver at a later point in the therapeutic process (i.e., *after* administration of an antiarrhythmic agent).

Carotid Sinus Massage (CSM)

As noted, the most commonly utilized vagal maneuver by medical personnel is CSM. Under *constant* ECG monitoring- the patient's head is turned to the left and the area of the *right* carotid bifurcation (near the angle of the jaw) is carefully but *firmly* massaged for 3-5 seconds. Carotid massage should *not* be continued for more than 5 seconds at a time. To be effective, *firm* pressure must be applied- so much so, that you may want to prewarn a conscious patient that the maneuver will be uncomfortable (and may even be a little painful). The amount of pressure that should be applied is comparable to that needed to squeeze (and indent) a tennis ball. Carotid massage must be applied in the correct location. All too often, pressure is applied too low (i.e., to the mid portion of the neck). The carotid sinus (bifurcation) lies *high* in the neck- *just below the angle of the jaw!*

If there is no response to an initial attempt at CSM, additional attempts may be made on the same side of the neck. *Always* be sure that *constant ECG monitoring* is ongoing during the procedure- and always be sure to limit the period of pressure application to *no more* than 5 seconds at a time. After several attempts on the right side, the left side may also be tried. *Never massage both carotids at the same time!*

> The reason many clinicians prefer to massage the *right* carotid first is that this side is believed to exert a greater influence on the sinus node, whereas the left carotid is believed to act more on the AV node.

Clinically- the efficacy of CSM may be increased (i.e., ***augmented*** **carotid massage**) by placing the patient in a Trendelenburg position of about -10°, having them take a full inspiration- followed by a full expiration- and then reapplying CSM in the Trendelenbug position if there has been no response (Pomeroy PR: Ann Emerg Med 21:1169, 1992).

CSM is *not* a completely benign maneuver- especially in older individuals. Complications that may occur include syncope, stroke (from dislodgement of a carotid plaque), bradyarrhythmias (such as sinus arrest, high-grade AV block, and prolonged periods of asystole), and ventricular tachyarrhythmias (especially in patients with digitalis toxicity). As a result, CSM should probably *not* be attempted in patients with a history of sick sinus syndrome (SSS), cervical bruits, cerebrovascular disease, or when the possibility of digitalis toxicity exists. For this reason it is important to listen to the neck for bruits *before* applying CSM!

As already emphasized- *continuous ECG monitoring must be ongoing while the maneuver is performed.* For documentation purposes (i.e., to *prove* that you didn't massage for *longer* than 5 seconds at a time)- and to assist in interpretation of the response to CSM, the onset and completion of the maneuver should be marked directly on the tracing. The person assigned to watch the monitor is there to alert the operator (and advise *immediate* cessation of massage) if significant slowing occurs (such as was seen in Fig. 2D-1).

Valsalva

A Valsalva maneuver is performed by having the patient forcibly exhale (bear down against a closed glottis- as if trying to go to the bathroom) for up to 15 seconds at a time. An obvious drawback of the Valsalva maneuver is that it requires the patient to be alert, cooperative, and able to understand instructions. However, it is often extremely effective- and may be preferred by many clinicians over CSM for patients who are able to perform the maneuver. If properly done- the Valsalva maneuver may produce even more potent vagal stimulation than CSM- simply because the maneuver produces *bilateral* baroreceptor stimulation (compared to the unilateral manual stimulation resulting from CSM).

It is important to emphasize that the Valsalva maneuver should always be performed with the patient in the *supine* position. This is because in the body's attempt to maintain a normal blood pressure- a compensatory increase in sympathetic tone may be produced if the procedure is performed when the patient is standing. Activation of sympathetic tone in this manner would at least partially *counteract* the vagotonic (parasympathetic) effect of Valsalva.

Finally- we draw attention to the fact that many otherwise healthy individuals with recurrent supraventricular tachyarrhythmias (such as PSVT) will have already taught themselves this maneuver by the time you see them- based on their own empiric experience that it "makes their palpitations go away". *Ask about self-application of Valsalva (or of other vagal maneuvers) in taking the history.*

Digital Rectal Massage (DRM)

A more recently described technique for increasing vagal tone is *digital rectal massage.* Although not usually thought of by health care providers as a potential therapeutic measure for the treatment of cardiac arrhythmias- DRM is effective (the rectum being richly supplied by sympathetic and parasympathetic nerve fibers), easy to perform, and probably *safer* than CSM when administered to older individuals who might have underlying carotid atherosclerosis (since it obviates the risk inherent with CSM of disloding a carotid plaque). DRM also offers the advantage of not interfering with resuscitative measures that may be ongoing at other anatomic sites. As with all other vagal maneuvers- *constant ECG monitoring* is advised while the procedure is performed.

"Chemical" Valsalva: Diagnostic Use of Adenosine

Although administration of Adenosine is technically *not* a vagal maneuver- we include it here because use of this drug may be helpful diagnostically in the evaluation of *selected* patients with supraventricular tachyarrhythmias of *uncertain* etiology. The almost immediate effect of Adenosine to produce *transient* slowing of AV conduction (and slowing of the ventricular response)- may reveal atrial activity in a similar way that application of CSM did in Fig. 2D-1 (i.e., ***"chemical" Valsalva***). This may allow definitive diagnosis of the arrhythmia.

The Precordial Thump

The precordial thump is a sharp, quick blow that is delivered with the fleshy part of the fist (hypothenar eminence) from a distance of 8-12 inches above the chest- to the mid-portion of the sternum. *It should not be so forceful as to break any ribs.*

The history of the precordial thump is interesting, and dates back to 1920 when the procedure was first used on a patient having Stokes-Adams attacks. Reports in the literature on the use of the thump had been limited since that time, until a resurgence was seen in the 1970's. Recent appreciation of the drawbacks of the procedure have again led to dramatic *deemphasis* of its use.

Mechanism/Clinical Effects

The precordial thump appears to be most effective in terminating rhythms that are dependent on a *reentrant* pathway. Perhaps the best example of an arrhythmia with this type of mechanism that responds to the thump is sustained ventricular tachycardia. Mechanical energy generated by the manuever produces a low amplitude depolarization (of approximately 2-5 joules) that may still be potent enough to interrupt a reentry-dependent arrhythmia- *if* it occurs at just the right moment during the cardiac cycle. The problem with the thump is that if inadvertently delivered at a point in the cardiac cycle that corresponds to the *"vulnerable"* period- the thump may precipitate deterioration of the rhythm to V Fib (in much the same way that the "R-on-T" phenomenon does). Unfortunately, there is no way to control at what point in the cardiac cycle the thump will occur. Clinical experience suggests a much greater likelihood of *worsening* the rhythm (and precipitating V Fib or asystole)- than successful conversion to sinus rhythm.

Indications

- *Pulseless* rhythms in a *witnessed* arrest- but *only* if no defibrillator is immediately available.

> AHA Guidelines emphasize that "when a defibrillator is available, it makes sense to go *directly* to that therapy- and *not* waste even a minimum of time with the thump" (AHA Text- Pg 1-15).

Special Points:

- Think of the thump as a ***"No-lose procedure"***. Reserve its use for treatment of patients who present with *pulseless* rhythms in which there is *nothing* to lose. This includes V Fib and pulseless ventricular tachycardia- especially when a defibrillator is not readily available. Because it appears that the amount of energy needed for successful defibrillation of V Fib increases dramatically (almost *exponentially*) within *seconds* after the onset of cardiac arrest- the thump *must* be delivered as soon as possible after the onset of this rhythm for there to be any realistic chance of terminating V Fib. Therefore, if out in the field *without* access to a defibrillator- there is really *nothing to lose* (and everything to gain) by attempting the thump on a patient with witnessed and *pulseless* cardiac arrest. *The patient will die without it.*

  On the other hand, if the patient is in sustained VT *with* a pulse- do *not* use the thump! There is simply too much to lose by risking the thump in this situation (i.e., you may *lose* the pulse). If the patient in sustained VT remains hemodynamically stable, a trial of medical therapy may be reasonable. If the patient is (or becomes) hemodynamically unstable- delivery of an electrical impulse at a *predictable* point in the cardiac cycle (i.e., on the upstroke of the R wave) with *synchronized cardioversion* is much safer- and offers a far greater chance for successful conversion to sinus rhythm than does the random delivery of electrical output provided by the thump.

Cough Version

The technique for cough version is simple: as soon as the arrhythmia is noted, instruct the patient to *"Cough hard, and keep coughing!"* Coughing should continue at 1 to 3 second intervals- either until the rhythm is converted, or until another appropriate intervention (i.e., cardioversion) can be tried.

Impetus for advocating the use of cough version resulted from observation in the cardiac catheterization laboratory that forceful and repetitive coughing (i.e., **"cough CPR"**) could sustain consciousness for surprisingly long periods of time (i.e., of *up to 90 seconds!*) in patients with pulseless VT, V Fib, or even asystole. Intrathoracic pressures of more than 100 mm Hg are produced by such coughing- and are somehow able to generate adequate blood flow *despite* the presence of an otherwise non-perfusing rhythm.

Mechanism/Clinical Effects

It is still *not* known whether the mechanism of action for cough version is the result of improved coronary perfusion (from the increase in intrathoracic pressure that it produces), stimulation of the autonomic nervous system, or conversion of mechanical energy from the cough into a small amount (≈2-5 joules) of electrical energy. What is known- is that *vigorous coughing* occasionally converts malignant arrhythmias to normal sinus rhythm.

Since the original description of cough CPR by Criley et al. in 1976, instructing patients to cough at the onset of nonperfusing rhythms has become a standard practice in many cardiac catheterization laboratories. However, the technique is still largely ignored by all too many other emergency care providers who rarely seem to invoke coughing at the onset of a malignant arrhythmia.

Indications

- At the *onset* of VT, V Fib, or asystole- *before* consciousness is lost.

Special Points:

- *Don't forget about cough version.* Consider using this technique at the bedside or in the field for *any* patient who remains conscious in the face of a sustained malignant arrhythmia. In contrast to the precordial thump- cough version appears unlikely to cause deterioration of the rhythm.
- The most common clinical situation for the use of cough version is in the treatment of VT *with* a pulse. Because of the rapidity with which some of these patients become hemodynamically unstable- it will often be impossible for the rescuer to react in time to instruct the patient to begin coughing. One might therefore consider formulating a *prearranged signal* with patients who experience repeated episodes of sustained VT to indicate that immediate coughing must begin. If cough version is successful- it will either convert the rhythm- or "buy time" (i.e., maintain perfusion) until definitive therapy can be administered.

Defibrillation

Electrical defibrillation is by far the most important treatment modality for the patient in ventricular fibrillation. Convincing studies have shown that if emergency medical service personnel are allowed to do nothing other than defibrillate victims of cardiac arrest, lives will be saved. By far, the most important determinant of survival for the patient who develops V Fib is *time.* Assuming there is no underlying irreversible condition, the likelihood that initial countershock will successfully convert V Fib to a rhythm with a pulse is *inversely proportional* to the time from patient collapse until delivery of the electrical discharge.

In discussion of the precordial thump, we noted how energy requirements for electrical conversion of V Fib increase dramatically *within seconds* after the onset of cardiac arrest. For this reason, realistic chances for survival drop off *exponentially* as time passes- and are already markedly reduced once delay in defibrillation surpasses several minutes. Unfortunately, even prompt performance of CPR- *in and of itself* - will not prevent deterioration of V Fib to asystole, although it may prolong the period of potential "viability" for a few additional minutes.

Survival statistics for victims of cardiac arrest are highly variable, and generally range from 5 to 15% for resuscitation of out-of-hospital V Fib. In addition to the inverse relationship that exists between long-term survival and time until the initial defibrillation attempt- other factors also affect the likelihood that resuscitation will be successful. These include whether the arrest was witnessed, if bystander CPR was promptly performed on the scene, and the underlying medical condition of the patient. For example- even *immediate* defibrillation will be ineffective in resuscitating a patient if the cause of arrest is a ruptured ventricular aneurysm. In contrast, the chance for successful defibrillation will increase dramatically if V Fib is witnessed, occurs in a medical setting where it can be promptly recognized and *immediately* treated (i.e., by defibrillation)- and occurs in a patient who does *not* have any underlying irreversible medical condition. This situation is best illustrated clinically by the experience accrued in carefully supervised cardiac rehabilitation programs. In this setting, more than 90% of patients who fibrillate are successfully resuscitated on the scene. This exceedingly high resuscitation rate is attributed to the fact that virtually all of these patients are potentially salvageable- and all are closely monitored while they exercise in the presence of trained personnel who have *immediate* access to a defibrillator. The message is clear- the *sooner* a patient who develops V Fib can be defibrillated- *the better the chance for successsful resuscitation.*

Indications

- V Fib, pulseless VT.

Mechanism/Clinical and Adverse Effects

The theory behind electrical defibrillation is simple: in an attempt to eliminate the chaotic asynchronous activity of the fibrillating heart- an electrical current is passed through the mass of myocardial cells. If defibrillation is successful, the mass of individual cardiac cells will be depolarized. Ideally, they will then *repolarize* in a uniform manner- with resumption of *organized* and coordinated contractile activity.

It is important to emphasize that defibrillation is *not* a benign process. Passage of electrical current through the heart has the potential to produce both functional and morphologic damage (AHA Text- Pg 4-6). This may result in severe conduction system abnormalities (such as 2° or 3° AV block) in the event that the patient is converted out of V Fib. It may also produce further deterioration of the rhythm to asystole that is then *resistant* to all attempts at treatment. Precipitation of asystole by defibrillation is most likely to occur in patients who had been unresponsive for a significant period of time *prior* to arrival of EMS personnel.

> Despite the potential of defibrillation to produce these adverse effects- the chance for *meaningful* survival from cardiac arrest (i.e., survival with *intact* neurologic function) is still greatest when defibrillation is carried out at the *earliest* possible moment. Delay of defibrillation for the purpose of intubating the patient, establishing IV access, and/or administering drugs is *not* advised (AHA Text- Pg 4-6).

In an attempt to *minimize* the chance of producing additional myocardial and/or conduction system damage- it therefore seems reasonable to try to limit the amount of energy used to the *lowest level possible* at which defibrillation will be successful. Unfortunately, it is extremely difficult clinically to predict the optimal amount of energy to use. Beginning at too low a level risks excessively delaying the process of defibrillation. Beginning too high may produce further damage to the conduction system (that might be deleterious if the patient is ever converted out of V Fib). Current recommendations for defibrillation (that are listed below) reflect the American Heart Association's attempt at achieving the optimal balance between these constraints.

Recommended Energy Levels for Defibrillation of Adults

- ***Initial defibrillation attempt***- 200 joules
- ***2nd defibrillation attempt***- 300 joules
- ***3rd defibrillation attempt***- 360 joules
- ***Subsequent defibrillation attempts***- 200-360 joules

Note- AHA Guidelines allow for a *range* (i.e., *between* 200-300 joules) as the accepted energy level for the **2nd shock**. However, because selection of the higher level (i.e., **300 joules**) offers the advantage of providing a "greater and more predictable increase in current" (AHA Text- Pg 4-6)- *routine increase in the energy selected within a given series of shocks is the approach we favor* (i.e., from **200**- to **300**- to **360 joules**).

AHA Guidelines also suggest that "if V Fib is initially terminated by a shock, but then *recurs* during the arrest sequence- shocks should be reinitiated at the energy level that previously resulted in successful defibrillation" (AHA Text- Pg 4-6). We favor modification of this guideline- and prefer to routinely *drop back* to 200 joules for our initial countershock attempt when V Fib recurs at a later point in the code. We tend to do so *regardless* of whether or not previous defibrillation required a higher energy to be successful. As already emphasized, significant structural damage to the heart is clearly more likely to occur when higher energies (i.e., ≥300-360 joules) are used. Moreover, just because a patient fails to respond to defibrillation with lower energy levels at one point in a code- *in no way* means that they won't respond to the *same* lower energy countershock later on. In the event that a patient with recurrent V Fib fails to respond to defibrillation with 200 joules- little is likely to be lost if one then rapidly increases the energy level to 360 joules for the next defibrillation attempt.

Pulse checks are *no longer* recommended in between shocks of the initial *stacked* sequence (of 200- 300- 360 joules)- provided that rescuers can be confident that the monitor is correctly hooked up, and that the rhythm being displayed is *truly* V Fib (AHA Text- Pg 1-15). Similarly, time should *not* be spent performing CPR or administering drugs during this crucial first series of rapidly applied countershocks. Instead, all efforts are best directed at ensuring prompt defibrillation.

AHA Guidelines now allow for continued delivery of shock attempts in "sets of 3" (i.e., ***stacked* defibrilation**)- *even after the initial sequence of the first 3 shocks.* Continued use of *stacked shocks* (in "sets of 3"- with energies from 200-360 joules)- is especially appropriate for treating persistent V Fib when administration of medication is delayed (AHA Text- Pg 1-18).

We emphasize that defibrillation is a procedure that must be performed with the upmost caution. Always be sure that the patient is properly positioned- that defibrillation paddles are correctly placed (i.e., sternal-apex location)- that appropriate conductive medium or adhesive defibrillator pads are used- that the appropriate energy level for defibrillation has been selected- and that 25 lbs of pressure is applied on both paddles when delivering the shock (AHA Text- Pg 1-8). AHA Guidelines go on to emphasize the importance of having rescuers call out some type of ***"Clearing Chant"*** *prior* to each defibrillation (i.e., *"I am going to shock on the count of three . . . - Everybody CLEAR!"*).

Theoretical Concepts: Electrical Defibrillation

Definition of several key terms will facilitate understanding the concept of defibrillation. These terms are energy, power, voltage (or electrical potential), current, and resistance (or impedance).

Defibrillation can most easily be thought of as the passage of an electrical ***current*** through the heart over a brief period of time. The strength (i.e., ***energy***) of a defibrillation attempt is most often expressed in ***joules*** (or *watt-seconds*), where:

$$\underset{\text{(Joules)}}{\text{Energy}} = \underset{\text{(Watts)}}{\text{Power}} \times \underset{\text{(Seconds)}}{\text{Duration}}$$

Current is defined as the flow of electrons in an electrical circuit. In the simplest electrical circuit, an electrical *potential* (measured in ***volts***) generates a flow of electrons (measured in *amperes*)- that passes through an electrical ***resistance*** (measured in ohms)- and which then returns to complete the circuit (Figure 2D-2).

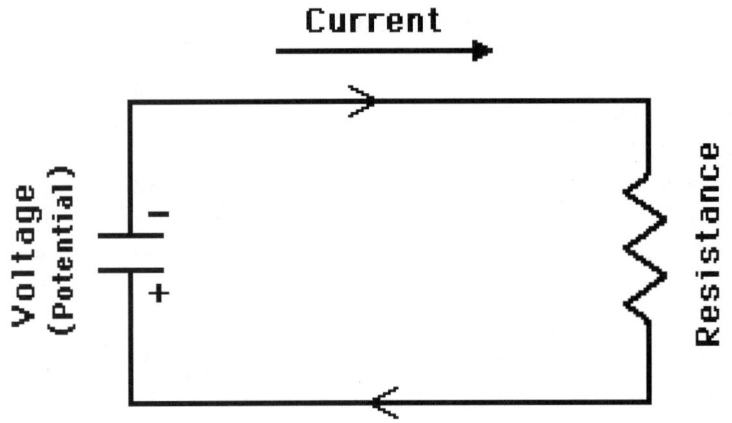

Figure 2D-2: Schematic illustration of the simplest electrical circuit. An electrical potential generates a *current* that flows through an electrical *resistance.*

The relationship between the parameters of current, voltage and resistance for the electrical circuit shown in Figure 2D-2 (as well as for *any* electrical circuit) are expressed by the following formula:

$$\underset{\text{(Volts)}}{\text{Potential}} = \underset{\text{(Amperes)}}{\text{Current}} \times \underset{\text{(Ohms)}}{\text{Resistance}}$$

Solving the above equation for *current* produces the following relationship:

$$\text{Current (Amperes)} = \frac{\text{Potential (Volts)}}{\text{Resistance (Ohms)}}$$

The point to emphasize clinically is that it is ***current*** passing through the chest (and *not* voltage!) that actually defibrillates. Appreciation of this concept is essential for understanding why (and how) various factors alter the effectiveness of defibrillation.

> Despite the fact that *current* defibrillates- convention still holds that calibration of defibrillators be designated in units of *energy* (i.e, ***joules***- or watt-seconds) rather than current. As might be expected, this practice is the source of some confusion.

From Figure 2D-2 and the above (boxed) formula- it can be seen that the amount of ***current*** flowing through a circuit for any given voltage- will vary *inversely* with the electrical ***resistance*** to the flow of that current. For example, if the resistance to flow increases- then *less* current will flow through the circuit. Conversely, if resistance decreases- then *more* current flows through the circuit.

This same relationship holds true in the clinical setting for electrical defibrillation. That is- the amount of current that will penetrate the chest wall to defibrillate the heart varies *inversely* with the *__T__rans__T__horacic __R__esistance* ***(TTR)*** to the passage of that current. If for *whatever* reason TTR is increased- *less* current will penetrate the chest (and the strength or energy for that defibrillation attempt will be correspondingly less). On the other hand, when TTR is lowered- current flow will increase. Thus, the most effective way to optimize current flow at any given voltage is to *minimize* TTR.

The final formula we present expresses the relationship between energy, voltage, and current:

$$\underset{\text{(Joules)}}{\text{Energy}} = \underset{\text{(Volts)}}{\text{Potential}} \times \underset{\text{(Amperes)}}{\text{Current}} \times \underset{\text{(Seconds)}}{\text{Duration}}$$

This equation further emphasizes the clinical importance of optimizing current flow. Because of the *direct* relationship between energy and current: the greater the current flow for any given shock- the greater the electrical energy for that defibrillation attempt.

The Importance of TTR

Return to the boxed formula we presented earlier that expressed the relationship between current and resistance.

$$\text{Current} = \frac{\text{Potential}}{\text{Resistance}}$$

Keep in mind that "resistance" to defibrillation in the human model is TTR. It should therefore be clear that clinical factors affecting TTR (i.e., transthoracic *resistance*) play a crucial role in determining the amount of *current* (and therefore *energy*) that penetrates the heart with each defibrillation attempt. Factors known to affect TTR include:

i) The amount of energy selected for defibrillation.
ii) The time interval *between* successive shocks.
iii) The total number of shocks delivered.
iv) Size of the paddle electrodes.
v) The interface used between the electrodes and the chest wall.
vi) Chest wall configuration.
vii) The pressure exerted on the electrodes against the chest wall.
viii) The phase of ventilation of the patient at the time of defibrillation.

The *number* of countershocks delivered to a patient in V Fib exerts a *cumulative* effect on TTR. TTR is also affected by the time interval *between* successive shocks. Thus, delivery of *multiple countershocks in rapid succession* is likely to significantly reduce TTR- and increase the amount of current flowing through the chest at any given energy level. This is the rationale for the recommendation to *minimize time* between countershock attempts.

Other factors that may affect TTR include *paddle size, paddle placement* and *pressure,* and the *interface* used. The recommended position for paddle placement is to put one paddle under the right clavicle (just to the right of the sternum)- while the other is placed lateral to the left nipple (in the anterior axillary line). Being sure to exert firm downward pressure (of approximately 25 pounds) on each paddle may reduce TTR by as much as 25%.

Chest wall configuration (especially chest *width*) may also play an important role in determining TTR. It is important to emphasize, however, that *TTR is not simply a function of body weight, size, and chest wall configuration.*

That TTR can *not* be predicted solely on the basis of physical appearance is evident from the finding by Kerber of a more than *fivefold* variation in TTR values among an unselected population of adults (of various body sizes) who were found in cardiac arrest (Kerber et al., Circulation 77:1038, 1988). *Even elderly, emaciated patients can occasionally have surprisingly high TTR values despite their seemingly negligible body mass.*

The final factor to consider regarding TTR is the *paddle-skin interface.* The skin serves as a potent electrical resistor between electrode paddles and the heart. Defibrillation without the use of a suitable interface is likely to result in a significant burn of the skin surface, and a lack of penetration of the defibrillator current.

A number of electrode gels are commercially available to optimize conductivity. In recent years, the problem of selecting a suitable conductive medium for defibrillation has been greatly simplified by development of *disposable electrode pads.* Routine use of these pads eliminates concern regarding the potential hazards of bridging and leftover electrode gel (leaving a slippery surface on the chest wall). It may also save precious time by eliminating a step (application of gel) in the defibrillation process.

Recent Developments: Potential Clinical Applications

Up until recently, there had been no practical way to clinically determine TTR (and adjust current delivery accordingly) at the scene of a cardiac arrest. Development of newer (current-based) defibrillators holds promise of being able to do so in the near future. Preliminary work with these devices has provided us with important clinical insights that may influence future practice when ***current-based* defibrillators** become more readily available. Among these insights are the following:

i) Realization of the fact that a significant percentage of patients with V Fib will respond to defibrillation at surprisingly low energy levels (of as little as 100 joules!). The chance of successfully defibrillating a patient at a low energy level is best when TTR is low (since a relatively greater amount of current will pass through the chest wall of such individuals at any given energy level).

ii) Awareness of the tremendous variation in TTR from one patient to the next. Although one might reasonably expect individuals of larger body size and frame to have relatively greater TTR- *body size and habitus are not reliable predictors of TTR values.* Thus, TTR might be *greater* in an 80 year old, 80 pound woman- than in a robust or muscular 200 pound man. There simply is *no way* to tell what TTR values will be from inspection of the patient. *Standard defibrillators provide no clue.*

iii) Appreciation that the amount of current that passes through the chest wall to defibrillate a patient will be very much influenced by the TTR value of that patient. Current flow at any given energy level will therefore also vary in direct response to *any* of the factors we discussed that affect TTR. Moreover, TTR values may *change* with time in a given patient as the code progresses (i.e., in response to the number of shocks delivered, the time between countershock attempts, and other factors in the code). Therefore- implementation of a *specified* defibrillating protocol (such as the AHA recommendation to administer 200- 300- 360 joules for successive countershock attempts)- will *not* necessarily standardize the amount of defibrillating current that a particular patient will receive.

iv) Understanding that more energy is *not* necessarily better. While it is true that in general, use of increasing energy levels enhances the likelihood of successful defibrillation- this relationship holds true *only up to a point.* Selection of higher energy levels *beyond* this point may paradoxically *decrease* the chance for successful defibrillation in a significant number of patients. In addition to reducing the chance for successful defibrillation- delivery of an excessively high defibrillating current may also be detrimental because it increases the likelihood of producing functional (conduction system) damage. Thus,

> The amount of defibrillating current should *ideally* be limited to the *lowest possible value* that is still capable of successfully converting the patient out of ventricular fibrillation.

As we have already indicated- the difficulty clinically is determining what the "lowest effective value" of current for successful defibrillation will be for any given patient at a particular moment in time during the resuscitation effort. Use of a defibrillator capable of *instantaneously* measuring TTR and *automatically adjusting* the amount of energy selected to ensure delivery of a pre-designated amount of current may provide the answer.

> Use of an ***automatic*** **current-based** (i.e., energy-adjusting) **defibrillator** should enable optimization of current flow delivery. Thus, for a patient who has an unexpectedly low TTR value, less energy will automatically be selected for the initial attempt at defibrillation than would be the case if a standard defibrillating protocol (beginning at 200 joules) was being followed. Conversely, a much higher initial energy level will be selected for defibrillation of a patient with an unexpectedly high TTR value. Moreover, knowing that TTR is unusually high in a particular patient suggests the need for continued use of high energy countershocks (of 360 joules or more) if ventricular fibrillation persists (or recurs).

Special Points:

At the present time, *current-based* defibrillators are not yet widely available for general use. As a result, determination of the energy level for defibrillation is still largely an *empiric* process. With this in mind, we emhasize the following points:

- Use of ***standardized*** **defibrillating protocols** (as recommended by **AHA Guidelines**) will select appropriate energy levels for defibrillation *most* of the time. Their use has the decided additional advantage of facilitating (and expediting) the decision-making process- and this is clearly the approach we favor.

- Many factors affect TTR (and therefore the amount of current flowing through the chest wall at any given energy level). This is why energy requirements for successful defibrillation vary so greatly from one patient to the next- and why surprisingly *low* energy levels will sometimes work.

- *Defibrillation is not benign.* While there are no suitable alternatives to defibrillating the patient who is in V Fib, the point to emphasize is that electrical countershock is *not* without risk- and may result in producing severe morphologic and/or functional damage (including the risk of precipitating asystole). In general, the higher the energy level selected for defibrillation- the greater the chance of producing such damage. Therefore- the *lowest* energy level that is likely to be successful in a given situation is the one that should be used.

- The *most* important determinant of successful defibrillation (*by far!*)- is *time.* Although attention to factors affecting TTR may help to optimize current flow delivery- *they are clearly no substitute for prompt defibrillation.*

- Finally- keep in mind that recommendations for defibrillation are likely to change when current-based defibrillators do become more widely available.

Synchronized Cardioversion

Synchronized cardioversion is a procedure that was born out of necessity. Following the successful use of closed-chest defibrillation in 1956, it became apparent that a therapeutic modality was needed for treatment of hemodynamically significant tachyarrhythmias that did not respond to pharmacologic therapy. Use of original defibrillating machines was unsafe for this purpose since the prolonged (150-250 msec) alternating current (AC) discharge they delivered was extremely likely to produce myocardial damage and/or precipitate postconversion cardiac arrhythmias (including asystole!). Development of direct current (DC) capacitors (able to deliver the electrical impulse in as little as 4-30 msec) and the ability to ***synchronize*** the discharge to the "nonvulnerable" period of the cardiac cycle made cardioversion a reality.

> The ***vulnerable*** **period** is the time during the cardiac cycle when the heart is most susceptible to developing ventricular fibrillation if stimulated by an electrical discharge. This period is approximately 30 msec in duration. Temporally, it just precedes the apex of the T wave on the surface ECG. By *synchronizing* the electrical impulse to the height of the R wave (which by definition occurs *before* the T wave- and therefore before the vulnerable period)- the risk of inducing a more malignant arrhythmia is minimized.

Cardioversion is most effective in the treatment of arrhythmias that depend on a *reentry* mechanism for their perpetuation (i.e., atrial flutter, PSVT, and ventricular tachycardia). The process works by producing a single, brief electrical discharge- that acts to terminate the arrhythmia by *interrupting* the reentrant circuit.

Definition of Terms

The term *cardioversion* is often the source of much confusion. This is because the term is commonly interchanged (and mistakenly equated) with two other terms- *defibrillation* and *countershock*.

As discussed earlier in this section, ***defibrillation*** is the process of passing an electric current through the heart with the express intent of completely depolarizing all myocardial cells. The electrical discharge that is delivered with defibrillation is *unsynchronized-* which means that it occurs at an entirely *random* point in the cardiac cycle.

In contrast, use of the term ***cardioversion*** implies that the electrical discharge has been timed (i.e., *synchronized*) to occur at a designated point in the cardiac cycle. Doing so not only facilitates conversion of certain tachyarrhythmias to sinus rhythm, but it also minimizes the chance that the electrical impulse will exacerbate the arrhythmia (as may occur if the stimulus happens to be delivered during the vulnerable period).

> To avoid confusion about terminology, as well as to clarify the mode of delivery of the electrical impulse, we frequently refer to this procedure as "***synchronized*** **cardioversion**" (rather than simply "cardioversion"). Although use of the combined term in this manner may engender an element of redundancy- *it leaves no doubt as to how the operator is about to proceed* (which is really the *KEY* for ensuring a coordinated team effort in resuscitation).

Among emergency care providers, the third term- ***countershock*** - and its diminutive, ***"shock"***- tend to be freely interchanged with the term, *defibrillation.* We favor this usage- and unless otherwise specified, generally treat these three terms synonymously. We therefore separate them from the term "cardioversion", and reserve our use of *defibrillation, countershock,* and *"shock"* for referring to delivery of an *unsynchronized* electrical impulse to a patient in ventricular fibrillation.

Emergency vs "Elective" Cardioversion

Distinction should be made between ***emergency* cardioversion** (which must be performed *immediately* because the patient is acutely decompensating)- and cardioversion that is *less* urgent. In this latter situation, the patient may still be symptomatic- but is at least able to maintain a pulse and measurable blood pressure (AHA Text- Pg 1-35). Cardioversion may therefore be performed in a *"more controlled"* manner (i.e., there should be at least enough time to *sedate* the patient and call anesthesia to the bedside).

At the other extreme is ***"elective" cardioversion***- in which the patient is *hemodynamically stable* but in a rhythm (such as A Fib or A Flutter) that has not responded to medical therapy. Discussion of the indications for *elective* cardioversion is beyond the scope of this book.

Indications for *Emergency* Cardioversion

- *Tachyarrhythmias* (VT and/or supraventricular rhythms) that are either hemodynamically *unstable*- or which fail to respond to other measures.

> **Note**- Practically speaking, it is highly *unlikely* that synchronized cardioversion will be needed on an *emergent* basis- if the heart rate of the tachyarrhythmia is *less than* **150 beats/minute** (AHA Text- Pg 1-33).

Most of the time when the heart rate is *less than* 150 beats/minute the patient will not be acutely unstable as a result of the rate. In such cases, optimal management can usually be achieved with one or more of the following actions:

i) *Medical therapy* (i.e., use of antiarhythmic drugs).
ii) Correction of *underlying conditions* that may be *causing* the tachycardia (i.e., hypotension, heart failure, hypoxemia, electrolyte disturbance, etc.).
iii) *Non-emergent* cardioversion (i.e., cardioversion performed at a *later* time under more stable conditions).

Suggested Energy Levels for Cardioversion

AHA Guidelines recommend use of the following ***Standard Sequence** of **Energy Levels*** for synchronized cardioversion of the various tachyarrhythmias (AHA Text- Pg 1-35):

- *1st attempt*- **100 joules**

- *If the 1st attempt is unsuccessful*- increase the energy level up to **200 joules**- then to **300 joules**- and finally to **360 joules**.

Clinically- it is of interest that many cases of VT will be responsive to synchronized cardioversion at relatively low energy levels (of 50 joules- or less). This should not be suprising given that VT is most often a *reentry* arrhythmia- and therefore susceptible to interruption of its cycle by an appropriately timed electrical stimulus (as is delivered with synchronized cardioversion). Despite awareness of the general responsiveness of VT to lower energy cardioversion- we fully support AHA recommendations to begin the process at 100 joules in the interest of standardizing the approach to cardioversion and providing extra assurance that adequate energy will be used to treat this potentially life-threatening arrhythmia.

Exceptions to Use of the Standard Sequence

For *ease of recall*- AHA Guidelines recommend the standard sequence of energy levels that are listed above for synchronized cardioversion. We draw attention to three important exceptions to use of this standard sequence:

- ***Polymorphic VT*** (i.e., VT with an *irregular* morphology and rate)- which often requires *higher* energy levels for successful cardioversion. AHA Guidelines therefore suggest *starting* with **200 joules**.
- ***Atrial Flutter***- which often responds to *lower* energy levels. AHA Guidelines allow for selection of **50 joules** as the *initial* energy level for attempts at converting A Flutter.
- ***Atrial Fibrillation***- which in our experience is also often a relatively difficult rhythm to successfully cardiovert when lower energy levels are used. We therefore prefer to *start* with **200 joules** for our *initial* attempt at cardioverting A Fib- and to increase this to 360 joules if a second attempt is needed.

A fine point to emphasize regarding the cardioversion of patients in A Fib relates to the importance of *closely* watching the monitor during the period *immediately after* delivery of the electrical impulse. "Non-responsiveness" (i.e., failure to convert to normal sinus rhythm) should be differentiated from *transient* successful conversion- in which sinus rhythm is *momentarily* restored, only to revert back to A Fib a few beats later. The former situation (i.e., "non-responsiveness") suggests that additional attempts at synchronized cardioversion (perhaps at higher energy levels) may be indicated. In contrast, momentary conversion to sinus rhythm with rapid reversion back to A Fib suggests that such additional attempts will also be unsuccessful at *maintaining* sinus rhythm (even if higher energy levels are used!). Electrical conversion to (and maintenance of) normal sinus rhythm may simply not be possible for such patients at that moment in time.

Cautions

Consideration of the following ideas may help in preparing for the procedure:

- *Try to anticipate potential problems that might be encountered.* Occasionally cardioversion can precipitate malignant arrhythmias (including V Fib or asystole). As a result, it is essential to have a fully equiped crash cart nearby. Should the patient suddenly develop V Fib- turn off the synchronizer switch and *immediately* defibrillate (with 200-360 joules). If cardioversion results in asystole- Atropine and/or immediate application of an external pacemaker are in order.
- Prior to cardioversion, a bed board should be placed under the patient in the event that CPR is needed. If the patient is awake and time permits, *sedation* (with IV Valium, Versed, or other agents) is strongly advised to minimize discomfort (and hopefully induce amnesia for the event). If possible (i.e., if time permits)- it may be preferable

to call an anesthesiologist/nurse anesthetist/respiratory therapist to the bedside to ensure the presence of qualified personnel to attend to the airway in the event that intubation is needed. Doing so *in advance* frees you to concentrate your efforts on directing resuscitation and managing any postconversion arrhythmias that occur.

- Be sure to *continually* monitor the patient throughout the procedure. Try to select an ECG monitoring lead that displays a tall R wave configuration if at all possible (since doing so may facilitate identification of both the QRS complex and synchronization spike).

- Remember that most defibrillators will not allow synchronized cardioversion to be performed when the rhythm displayed is obtained by means of quick look paddles. Instead, the patient must be hooked up to hard wire monitoring leads for synchronization to be possible.

- Keep in mind that even though a decision to cardiovert the patient may have been made, medications *may* still be administered- if the medications are immediately available and appropriate for the situation (AHA Text- Pg 1-35). *Delay is the issue.* AHA Guidelines emphasize that Lidocaine (or other drugs, as appropriate) may be given *at the same time* as preparations are made to cardiovert. If medication administration is delayed, however (for *whatever* reason) and the patient is hemodynamically unstable- *immediate* cardioversion takes precedence!

Technique for Cardioversion

Emergency cardioversion may be performed as follows:

i) Apply conductive medium to the electrode paddles (or use disposable electrode pads), and place the paddles on the patient's chest in the same manner as for unsynchronized defibrillation.

ii) Turn on the "synch" switch- and verify that the defibrillator is sensing the QRS complex.

iii) Charge the defibrillator, making sure everyone is clear from the bed.

iv) Apply 25 pounds of pressure on both paddles (as for defibrillation).

v) Simultaneously depress the buttons on each paddle. Unlike the case for defibrillation- the buttons on each paddle must *remain* depressed until the machine has discharged.

vi) Recheck the patient, the pulse, and the ECG monitor *immediately after* discharge to assess hemodynamic status and determine the post-conversion rhythm. If the arrhythmia persists- consider *increasing* the energy level (as per protocol) if another attempt at cardioversion is indicated. Remember to *reset* the sync mode if needed (as many defibrillators *automatically* default back to the unsynchronized mode after energy delivery!).

Special Points:

- Although certain cardiac arrhythmias are clearly more responsive to synchronized cardioversion than others (and require lower energy levels for success)- three concepts are even *more important* than the specific number of joules to use for the procedure:

  i) Awareness of ***when*** the procedure is *immediately* needed (and when it is safe and appropriate to proceed with medical therapy).

  ii) Knowing ***how*** to use the machine (on your floor or in your area- *in your particular institution!*) for delivery of synchronized cardioversion.

  iii) Remembering that if *for any reason* synchronization is delayed and the patient is acutely unstable- that you should ***abort* synchronization attempts**- and *immediately defibrillate* the patient (i.e., with an *unsynchronized* shock)!

> Despite the best of intentions (and the most diligent preparation)- we stress the importance of *accepting* the clinical reality that there may be times when the synchronized electrical impulse will simply not discharge. If a rapid attempt at troubleshooting does not resolve the problem- *do NOT persist in trying to cardiovert the patient.* Admittedly, an unsynchronized countershock is less optimal than synchronized cardioversion for treatment of VT with a pulse. Nevertheless- *delivery of an unsynchronized discharge is far preferable to delivery of no discharge at all.* Practically speaking, unsynchronized countershock will work equally well most of the time *without* excessively increasing the risk of exacerbating the arrhythmia. If you therefore find yourself *unable* to cardiovert a patient with a potentially life-threatening and hemodynamically unstable tachyarrhythmia (for *whatever* reason)- we favor delivery of an *unsynchronized* countershock instead.

- Realize that it will *not* always be possible to determine (with certainty) the etiology of every cardiac arrhythmia. Acceptance of this clinical reality is particularly important when confronted with a *WCT* (*Wide-Complex Tachycardia*) of *uncertain* etiology. Practically speaking, if the patient is (and/or becomes) hemodynamically unstable- *the etiology of the arrhythmia no longer matters.* This is because in this situation synchronized cardioversion is *immediately* indicated regardless of whether the WCT is due to VT or SVT with aberrant conduction.

  On the other hand, if the patient *remains* hemodynamically stable- an initial trial of medical therapy may be preferable. If this is unsuccessful, synchronized cardioversion (on a somewhat less emergent basis) may then become indicated.

Pacemaker Therapy

The topic of cardiac pacing is a comprehensive one that extends well beyond the scope of this book. We therefore limit our comments in this section to those aspects of cardiac pacing that are pertinent to the emergency care provider in charge of an acutely unstable patient (and/or in the setting of cardiac arrest).

Pacemaker Options

Three types of cardiac pacemakers have been used in the emergency care setting: *transvenous* pacemakers, *transthoracic* pacemakers, and *transcutaneous* (external) pacemakers.

- ***Trans-VENOUS* Pacing-** is "best suited for use in urgent situations in which there is adequate time for fluoroscopy" (AHA Text- Pg 5-6). Insertion of a transvenous pacemaker is accomplished through a major vein such as the brachial, subclavian, internal jugular, or femoral vein. The pacemaking wire is advanced by means of a flow-directed, balloon-tipped catheter (with electrocardiographic monitoring)- and/or by fluoroscopic guidance (if time allows and skilled personnel and equipment are on hand). In its final position, the pacemaker lies in the right ventricular apex.

  Drawbacks of transvenous pacing are that the procedure is invasive- it requires more time to implement than other emergency pacing procedures- and it mandates the need for an operator skilled in the technique. Its advantages compared to transcutaneous pacing reside in its greater reliability in achieving ventricular capture and better patient tolerance (once the device is in place).

- ***Trans-THORACIC* Pacing-** is accomplished by passage of a transthoracic needle through the skin at a point just to the left of the subxiphoid notch. The transthoracic needle is then advanced while aiming toward the right ventricular cavity. Correct anatomic placement within the right ventricle is confirmed by withdrawing the inner trocar of the needle and aspirating blood- after which the pacing wire can then be introduced, and hookup completed to an external energy source.

  In the past, the principal advantage of transthoracic pacing was speed of insertion. Skilled operators could complete the procedure in *less* than one minute. Unfortunately (as might be imagined)- the risk of complications (including pneumothorax, hemothorax, and/or hemopericardium) was extremely high. Moreover, the reliability of pacing with this device was far from optimal. With development (and refinement) of transcutaneous pacing- *transthoracic pacing is now almost obsolete.*

- ***Trans-CUTANOUS* Pacing-** has become the *initial pacing method of choice* in the emergency setting (*See below*). Even when transvenous pacing is preferred- use of a TCP may serve as a *"bridge"* to stabilize the patient until such time that a transvenous pacemaker may be safely inserted under more controlled circumstances (AHA Text- Pg 5-6).

Transcutaneous Pacing

The most exciting advance in emergency pacemaker therapy has been development of the ***T****rans****C****utaneous* ***P****acemaker* **(*TCP*).** First introduced by Zoll in 1952, this device fell out of favor when transvenous pacing became popular during the 1960s. Problems caused by the original TCP model were severe patient discomfort (from cutaneous sensory nerve and skeletal muscle stimulation) and significant stimulus artifact (from involuntary skeletal muscle contraction) that made interpretation of the surface ECG exceedingly difficult.

The device was modified and reintroduced in 1981. Continued refinements in technology have greatly reduced patient discomfort (from cutaneous sensory nerve stimulation and skeletal muscle contraction), and now provide an easily interpretable ECG recording. Three additional features contribute to making TCP the emergency pacing procedure of choice (AHA Text- Pg 5-2):

i) *Lack* of invasiveness.
ii) Easy and *rapid* application.
iii) *Effective* cardiac pacing in a majority of cases.

It should be emphasized that transcutaneous pacing is only a *temporizing* measure. Transvenous pacing remains the treatment of choice for patients who develop a severe conduction disorder that is likely to require a prolonged period of pacemaker support. However, when time is of the essence (as for a patient with bradyasystolic cardiac arrest)- and/or when transvenous pacing is not readily available- then transcutaneous pacing may be a suitable (and much more rapidly instituted) alternative.

Another application for TCP is in less critical situations when the need for transvenous pacing may be uncertain. For example, a patient with acute *inferior* infarction may present with 2° or 3° AV block and an acceptable ventricular response that renders them hemodynamically stable. Immediate insertion of a transvenous pacemaker might not necessarily be needed in this situation- especially in view of the fact that AV conduction disturbances that occur in association with acute *inferior* infarction often resolve spontaneously (and/or readily respond to administration of Atropine). Ready availability of a *noninvasive* pacing modality (i.e., the transcutanous pacemaker) to serve as a *backup* (in the event that the patient does decompensate)- may be preferable to routine (and invasive) prophylactic insertion of a transvenous pacemaker. This application of transcutaneous pacing is known as ***Anticipatory Pacing Readiness***.

In contrast- development of Mobitz II 2° AV block and/or 3° AV block in association with acute *anterior* infarction are much more likely to be persistent conduction disorders that will not respond to medical therapy (and which may suddenly deteriorate to profound bradycardia or even ventricular standstill). Immediate insertion of transvenous pacing at its *earliest* availability is appropriate treatment for these more ominous conduction disorders.

Note- Strictly speaking, transcutaneous pacing is *not* a truly "non-invasive" procedure- since current (with the potential to cause cardiac and tissue damage) *is* introduced into the body (AHA Text- Pg 5-2). However, TCP is clearly the *least* invasive of the pacing modalities.

AHA Guidelines also note that *transcutaneous pacing* is the preferred term for this modality (AHA Text- Pg 5-2). Use of the previously popular term, *"external pacing"* may be misleading and is no longer recommended. This is because in pacemaker terminology- *any* pulse generator that is not implanted in the body may be described as an "external" pacer (including transvenous, transthoracic, and transesophageal pacing devices.

Indications for *Emergency* Pacing (*and/or* Pacing Readiness)

- Bradycardia that is *hemodynamically significant* or *compromising* (meaning that the patient is symptomatic *because of* the *slow* heart rate). This is a **Class I** indication for emergency pacing (AHA Text- Pg 5-2).
- *Bradycardia* with an *escape rhythm* that has *not* responded to pharmacologic therapy. This is a **Class IIa** (i.e., *probably* helpful) indication for emergency pacing.
- *Bradyasystolic cardiac arrest* (including asystole/PEA). This is a **Class IIb** (i.e., *possibly* helpful) indication for emergency pacing- *provided that* pacing can be instituted relatively soon after the onset of arrest. Otherwise, pacing is *not* routinely recommended for such patients because of their exceedingly bleak prognosis- which is almost uniformly fatal when pacing is delayed (AHA Text- Pg 5-2).
- Overdrive pacing of *selected* tachycardias *not* responding to drugs or cardioversion (a Class IIb indication- *although not yet commonly used*).
- Consideration of ***Anticipatory Pacing Readiness*** (i.e., application of TCP with the device set on "standby")- for the patient with acute myocardial infarction (or other emergency situation) who develops a bradyarrhythmia or other conduction system disorder that *might* require emergency pacing- but which is initially associated with a *stable* hemodynamic condition.

  Specific conduction disorders that are most likely to require pacing (either immediately if the patient is symptomatic- or on *standby* if the patient is stable)- include Mobitz type II 2° AV block and 3° AV block with QRS widening).

Futility of Pacing in Bradyasystolic Cardiac Arrest

Despite numerous technological improvements- *pacemaker therapy is rarely a lifesaving procedure in the setting of cardiac arrest.* The sombering clinical reality is that overall prognosis for patients with bradyasystolic cardiac arrest is dismal- *regardless* of whatever interventions are undertaken.

Time is a critical factor. In the past, most studies on the use of pacing for cardiac arrest were *retrospective-* in which pacemaker insertion was only attempted after all other resuscitative measures had been tried and failed. One could not reasonably expect *any* intervention to work under such circumstances.

Unfortunately- even when used in more timely fashion, transcutaneous pacing has *not* been shown in the prehospital setting to significantly improve long-term prognosis. Whether to attempt TCP in such patients is a matter of individual judgement *if* rescue personnel arrive *promptly* on the scene. If pacing is delayed (especially if for *more* than 20 minutes)- AHA Guidelines now advise that the procedure becomes *relatively contraindicated* because of the well documented dismal prognosis of these patients (AHA Text- Pg 5-2).

In contrast to the prehospital setting where the finding of bradyasystolic cardiac arrest most often implies *irreversible* myocardial damage (and *inability* of the myocardium to generate effective contraction even if appropriately stimulated)- early application of transcutaneous pacing may be effective as treatment if the patient is *not* in cardiac arrest. Thus, the procedure may be *lifesaving* when meaningful (albeit slow) contractile activity is present (i.e., for treatment of hemodynamically significant bradyarrhythmias in the patient who is *not* in cardiac arrest).

Pacing may also be potentially lifesaving if applied as a *supportive measure* to patients with bradyasystolic arrest that occurs in association with *special circumstances* (i.e., as a result of profound hypothermia, electrocution, drowning, or drug overdose). Underlying the rhythm disorder, the myocardium in such patients may be relatively normal- so that resuscitation may be possible if the patient is paced until the precipitating cause can be appropriately treated.

Special Points

- As a modality, pacing is most effective when used to treat patients who *do* have a pulse- but who have bradyarrhythmias that are *hemodynamically unstable*. Although pharmacologic treatment (i.e., with Atropine or a pressor agent) may increase heart rate and improve perfusion of patients with hemodynamically compromising brady-arrhythmias- *"Pacing should not be delayed if drug therapy is not immediately available"*. Moreover- "it *may* be appropriate to initiate pharmacologic therapy *and* pacing *simultaneously* to stabilize the patient as rapidly as possible" (AHA Text- Pg 5-1).

- Realistically speaking- pacing is *unlikely* to be effective when used to treat patients with bradyasystolic cardiac arrest. In acknowledgement of this clinical reality, AHA Guidelines *no longer* routinely recommend emergency pacing as part of the treatment protocol for asystole (AHA Text- Pg 1-24). If used at all in this setting- attempts at pacing should be tried *as early as possible* after onset of arrest- and should occur in association with *simultaneous* administration of drugs (such as Epnephrine). If more than 20 minutes have elapsed since the onset of bradyasystolic arrest, the chance for successful resuscitation is almost negligible- and attempts at pacing become *relatively contraindicated* (AHA Text- Pg 5-2).

- Possible exceptions to the general rule that asystole/PEA do not respond to pacing include patients for whom the cause of arrest is drug overdose, acidosis, and/or an electrolyte disorder. Underlying the rhythm, such patients will often have a *normal* heart- that *may* respond to the stimulation of pacing (AHA Text- Pg 1-23).

- Severe hypothermia is one of the few *relative contraindications* to pacing (AHA Text- Pg 5-2). The profound bradycardia that is so commonly seen in such patients is often *physiologic* (as a result of the reduction in metabolic rate)- and will usually resolve with gradual rewarming as core temperature increases. Stimulating the heart with cardiac pacing in this situation may be counterproductive- and even precipitate V Fib in the severely hypothermic patient (which may be refractory to defibrillation until rewarming occurs).

- Finally- keep in mind the three major pitfalls associated with use of TCP. These are: 1) Failure to recognize that the pacer is *not* capturing; 2) Failure to recognize that underlying V Fib is present (and that the patient should be defibrillated); and 3) Patient discomfort from the device. For patients who are conscious and extremely uncomfortable from the skeletal muscle contractions produced by pacing stimuli, judicious use of a *benzodiazepine* (for treatment of anxiety/muscle contractions)- and/or *Morphine* (for pain relief) may be invaluable adjuncts.

Section 2E: *Additional Drugs*

Digoxin

How Dispensed:

- **IV Use**- 0.25 mg/ml (2 ml amp = 0.5 mg)
- **Oral Use:**
    - **Lanoxin**- tablets of 0.125 mg, 0.25 mg, and 0.5 mg
    - **Lanoxicaps**- capsules of 0.05 mg, 0.1 mg, and 0.2 mg

Indications

Indications for the use of Digoxin are relatively *limited* in the acute care setting!

- *Rapid A Fib/Flutter*- Digoxin may help with *rate control* (especially if the patient is also in heart failure).
- *PSVT* (although Adenosine, Verapamil, Diltiazem, and/or IV beta-blockers all work faster and are more effective in the acute care setting).

Mechanism/Clinical Effects:

Despite being the source of continued controversy- digitalis preparations have been a mainstay in the treatment of congestive heart failure ever since William Withering's first description of the foxglove in 1785.

The drug has several actions. It increases the force and velocity of myocardial contraction (positive *inotropic* effect). When used in patients with congestive heart failure- heart size decreases and overall cardiac performance is improved. Digoxin also *prolongs* the refractory period of the AV node- an effect that helps to slow the ventricular response to most supraventricular tachyarrhythmias.

Despite these beneficial effects- *indications for the use of Digoxin in the emergency care setting remain quite limited.* This is because the increase in cardiac contractility that the drug produces tends to be relatively modest (and is at least partially offset by an increase in myocardial oxygen consumption). Other more rapidly acting (and more easily controlled) medications (i.e., IV Nitroglycerin, Dobutamine, diuretics, ACE-inhibitors, etc.) are therefore preferable for treatment of the patient in sinus rhythm who develops heart failure in the acute care setting. On the other hand, Digoxin remains an agent of choice when supraventricular tachyarrhythmias (especially rapid A Fib) complicate acute myocardial infarction and/or occur in association with acute left ventricular failure.

It is important to appreciate that the principal mechanism by which Digoxin slows the ventricular response to rapid A Fib is through an increase in vagal (i.e., *parasympathetic*) tone. As a result, even high doses of the drug will sometimes fail to control the ventricular rate in certain acutely ill patients for whom the tachyarrhythmia primarily reflects catecholamine excess from sympathetic stimulation. For the same reason, Digoxin may be less than optimally effective in controlling the ventricular response of patients receiving a pressor (i.e., catecholamine) infusion with agents such as Epinephrine or Dopamine. For such individuals, the direct catecholamine inhibiting effect of *beta-blockade*- and/or the more direct AV nodal slowing action brought about by *IV Verapamil/Diltiazem* will be much more likely to control the ventricular response to rapid A Fib than the vagotonic effect of digitalis.

Alternatively, *combination therapy* (i.e., concomittant use of IV Digoxin *and* IV Verapamil/Diltiazem) may produce a *synergistic* effect on heart rate control in the emergency setting. Combined use of these drugs in this manner may also reduce adverse effects because lower doses of each agent can often be used.

> It should be emphasized that although Digoxin slows the ventricular response to A Fib/Flutter- the drug *by itself* does not help in converting these arrhythmias to sinus rhythm. Many patients who present with new-onset A Fib/Flutter do *not* persist with the arrhythmia, but instead *spontaneously* convert to sinus rhythm- especially if precipitating factors (i.e., hypoxemia, heart failure, ischemia, and/or electrolyte disturbances) are corrected.

Dose & Route of Administration:

- **IV Loading**- For patients not previously digitalized, consider IV loading with an initial dose of 0.25- 0.50 mg. This may be followed with 0.125- to 0.25 mg IV increments given every 2-6 hours until a *total* loading dose (of 0.75- to 1.50 mg) has been administered over the first 24 hours. One may then begin the next day to administer a daily maintenance dose (either orally or IV- depending on the patient's clinical condition).

- **Maintenance Dosing**- The *average* daily **oral *maintenance* dose** of Digoxin for adults under 60 years of age who have normal renal funciton is **0.25 mg/day**. Lower doses (i.e., **0.125 mg daily**- or every *other* day) are recommended for older individuals and/or in those with renal impairment.

  Occasionally, IV dosing may need to be continued beyond the initial loading phase. This is especially true for acutely ill patients who are unable to take medication orally- and/or for those with persistent tachyarrhythmias in need of a more rapid onset of action than afforded by oral Digoxin. The point to emphasize is that oral Digoxin is *only* 65-70% bioavailable- which means that IV dosing should be *reduced* (by about 30-35%) in order to administer a corresponding amount of active drug (*See section on Relevant Pharmacokinetics below*).

> When doubt exists as to the appropriate amount of Digoxin to administer- obtaining a *stat* serum Digoxin level may prove invaluable in resolving the dilemma (*See below*).

Relevant Pharmacokinetcis of Digoxin:

It is important to emphasize that the dosing schedule suggested above provides no more than a rough guideline. It may need to be varied according to patient tolerance, underlying medical conditions (especially renal function), and the resultant ventricular response.

- The effects of **IV Digoxin** occur more rapidly than is generally appreciated. Onset of action may begin *within* 5-10 minutes! An initial peak of action is typically seen at about 30 to 60 minutes, with a maximum peak effect in about 4 to 6 hours.

- Digoxin is equally effective when administered orally- albeit with a slightly delayed onset of action. The most commonly used oral preparation of the drug is **Lanoxin** which has a ***bioavailability*** of between 65-70%. Therefore (as noted above in the section on dosing)- when using this oral form of the drug, one would have to prescribe approximately one third *more* than the amount prescribed with the IV form to obtain the same effect. That is, an oral dose of 0.325- 0.350 mg of Digoxin will be comparable to an IV dose of ≈0.25 mg. In contrast, bioavailability of the less commonly used Lanoxicaps is much better (90-100%), and probably no correction at all need be made when switching from IV Digoxin to this oral form.

- The ***therapeutic range*** that is cited for serum Digoxin levels varies from one laboratory to the next- but usually falls between **0.8-2.0 ng/ml**. Several additional points should be kept in mind when interpreting the clinical significance of the level:

    i) Considerable *overlap* exists between levels that are therapeutic and toxic. For example, elderly patients may derive significant benefit from the drug at serum levels as low as 0.5 ng/ml. Conversely, if clinical features and/or suggestive arrhythmias are present, a patient may be toxic despite a serum level as low as 1.5 ng/ml!

    ii) The time of the *last* dose is a critical determinant of the serum Digoxin level. Serum levels may be falsely increased by 50% (or more!) if obtained within 2-3 hours of taking the last oral dose. Usually, it is best to wait *at least* 4 hours after the last IV dose- and 6-8 hours after the last oral dose- *before* drawing blood to check a serum level.

    iii) In general, relatively higher serum levels of Digoxin are needed to achieve optimal rate control than are needed to produce its positive inotropic effect. Thus, less drug may be needed when treating a patient with heart failure than when trying to slow the ventricular response of a patient with rapid A Fib or Flutter.

- The ***half-life*** of a drug is the amount of time it takes for 50% (i.e., "half") of that drug to be eliminated from serum. For Digoxin, the half-life varies *between* **36 hours** (for a healthy, young adult)- and **5 days** (for an elderly patient with severe renal failure). Awareness of this range allows you to *estimate* the *half-life* duration of Digoxin for your particular patient (provided you also know the patient's age and renal function). For example, a middle-aged adult with normal renal function probably has a half-life of approximately 2 days. In contrast, an elderly patient with end-stage renal failure is likely to have a near maximally prolonged half-life of between 4-5 days.

- **Digoxin pharmacokinetics are *linear*.** This means that when you *double* the daily dose of the drug- the steady state serum drug level will similarly double. It also means that if an elderly patient with renal failure has an estimated *half-life* of 4 days- it should take approximately this long for a toxic level of 4 ng/ml to decrease by *half* (i.e., to 2 ng/ml)- and 4 *more* days for it to come down to a normal value of 1 ng/ml.

- As a rule of thumb- it generally takes between **3** to **5 half-lives** of a drug to *either* work up to a therapeutic level (if beginning a patient on the drug and giving the expected daily maintenance dose)- or when *stopping* the drug (to eliminate it from the system). Clinical applications of this pharmacokinetic principle are abundant. For example, less severely ill patients who are treated for heart failure in an ambulatory setting may be slowly (and *safely*) loaded with Digoxin over a more gradual period (of about 1 to 2 weeks) simply by starting them on their regular expected maintenance dose. The patient and serum Digoxin level should be checked at the end of this time- realizing that full steady state levels might not be reached for 3 weeks or more if the patient was elderly and had significant renal impairment. Similarly, if *discontinuing* Digoxin in a patient who had been therapeutic- it may take up to 2 to 4 weeks (i.e., 3 to 5 half-lives of drug for that patient) for the drug to be cleared from the body.

Digitalis Toxicity:

By far, the biggest potential drawback to the use of Digitalis is the ever present risk of developing *toxicity*. The very narrow "therapeutic window" that exists between beneficial effects of the drug and toxicity makes it essential to carefully monitor patients on this medication. Clinically, one should be alert to the possibility of ***digitalis toxicity*** whenever any of the signs or symptoms listed below occur in a patient taking the drug:

- nausea, vomiting, or anorexia
- disturbanes in color vision (especially of red-green color perception, or seeing halos around light bulbs)
- new-onset symptoms of psychosis
- new-onset of non-specific complaints of weakness, fatigue, or dizziness
- development of certain cardiac arrhythmias suggestive of digitalis toxicity (i.e., frequent and/or multiform PVCs, ventricular tachycardia, atrial tachycardia with block, accelerated junctional rhythms, Wenckebach rhythms, A Fib with a slow or "regular" ventricular response.

Lower doses of Digoxin are recommended for patients who are likely to be more susceptible to developing toxicity. Such individuals include patients with chronic obstructive pulmonary disease (who may be hypoxemic), patients with electrolyte disturbances (especially hypokalemia, hypomagnesemia, or hypercalcemia), the elderly, patients with renal impairment, hyperthyroidism, and/or in the setting of acute ischemia. In addition, patients who are taking certain medications (such as Quinidine or Verapamil) may experience a drug interaction that significantly increases their serum Digoxin concentration. Steady state levels of drug may be increased by up to 100% (or more!) by concomittant use of Quinidine- and by up to 50% with Verapamil.

> As noted earlier, patients who are particularly sensitive to the effects of Digoxin may sometimes manifest signs of toxicity at serum levels that are still within the "therapeutic range" (i.e, at serum Digoxin levels between 1.5- 2.0 ng/ml). The diagnosis of digitalis toxicity must be a *clinical* one- and should *not* be made exclusively on the basis of the serum Digoxin level.

Treatment of Digitalis Toxicity

A number of interventions should be considered in the treatment of digitalis toxicity- depending on predisposing/associated medical factors and the severity of the patient's clinical condition. These interventions include:

i) Withdrawing digoxin
ii) Telemetry monitoring
iii) Correcting electrolyte abnormalities (especially hypokalemia and hypomagnesemia)
iv) Optimizing the patient's underlying medical condition (i.e., normalizing acid-base and volume status, correcting hypoxemia, treating ischemia, etc.)
v) Consideration of antiarrhythmic therapy (i.e., with Lidocaine or Dilantin) as needed if worrisome ventricular arrhythmias develop
vi) Consideration of *Digoxin antibody fragments* (Digibind).

In many cases of digitalis toxicity, *little more than withdrawing the drug is needed.* Telemetry monitoring is advised if symptoms are associated with significant arrhythmias. It is important to appreciate that because the half-life of Digoxin is commonly prolonged to 3-5 days in older individuals with impaired renal function- it may take *at least* several days (or even a week or more!) for markedly elevated levels in such patients to return to the normal range.

Correction of electrolyte abnormalities is an important component of the treatment of digitalis toxicity. However, care should be taken *not* to administer IV potassium or magnesium too rapidly- since doing so may temporarily exacerbate cardiac arrhythmias.

Lidocaine (in standard doses) and/or Dilantin have been recommended as the antiarrhythmic agents of choice for digitalis-induced cardiac arrhythmias. **Dilantin** is administered in 100 mg incremental doses by *slow* IV infusion (over a period of *at least* 5 minutes for every 100 mg dose)- until the arrhythmia is controlled, a total of 600-1,000 mg have been given, or Dilantin toxicity develops.

At the present time, the principal indication for administration of ***Digibind*** is for treatment of potentially *life-threatening* arrhythmias (i.e., sustained ventricular tachycardia, V Fib, and/or severe bradyarrhythmias not responsive to Atropine) that are the direct result of digitalis toxicity. Use of this modality will *not* be needed for most cases of digitalis toxicity. It should be noted that once Digibind is given, the serum Digoxin level can no longer be used for monitoring the patient (so that it will be difficult to know when to restart the drug).

Special Points:

- The role of Digoxin in the treatment of supraventricular tachyarrhythmias continues to evolve. While fully acknowledging that the drug has withstood the test of time and retains a place in the treatment of certain arrhythmias (especially rapid A Fib/Flutter)- *other* treatment modalities (i.e., use of Verapamil/Diltiazem and/or beta-blockers) may be preferable in many instances. This is especially true in the treatment of patients who are not in heart failure and who are likely to have increased sympathetic tone.

- Digoxin is *not* a benign medication. Caution in dosing is needed to prevent development of toxicity.

- The principal mechanism by which Digoxin slows the ventricular response to A Fib/Flutter is by enhancing vagal tone. The drug may not work well when given to patients with catecholamine excess from sympathetic stimulation. If the decision is made to use Digoxin- the possibility of less than optimal arrhythmia control should be kept in mind. Consideration should then be given to alternative therapy (i.e., swsitching to or adding Verapamil/Diltiazem or beta-blockers) if the desired clinical response is not achieved.

- It appears that Digoxin per se does *not* facilitate conversion of A Fib/Flutter to sinus rhythm. If these arrhythmias persist- other drugs (i.e., Quinidine, Procainamide, etc.) may be added in an attempt to convert the rhythm- and/or synchronized cardioversion may be used.

- If needed, synchronized cardioversion *can* usually be carried out safely in patients who have received therapeutic amounts of Digoxin. However, this procedure is potentially dangerous (*and should be avoided if at all possible!*) when there is a chance of digitalis toxicity.

- Digoxin should only be used with great caution (*if at all*) for treatment of MAT. Not only is the drug relatively ineffective in slowing the ventricular response to MAT- but such patients are particularly prone to developing digitalis toxicity.

- Digoxin is *contraindicated* for use in the treatment of A Fib that occurs in association with WPW. Because Digoxin speeds conduction in the forward direction over the accessory pathway- it may further accelerate the ventricular response to A Fib in such patients, and therefore precipitate development of V Fib. Suspicion that a patient in A Fib may have WPW is suggested by the presence of QRS widening and an *excessively* rapid ventricular response (of 220-250 beats/minute- or more!).

Esmolol

How Dispensed → Ampules containing 10 mg/ml and 2.5 g/10 ml.

Indications:

Indications for the use of IV Esmolol are generally similar to those presented for the use of IV Propranolol (page 155):

- *Refractory ventricular arrhythmias*- especially if acute ischemia, excessive sympathetic discharge, digitalis toxicity, and/or cocaine overdose are suspected as contributing factors.
- *Supraventricular tachyarrhythmias*- as an alternative agent to IV Verapamil/Diltiazem, Adenosine, and/or Digoxin.

In addition, the rapid onset of action of this drug, its short half-life, and availability as a continuous IV infusion make Esmolol ideally suited for treatment of hypertensive urgency/emergency and treatment of patients with acute myocardial infarction.

Mechanism/Clinical Effects

Esmolol is a cardioselective beta-adrenergic blocking agent with a rapid onset of action following IV administration, and a short duration of action. Because its elimination phase half-life is *less* than 10 minutes- adverse effects are generally short-lived and pharmacologic effects will usually dissipate within 15-30 minutes of discontinuing the drug. This confers the drug with a decided advantage compared to other IV beta-blocking agents such as Propranolol, Metoprolol, and Atenolol- which have a significantly longer duration of action (of several hours or more).

IV Esmolol effectively slows the ventricular response to rapid A Fib/Flutter- and it appears to be more effective than IV Verapamil/Diltiazem in converting these arrhythmias to sinus rhythm. The drug is also an effective alternative agent (to IV Verapamil/Diltiazem or Adenosine) for treatment of *reentry* supraventricular tachyarrhythmias such as PSVT.

IV Esmolol is generally safe to administer to patients with acute myocardial infarction- even in the presence of mild to moderate left ventricular dysfunction. Because adverse effects are rapidly reversed, the drug has developed a special role for use in this setting when it becomes important to determine whether a beta-blocking agent can be tolerated. The relative cardioselectivity of Esmolol makes it less likely than other beta-blockers to precipitate bronchospasm in potentially susceptible patients.

Dose & Route of Administration:

Dosing recommendations for use of IV Esmolol are somewhat complex- and this is a decided drawback of using the drug. AHA Guidelines suggest the following protocol (AHA Text- Pg 8-12):

i) Administer an ***initial*** **IV Loading Dose** (of **250-500 µg/kg**) over a 1 minute period.
ii) Follow with a 4 minute infusion at **25-50 µg/kg/minute**.
iii) If the desired response is not obtained- titrate the rate of infusion *upward* by **25-50 µg/kg/minute** at 5-10 minute intervals (up to a *maximal* dose of 200-300 µg/kg/minute).
iv) May then begin oral antiarrhythmic therapy (and *gradually* taper IV Esmolol).

More rapid attainment of optimal therapeutic effect can be achieved with IV Esmolol by readministering the loading dose (of 250-500 µg/kg- given over a 1 minute period) *before* each incremental increase in the rate of infusion. Be sure to continue the maintenance infusion for *at least* 5 minutes after each incremental increase in rate.

Most patients who respond to IV Esmolol do so at maintenance infusion rates of between 50-150 µg/kg/minute. Infusion rates greater than 200 µg/kg/minute are generally *not* advised- because additional clinical benefit is unlikely, and the risk of producing significant hypotension may be unduly increased.

Contraindications/Cautions

As is the case for IV Propranolol (and other IV beta-blockers)- use of IV Esmolol is *contraindicated* in the treatment of patients with acute bronchospasm, and/or significant conduction system abnormality. However, relative cardioselectivity of the drug may make it somewhat less likely than IV Propranolol to precipitate bronchospasm in susceptible patients who are not initially wheezing.

Special caution is urged when contemplating use of a beta-blocking agent in a patient who has (or may have) left ventricular dysfunction. Because beta-blocking drugs all exert a negative inotropic effect, they all have the potential to exacerbate the condition of patients with heart failure. However, two pharmacologic properties of Esmolol make it *less* likely than other IV beta-blockers to precipitate frank cardiac decompensation. As noted earlier, the short half-life of action results in rapid dissipation of clinical effects (usually *within* 15-30 minutes) after infusion of the drug is stopped. Availability of a continuous IV infusion allows moment-to-moment dose titration- with the hope that small incremental increases in dosing will alert the wary clinician when additional dosing may not be tolerated.

IV Esmolol should *not* be used with 30 minutes of giving IV Verapamil/Diltiazem- because the combination of these agents may result in excessive bradycardia (or even asystole).

Special Points:

IV Esmolol is a *cardioselective* beta-blocking drug that is the agent of choice for use in those situations in which it is desirable to administer a *rapidly* acting beta-blocker whose actions reverse promptly if an adverse effect does occur. Unfortunately, three major *drawbacks* make it less likely that this agent will establish a niche in the routine treatment of cardiac arrhythmias:

- The relatively complex nature of its dosing regimen.

- A high incidence of hypotension (especially when dosing increments are made too quickly and the rate of infusion exceeds 200 µg/kg/minute).

- The need to avoid concomitant administration of IV Verapamil/Diltiazem (for *at least* 30 minutes).

Amiodarone

Indications:

- **In the setting of Cardiac Arrest-** *Refractory VT/V Fib* (i.e., that has not responded to standard therapy).

- **In Emergency Cardiac Care-** selected patients with *refractory* supraventricular arrhythmias (including tachyarrhythmias associated with WPW).

> **Note-** IV Amiodarone has recently been approved for general use in this country. However, as of this writing- the drug is *not* yet included in AHA ACLS Guidelines.

Mechanism/Adverse Effects

Amiodarone is a class III antiarrhythmic agent. As such, it prolongs the duration of the myocardial action potential and increases the refractory period without affecting the resting membrane potential of myocardial cells. The drug depresses sinus node function and prolongs the PR, QRS, and QT intervals. The drug also slows AV nodal conduction and exerts an anti-adrenergic effect. Overall, Amiodarone may be the most potent antiarrhythmic agent available for treatment of ventricular arrhythmias, supraventricular arrhythmias, and tachyarrhythmias associated with accessory pathway conduction (i.e., WPW). We feel that the principal use of this drug in the treatment of cardiac arrest will be for patients with refractory V Fib that fails to respond to standard measures- and/or for the patient with recurrent VT who is unable to maintain sinus rhythm with conventional therapy.

The most common adverse effect of IV Amiodarone in the patient who is not in cardiac arrest is hypotension (which presumably results from the drug's vasodilating and negative inotropic actions). This problem sometimes resolves with slowing the rate of IV infusion- but in some patients the drug may need to be stopped.

Dose & Route of Administration:

Until results from additional studies become available, dosing recommendations in the setting of cardiac arrest will be largely *empiric*. The Medical Letter recommends the following regimen (Vol 37:114-115, 1995):

- Consider rapid **IV loading** of **150 mg** of drug over a 10-minute period. This dose may be repeated one or more times (each time over a 10-minute period) for the patient with recurrent VT/V Fib.

- After initial stabilization- follow with slow IV infusion at a rate of **1 mg/minute** over the next **6 hours** (= 60 mg/hour X 6 hours = 360 mg).

- Then continue with a slower IV *maintenance* infusion at a rate of **0.5 mg/minute** over the next **18 hours** (= 30 mg/hr X 18 hours = 540 mg)- or longer, if needed. IV Amiodarone is usually infused for no more than a 2-4 day period. Transition to oral Amiodarone (if indicated) must take into account the very different and highly variable oral pharmacokinetics of the drug.

Special Points:

Although not yet included in AHA Guidelines, IV Amiodarone holds promise of fulfilling an important role in the treatment of refractory cardiac arrest. Clearly the efficacy of Lidocaine and Bretylium has been disappointing as antifibrillatory therapy for patients who fail to respond to initial attempts at defibrillation. Preliminary work with IV Amiodarone suggests that this drug may provide a more effective alternative for antifibrillatory therapy in this situation.

Discussion of the use of Amiodarone (either IV or oral) outside of the setting of cardiac arrest extends beyond the scope of this book. Pharmacokinetics of the drug with oral dosing are both fascinating and problematic. For example, the half-life of oral Amiodarone is estimated to be between 20 to 100 days- which means that clinical (or toxic!) effects of the drug could still be present for literally *months* after Amiodarone was discontinued! Potential side effects with long-term dosing are numerous, and necessitate careful monitoring. Nevertheless, the drug *is* extremely effective- and its ultimate role both in emergency and non-emergency cardiac care remains to be determined.

Aminophylline

How Dispensed:

- **IV Use**- Vials containing 2.5 g- at a concentration of 25 mg/cc.

Suggested Indications

- *Bradyasystolic arrest* (or *severe* hemodynamically significant bradycardia)- that has been *refractory* to standard measures.

> **<u>Note</u>**- As of this writing- *Aminophylline is not yet included in AHA ACLS Guidelines.* We therefore emphasize that use of this drug in the treatment of cardiac arrest is *not* yet generally accepted. Nevertheless, preliminary studies are promising, and suggest that Aminophylline *may* be worth trying- <u>*IF*</u> you have *already* tried Epinephrine, Atropine, pacing- and the patient has failed to respond (i.e., *"You can't be deader than dead"*).

Mechanism/Clinical Effects

The theory proposed to account for the beneficial effect of Aminophylline in asystolic cardiac arrest is both plausible and fascinating. It relates to potential mediation of severe ischemia and bradycardia/asystole by release of *endogenous adenosine* (in the body's attempt to vasodilate and restore myocardial oxygen supply). As a result, endogenous adenosine may accumulate- leading to further exacerbation of ischemia (by a "coronary steal" phenomenon), and/or contributing to (or causing) more profound bradycardia/asystole. The mechanism by which Aminophylline works may therefore result from the known *antagonistic* effect that this drug exerts on adenosine.

> Although clearly more data are needed, it is hard to imagine how administration of Aminophylline could worsen the prognosis of refractory asystolic cardiac arrest. *Consideration might therefore be given to empiric use of this drug for this otherwise almost certainly lethal condition.*

Dose & Route of Administration:

- **<u>IV Bolus</u>**- Give **250 mg IV** (over 1-2 minutes)- which may then be repeated if needed in several minutes.

Adverse Effects

Practically speaking- there are *no* adverse effects to giving Aminophylline to a patient with refractory bradyasystolic arrest- *because this is an otherwise uniformly fatal condition!*

Special Points

Although administration of Aminophylline has admittedly not yet received general acceptance as a recommended intervention in the management of asystolic cardiac arrest- use of the drug *may* offer a potential life-saving treatment for a condition that previously was associated with near-certain death. Preliminary work is encouraging (Viskin et al: Ann Int Med 118:279, 1993). Clearly more studies are needed to determine the ultimate role of this drug in the setting of cardiac arrest.

<u>Section 2F:</u> *Deemphasized Drugs*

Sodium Bicarbonate

<u>How Dispensed</u> → 50 mEq per 50 ml ampule.

Indications

Indications for the use of Sodium Bicarbonate are *limited* in the setting of cardiac arrest. Practically speaking they include:

- Severe *metabolic acidosis* that persists beyond the initial phase (i.e., *beyond* the first 5-15 minutes) of the arrest.
- Cardiac arrest in a patient *known* to have a severe *preexisting* metabolic acidosis *prior* to the arrest-

- *<u>IF</u> any Bicarb is indicated at all during cardiac arrest . . . .*

AHA Guidelines emphasize that in general- ***"Good CPR is the best buffer therapy"*** (AHA Text- Pg 7-15). Several special resuscitation situations exist however, in which use of Sodium Bicarbonate is both appropriate and *likely* to be helpful. These include:

- *Hyperkalemia-* for which Bicarb facilitates potassium entry *into* body cells (and therefore *out of* the extracellular fluid or blood compartment).
- *Tricyclic antidepressant overdose-* with the goal of alkalinizing the serum (ideally to achieve an arterial pH of between 7.45-7.55). Alkalinization of serum pH increases protein binding of these drugs- which may significantly *lessen* the potential for drug toxicity (by reducing the amount of unbound or "active" drug in the serum).
- *Phenobarbital overdose-* with the goal of alkalinizing the urine to facilitate drug elimination.
- *After the arrest is over-* administration of Bicarb *may* be appropriate if *severe* metabolic acidosis persists. In this situation Bicarb may help to buffer the acid washout that is commonly seen with restoration of spontaneous circulation after prolonged arrest (AHA Text- Pg 7-15).

Dose & Route of Administration:

- *<u>IF Sodium Bicarbonate is indicated at all</u>-* an *initial* **IV dose** of **1 mEq/kg** (≈1-1.5 amps) has been recommended for use in cardiac arrest (AHA Text- Pg 7-15). No more than half this amount should be given every 10 minutes. In the postresuscitation phase, ABGs should guide therapy.

> **<u>Note</u>**- Sodium Bicarbonate may be given by ***continuous* IV infusion** when the therapeutic objective is more gradual correction of acidosis and/or alkalinization of serum or urine (AHA Text- Pg 7-15).

Mechanism/Clinical and Adverse Effects

Despite the seemingly intuitive logic that administration of Sodium Bicarbonate to buffer acid should be beneficial during cardiopulmonary arrest- there is little objective data to back this up. During the early minutes of an arrest, the *primary* acid-base disturbance is ***respiratory* acidosis**. This results from hypoventilation. If a victim of cardiopulmonary arrest can be adequately ventilated and perfused during this critical period- *the need for Sodium Bicarbonate should be minimal (at most).*

It appears that significant metabolic acidosis does *not* develop in cardiopulmonary arrest for *at least* some of time (5-15 minutes?) after patient collapse. Since the primary abnormality during these initial minutes is *hypoventilation* (i.e., *respiratory* acidosis)- it would seem far more appropriate to correct this acidosis by improving ventilation (i.e., *hyperventilating* the patient) than by administering Bicarb.

Sodium Bicarbonate therapy is NOT benign. Adverse effects of excessive administration of this agent include extreme alkalosis, hyperosmolality, hypokalemia, sodium overload, shifting of the oxyhemoglobin dissociation curve leftward (with consequent impaired oxygen release to the tissues), and precipitation of convulsions, ischemia, and/or arrhythmias. Moreover, unless adequate ventilation is achieved, carbon dioxide (CO_2) will tend to accumulate. Since CO_2 is *freely diffusable* across cellular and organ membranes- it readily enters the brain and heart where it is likely to further depress function by producing a **paradoxical *intracellular* acidosis**. Administration of Bicarb only serves to aggravate this process.

The manner in which a paradoxical intracellular acidosis may be produced by Sodium Bicarbonate therapy can best be explained by means of the following equation:

$$H^+ + HCO_3^- \leftrightarrow H_2CO_3 \leftrightarrow H_2O + CO_2$$

According to this equation, acid (i.e., *hydrogen ion* = $\mathbf{H^+}$) is neutralized by *bicarbonate ion* (= $\mathbf{HCO3^-}$)- which is provided by administered Sodium Bicarbonate. This results in formation of a weak acid (carbonic acid = $\mathbf{H_2CO_3}$), which subsequently breaks down into *water* ($\mathbf{H_2O}$) and *carbon dioxide* ($\mathbf{CO_2}$).

The source of the problem in the above equation is the $\mathbf{CO_2}$- because this gas is freely diffusable across cellular membranes. Once inside the various body cells- *CO_2 combines with H_2O to drive the above reversible equation back to the left.* That is, CO_2 and H_2O combine to form H_2CO_3 - which then breaks down to produce HCO_3^- and H^+.

Thus, the end result of trying to neutralize *extracellular* acidosis (i.e., the excess concentration of H^+ ions in blood) by IV administration of Bicarb (i.e., HCO_3 -) will be to generate *additional* CO_2. This CO_2 readily diffuses into body cells (*including* the cells of the heart and brain). Excess CO_2 accumulates *within the cells-* and results in a *reversal* of the process whereby the above equation is now driven back to the left- ultimately leading to production of an excess concentration of *intracellular* H^+ ions. This results in a lowering of intracellular pH- and production of the *paradoxical intracellular acidosis.*

In the setting of cardiac arrest, the old standby- ***arterial blood gas (ABG) studies***- is *not* the dependable predictor of intracellular acid-base status that we used to think. Instead, it is the pH of mixed *venous* blood that most closely reflects the true pH within the cells. Unfortunately, there is no *practical* way to rapidly determine the pH of mixed venous blood during a code.

With the onset of cardiac arrest a significant discrepancy (of up to several pH units) *rapidly* develops between arterial and mixed venous blood. As a result, severe venous hypercarbia and acidosis may *simultaneously* exist with arterial alkalosis. Fortunately, mixed venous acidosis (and hence *intracellular* acidosis) can usually be corrected for the most part simply by hyperventilation. Elimination of excess CO_2 by hyperventilation helps to prevent the above cited equation from being driven back to the left.

In the past, one or more ampules of Sodium Bicarbonate were almost always *reflexively* given at the onset of cardiopulmonary arrest, and repeated liberally thereafter until arterial blood pH values normalized. While this practice often succeeded in correcting arterial pH (and made the emergency care provider feel better because ABG values "improved")- in the long run it *exacerbated* the situation by increasing the degree of *intracellular* acidosis. We now appreciate that additional CO_2 generated as a result of IV-adminstered Sodium Bicarbonate readily diffuses into body cells- and produces an *intramyocardial* and *intracerebral* acidosis. This effect ultimately leads to *depression* of both myocardial and cerebral function.

> Surprisingly, ABGs obtained during cardiopulmonary resuscitation often demonstrate relatively normal PaO_2 readings. *Such readings may well be misleading.* Pulmonary blood flow is dramatically reduced in patients with cardiac arrest who are being resuscitated. High oxygen saturation values may result. It is important to realize that near "perfect" oxygen saturation in this situation is primarily a reflection of the markedly *prolonged* time required for passage of blood through the pulmonary circuit. It indicates *little* about the much larger pool of stagnant, acidotic, hypercarbic, and hypoxic blood that resides in most body tissues.

Traditionally, the rationale for administering Bicarb to patients in cardiac arrest has been based on a number of assumptions:

i) that such treatment would limit lactate production.
ii) that intracellular pH could be corrected in a predictable manner
iii) that survival would be improved.

None of the above assumptions have proven to be true. Instead, we now know that Bicarb administration *impairs* tissue oxygenation- an effect that leads to development of anaerobic metabolism and an *increase* in lactate production. Intracellular acidosis is exacerbated by Bicarbonate therapy, and myocardial contractility is reduced. Finally, the hypertonicity of Sodium Bicarbonate has been shown to *reduce* aortic diastolic pressure and increase right atrial pressure. This leads to an overall reduction in coronary perfusion pressure (which is the critical determinant of survival during cardiopulmonary resuscitation). In summary- *survival of patients with cardiac arrest is not improved by treatment with Sodium Bicarbonate.* Clinically- there appears to be little (or no) justification for rapid correction of arrest-induced metabolic acidosis- especially if arterial pH is 7.15-7.20, or higher. Even when arterial pH is lower than this- *trying to correct intraarterial pH with Sodium Bicarbonate may be harmful.*

Special Points:

- With the usual scenario that occurs during cardiopulmonary arrest- the acidosis that develops appears to be primarily *respiratory* in nature during the *early* minutes after patient collapse. *Appropriate initial therapy should therefore be aimed at optimizing ventilation.* Bicarb administration is probably *not* indicated for *at least* the first 5-10 minutes of the resuscitation effort- *if it is ever indicated at all . . .*

- The only exceptions to the above generality (when earlier Bicarb administration may be appropriate)- is for patients who are *known* to have a severe *preexisting* acidosis prior to the arrest- and/or for patients with special resuscitation situations (such as hyperkalemia and drug overdose from tricyclic antidepressants or phenobarbital).

- Standard ABG studies in cardiac arrest cannot be relied upon because they do *not* accurately reflect the true state of *intracellular* homeostasis. Even if mixed venous blood gas studies were routinely available to emergency care providers, one would still be faced with the dilemma of knowing that Bicarb administration may paradoxically *exacerbate* the degree of intracellular acidosis- and ultimately result in depression of cerebral and myocardial function.

- ABG studies do become a reliable indicator of intracellular homeostasis *after* restoration of spontaneous circulation. If treatment of persistent severe metabolic acidosis is contemplated in the post-resuscitation phase (after restoration of spontaneous circulation)- Bicarb therapy should be guided by ABG results.

Calcium Chloride

How Dispensed → The 10% solution of Calcium Chloride contains 1,000 mg (=13.6 mEq) of calcium per 10 ml syringe.

Dose & Route of Administration:

- **IV Bolus**- Give **500-1,000 mg** (5-10 ml) by ***slow* IV** (over 5-10 minutes). May repeat every 10 minutes if needed up to 1-2 g. Lower doses of drug (i.e., 250-500 mg IV) may be adequate for calcium pre-treatment (i.e., prior to use of IV Verapamil/Diltiazem). In contrast, as much as 4 g may be needed for treatment of refractory calcium channel blocker toxicity (AHA Text- Pg 10-23).

Indications

In the acute care setting the indications for Calcium Chloride are primarily limited to 4 clinical situations:

i) *Hypocalcemia*
ii) *Hyperkalemia*
iii) As *PRE-Treatment* prior to IV use of Verapamil/Diltiazem
iv) Treatment of *calcium channel blocker toxicity* (i.e., if marked bradycardia/asystole occurs following use of Verapamil/Diltiazem.

Mechanism/Clinical and Adverse Effects

In the past, Calcium Chloride had been routinely recommended for treatment of asystole and EMD. *No longer.* Clinical data in support of these indications in the setting of cardiac arrest are lacking. Previous reports on the use of Calcium Chloride in the setting of cardiac arrest were largely anecdotal, and included surgical patients (who were likely to be hypocalcemic from multiple blood transfusions) and patients with pulseless intraventricular conduction defects that were the result of hyperkalemia. Both of these conditions should have been *expected* to respond to Calcium administration. If anything, experience with the use of Calcium Chloride for patients with prehospital cardiovascular collapse and asystole have suggested an *adverse* effect on ultimate outcome. Undesirable clinical actions of the drug include stimulation of ventricular excitability, suppression of sinus impulse formation, and possibly precipitation of spasm in the cerebral microvasculature. Given too rapidly or in excess amount, IV administration of Calcium may produce marked heart rate slowing or even asystole.

At the present time, indications for the use of Calcium Chloride in the emergency care setting relate principally to those situations for which administration may reverse (or prevent) deficiency states of this cation and for acute treatment of hyperkalemia. In the normal heart, the positive inotropic and vasoconstricting effect of the drug raises systolic blood pressure. This accounts for its beneficial effect as *pre-treatment* prior to use of Verapamil/Diltiazem. Infusion of Calcium *minimizes* the hypotensive response of these drugs *without* diminishing their efficacy in converting/controlling the ventricular response of supraventricular tachyarrhythmias. Calcium pre-treatment might be considered particularly for patients with borderline hemodynamic status (i.e., systolic blood pressure of *less* than 100 mm Hg) in association with their tachyarrhythmia.

In hyperkalemia, the mechanism of Calcium Chloride is not the result of affecting an actual lowering of the serum potassium level- but rather of *antagonizing* the toxic effects of excess potassium. Because onset of action of Calcium in this situation is extremely rapid (i.e., *within* minutes)- it is probably the best *initial* agent to administer for true hyperkalemic emergencies. Following this with glucose/insulin infusion and/or administration of Sodium Bicarbonate may then be appropriate to facilitate potassium uptake into body cells (which will acutely lower serum potassium levels). Removal of potassium from the body may then be accomplished (over the next day) with use of cation exchange resins such as Kayexalate.

Special Points:

- The dose of Calcium Chloride should be individualized depending on the condition being treated and the patient's clinical response. In general, dosing is begun with 500-1,000 mg of a 10% solution of Calcium Choride infused IV over a 5-10 minute period. Too rapid IV infusion may produce a generalized sensation of "heat" to the patient- which usually resolves if the rate of infusion is slowed or temporarily stopped.

- If the indication for replacement is less urgent (i.e., less severe hypocalcemia in a hemodynamically stable patient)- Calcium Chloride may be added to the patient's IV solution and more gradually infused over a period of several hours.

- Although Calcium Chloride is the most commonly administered form of this cation- *other* calcium preparations are available. The point to emphasize is that the amount of *elemental* calcium (i.e., the potency) of each preparation may vary significantly. For example, *three* times as much elemental calcium is contained in one 10 ml ampule of ***Calcium Chloride*** as in one 10 ml ampule of ***Calcium Gluconate*** (i.e., 270 mg compared to 90 mg). Thus, compared to Calcium Chloride- *larger amounts of Calcium Gluconate are needed to obtain the same therapeutic effect.* Awareness of the particular preparation being administered is therefore essential.

- Calcium should *not* be administered in association with Sodium Bicarbonate (because combination of these two drugs may precipitate out).

- Calcium must be carefully administered to patients receiving Digoxin (because the drug increases ventricular irritability and may facilitate development of digitalis toxicity).

- Finally, although indications for the use of Calcium Chloride are clearly limited in emergency cardiac care- it is important *not* to forget about this drug in situations such as calcium channel blocker-induced bradycardia/asystole for which Calcium administration may be lifesaving.

Isoproterenol

How Dispensed → 1 mg vials.

Indications:

Indications for Isoproterenol have been dramatically reduced in recent years:

- AHA Guidelines allow that Isoproterenol "can be used" for *temporary* control of hemodynamically significant bradycardia in the patient with a pulse. However, they emphasize that Atropine, pacing, Dopamine, and Epinephrine should all be used *before* Isoproterenol for treatment of symptomatic bradycardia (AHA Text- Pg 8-6).

- AHA Guidelines suggest that the major remaining indication for Isoproterenol at this time is for the transplant patient with a denervated heart (AHA Text- Pg 8-6).

Dose & Route of Administration:

- **IV Infusion**- Mix 1 mg in 250 ml of D5W, and *begin* drip @ 30 drops/min (=2 μg/minute). Titrate infusion to clinical effect (but do *not* exceed 10 μg/minute).

At low doses (i.e., <10 μg/minute)- Isoproterenol is designated a **Class IIb** drug for providing *pure* chronotropic support to *selected* bradycardic patients who are not hypotensive. *The drug should not be used at higher doses.*

Mechanism/Clinical and Adverse Effects

Isoproterenol is a pure beta-adrenergic receptor stimulating agent which exerts an equipotent effect on beta-1 and beta-2 receptors. The former action results in enhanced myocardial contractility and an increase in heart rate (i.e., positive inotropic and chronotropic effects)- whereas the beta-2 adrenergic stimulating effect results in vasodilatation and a reduction in systemic vascular resistance.

Although in the past, Isoproterenol had been recommended as a vasopressor of choice in the setting of cardiac arrest- use of the drug has been greatly *deemphasized* in recent years. There are many reasons for this deemphasis. Adverse effects that are likely to be seen with the use of Isoproterenol include excessive acceleration of heart rate, arrhythmogenicity, increased myocardial oxygen consumption, hypotension, and decreased myocardial and vital organ perfusion.

The excessive tachycardia so commonly seen in association with Isoproterenol infusion may be deleterious in several ways. Because of disproportionate shortening of the period of diastole, left ventricular filling time is curtailed. Tachycardia also increases myocardial oxygen consumption and predisposes the patient to myocardial ischemia and cardiac arrhythmias.

Hypotension is likely to result from the reduction in systemic vascular resistance. The effect is likely to further reduce aortic diastolic pressure and coronary perfusion. As a result, Isoproterenol is now felt to be *contraindicated* as a treatment measure in the arrested heart (i.e., for ventricular fibrillation, asystole, or EMD). In the patient with a spontaneous circulation, the vasodilatory effect of Isoproterenol tends to redistribute blood flow to *nonvital* organs (i.e., skin and skeletal muscle). This further compromises oxygen delivery to the heart, brain, and kidneys. Thus, when confronted with a patient in cardiac arrest or in a hemodynamically significant bradyarrhythmia- use of a pressor agent with alpha-adrenergic (vasoconstrictor) activity (i.e., Epinephrine or Dopamine) is far preferable to the use of Isoproterenol. The drug could be of benefit in providing pure chronotropic support (i.e., for the severe bradycardia patient who is not hypotensive)- but normotension in this situation is distinctly uncommon.

Special Points:

- Isoproterenol has become a *deemphasized* drug. It is now *contraindicated* (i.e., **Class III**- or possibly *harmful!*) for treatment of asystole, EMD, and V Fib because it increases myocardial oxygen consumption and its pure beta-adrenergic effect results in vasodilatation (which *lowers* aortic diastolic pressure and *reduces* coronary flow!). Isoproterenol might still be of some use for selected bradycardic patients in providing *pure* chronotropic support- but Atropine, pacing, and *other* vasopressors (i.e., Epinephrine and Dopamine) should clearly be used first.

Section 2G: *Pediatric Resuscitation*

Pediatric resuscitation is a topic unto itself. Although full discussion of this issue is best reserved for comprehensive review in an AHA/AAP (American Academy of Pediatrics) course in ***P**ediatric **A**dvanced **L**ife **S**upport* (i.e., ***PALS***)- we have included a brief section in this book on the most important drugs used in pediatric resuscitation because: 1) Adult ACLS providers are likely to at least *occasionally* encounter cardiopulmonary emergencies in children; and 2) Dosing considerations for the drugs used in pediatric resuscitation are very different than for use of the same drugs in adults. Ready reference to a source of information on drugs used in pediatric resuscitation may greatly facilitate dose determination at the time of emergency.

Dosing recommendations cited in this section are based on weight of the child in kilograms (kg)- with specific values provided for a **10 kg**- **20 kg**- and **30 kg** patient- and inclusion of the recommended adult dose for comparison.

Reference is periodically made in this section to the American Heart Association (AHA) Textbook in ***P**ediatric **A**dvanced **L**ife **S**upport* (***PALS***)- Chameides L, Hazinski MF (Eds), American Heart Association, Dallas, 1994.

Overview of KEY Concepts in Pediatric Resuscitation

Inadequate oxygenation is the *most* common cause of cardiac arrest in children! As a result, the most important *initial focus* of cardiopulmonary resuscitation in pediatric patients *must* be to optimize ventilation/oxygenation- *rather than* administering drugs.

- The pediatric heart most often responds to hypoxemia by *slowing* the heart rate. This is why ***asystole*** and ***bradyarrhythmias*** (i.e., *sinus bradycardia- sinus node arrest* with a slow *escape* rhythm- severe bradycardia from *advanced AV block*)- are the most common ***preterminal* rhythms** to be seen in association with cardiopulmonary arrest in children.

- Establishing a patent airway that allows adequate ventilation and oxygenation (*enhanced* by supplemental oxygen) is the *KEY* to success- *and will often be all that is needed.* Practically speaking then- **Oxygen** is the *most important drug* in pediatric resuscitation.

- In addition to hypoxemia, other factors that are likely to contribute to causing pediatric cardiopulmonary arrest/arrhythmogenesis include *acidosis- hypotension- electrolyte* disturbance- *hypoglycemia- hypothermia-* and/or the presence of an *underlying illness* (i.e., sepsis, pneumonia, dehydration, etc.). Correction of ***underlying disorders*** is therefore the second important *KEY* for successful resuscitation in children.

- If pharmacologic therapy *is* needed for treatment of pediatric bradycardia/asystole- ***Epinephrine*** is the drug of choice (*See below*). Atropine is a *second-line* agent that should probably be used *only* when symptoms are *severe* and the patient has *not* responded to other measures (*including* adequate oxygenation and Epinephrine).

Arrhythmia Interpretation: KEY Concepts

The intricacies of arrhythmia interpretation are far less important in the treatment of pediatric resuscitation than they are in the treatment of adults. This is because specific treatment of the rhythm per se is far less likely to be needed.

- Practically speaking- most arrhythmias seen during pediatric resuscitation are *SUPRAventricular.* By far, the most common *mechanism* is ***sinus***- and the most common rhythms seen are sinus *bradycardia- tachycardia-* or *normal* sinus rhythm.

- Differentiation between the sinus mechanism rhythms depends *both* on the patient's age as well as on the clinical condition. For example- a heart rate of 120 beats/minute should be considered as normal for children up to 2 years of age. Mean heart rate in children does not drop below 100 beats/minute until about 8 years of age. On the other hand, a seemingly "normal" heart rate of 80 beats/minute most probably reflects a *relative* bradycardia when it occurs in the setting of a cardiopulmonary arrest in a child.

- Unlike the situation in adults- ***Pulseless VT/V Fib*** are extremely *uncommon* arrhythmias in pediatric arrests. As a result- *defibrillation is only rarely needed in pediatric resuscitation.* (In cases when V Fib *does* occur in a child- it is almost always associated with congenital heart disease- and/or following a *prolonged* period of hypoxemia from a preceding respiratory arrest.)

- *In infants-* the most common tachyarrhythmia to produce hemodynamic instability is ***PSVT*** (*Paroxysmal SupraVentricular Tachycardia* . Heart rates of infants with this rhythm may be as fast as 250-300 beats/minute. However, because sinus tachycardia may also attain heart rates of over 200 beats/minute in this age group- differentiation between sinus tachycardia and PSVT will *not* always be easy.

Epinephrine

Next to Oxygen- ***Epinephrine*** is the most important drug used in pediatric resuscitation. Unfortunately, the optimal dose of Epinephrine for use in pediatric resuscitation remains uncertain. Two principal factors account for this uncertainty: 1) the limited number of clinical trials that have been performed on the use of this drug in the treatment of pediatric cardiopulmonary arrest; and 2) the clinical reality that *regardless* of whatever interventions are tried- the likelihood of achieving meaningful *long-term survival* (i.e., with intact neurologic function) is exceedingly small.

Recommendations for ***Dosing of Epinephrine*** for pediatric resuscitation are based on the following premises:

- *Lower doses* of Epinephrine (i.e., **0.01 mg/kg**) may be effective in the treatment of symptomatic bradycardia- *and should be tried first.*
- Significantly *higher doses* of Epinephrine are likely to be needed for more severe bradycardia- especially for treatment of children with asystolic or pulseless cardiac arrest. As a result, a higher dose of IV Epinephrine (i.e., **0.1 mg/kg**) should be tried after 3-5 minutes- *IF* the patient fails to respond to the lower (i.e., 0.01 mg/kg) dose.
- Epinephrine (in appropriate doses) should be repeated on a *regular* basis (i.e., *every* ***3-5 minutes***- as needed)- *throughout* the resuscitative effort if the patient fails to respond to other measures.
- *If IV access cannot be achieved*- Epinephrine (as well as *Lidocaine* and *Atropine*)- can be given by the ***EndoTracheal (ET) route.*** Because absorption following ET administration is *less* reliable- *higher doses* of drug should be used than for IV administration (*See below*).
- Epinephrine (as well as *other drugs, fluids,* and *blood*) may also be given by the ***IntraOsseous (IO) route.*** Because absorption of drugs and fluids is *excellent* by this route (with onset of action and peak serum levels being *comparable* to that achieved following IV administration)- recommendations for dosing (*of both drug boluses and continuous infusions*) by the **IO route** are virtually the *same* as recommendations for **IV dosing**.

> **Note**- Absorption of Epinephrine following *either* **IV** *or* **IO** administration is superior to absorption of drug following administration by the **ET** route. As a result, *both* IV and IO access are preferred over the ET route for drug administration. In general, if reliable IV access cannot be achieved in a child *less* than 6 years of age *within* 3 attempts (and/or *within* ≈90 seconds)- *then an attempt should be made to establish* ***IO*** *access* (AHA Text- Pg 1-64).

Epinephrine Dosing- Treatment of Symptomatic Bradycardia:

- ***Dose** for **IV** or **IO** administration* = **0.01 mg/kg** (0.1 mL/kg of 1:10,000 solution). This dose may be repeated every 3-5 minutes (AHA PALS Text- Pg 6-6).
- ***Dose** for **ET** administration* = **0.1 mg/kg** (0.1 mL/kg of 1:1,000 solution). This dose may be repeated every 3-5 minutes (AHA PALS Text- Pg 6-6).

> **Note**- The dose of ***Epinephrine*** recommended for ***ET*** administration is now **10 times greater** than the dose recommended for either IV or IO administration (0.1 mg/kg *compared to* 0.01 mg/kg). However, because the *concentration* of the Epinephrine solution recommended for ET administration *also* differs by a factor of 10 (i.e., 1:1,000 soln. *instead* of 1:10,000)- the *total* amount of fluid delivered to a child of any given body weight should be the same- *regardless* of whether the drug is given by the IV, IO, or ET routes (*See Table below*).

Epinephrine Dosing: ***For Treatment of Symptomatic Bradycardia***

Weight of Patient	Dose for IV or IO Bolus Administration (= 0.01 mg/kg) (= 0.1 mL/kg of 1:**10,000** soln.)	Dose for ET Administration (= 0.1 mg/kg) (= 0.1 mL/kg of 1:**1,000** soln.)
10 kg	**0.1 mg** (1 ml of 1:10,000 soln.)	**1 mg ET** (1 ml of 1:1,000 soln.)
20 kg	**0.2 mg** (2 ml of 1:10,000 soln.)	**2 mg ET** (2 ml of 1:1,000 soln.)
30 kg	**0.3 mg** (3 ml of 1:10,000 soln.)	**3 mg ET** (3 ml of 1:1,000 soln.)
Adult Dose	1.0 mg IV (= SDE)	≈ **2-2.5 mg ET** (*as initial dose*)

> **Note**- New AHA recommendations that we cite on these pages advise use of *differing concentrations* of Epinephrine (i.e., use of a **1:10,000 soln.** and **1:1,000 soln.**- when giving *lower* and *higher* doses of drug, respectively). As a result- *extreme care must be taken to avoid errors in dosing* !!!

Epinephrine Dosing- Treatment of Asystole/Pulseless Arrest:

- ***Initial Dose*** *for* **IV** *or* **IO** *administration* = **0.01 mg/kg** (0.1 mL/kg of 1:10,000 solution)- *which is the SAME dose recommended for use of IV (or IO) Epinephrine in treating symptomatic Bradycardia!*
- ***Initial Dose*** *for* **ET** *administration* = **0.1 mg/kg** (0.1 mL/kg of 1:1,000 solution)- *which is the SAME dose recommended for use of ET Epinephrine in treating symptomatic Bradycardia!*
- ***2nd (and subsequent) Doses*** *for* **IV**, **IO**, *or* **ET** *administration* = **0.1 mg/kg** (0.1 mL/kg of 1:1,000 solution)- *given every* ***3-5 minutes*** *as needed.*

Epinephrine Dosing: ***For Treatment of Asystolic or Pulseless Arrest***

Weight of Patient	***Initial Dose*** **for IV or IO Bolus Administration*** (= 0.01 mg/kg) (= 0.1 mL/kg of 1:**10,000** soln.)	**2nd (and Subsequent) Doses for IV, IO, or ET* Bolus Administration** (= 0.1 mg/kg) (= 0.1 mL/kg of 1:**1,000** soln.)
10 kg	**0.1 mg** (1 ml of 1:10,000 soln.)	**1 mg** (1 ml of 1:1,000 soln.)
20 kg	**0.2 mg** (2 ml of 1:10,000 soln.)	**2 mg** (2 ml of 1:1,000 soln.)
30 kg	**0.3 mg** (3 ml of 1:10,000 soln.)	**3 mg** (3 ml of 1:1,000 soln.)
Adult Dose	1.0 mg IV (= **SDE**)	*Highly variable* (i.e., *SDE to HDE*)

* **Note**- For simplicity, *we have not indicated the Initial Dose for ET Bolus administration in this Table.* The *initial dose* of **Epinephrine** recommended for **ET bolus administration** of *asystolic or pulseless arrest* is the *SAME* as that recommended for treatment of *symptomatic bradycardia* (= **0.1 mg/kg** = 0.1 mL/kg of 1:1,000 solution).

IV Infusion of Epinephrine

The recommended range for ***IV Infusion of Epinephrine*** in pediatric patients is *between* **0.1- 1.0 μg/kg/minute**. Preparation for IV infusion may be accomplished as follows:

- Mix [0.6 mg X body weight (kg)] of drug in 100 ml of **diluent** (D5W, NS, or Ringer's lactate). At this concentration:

  - 1 drop/minute = 0.1 μg/kg/minute. *Titrate to effect.*

Weight of Patient	**How to Mix *EPINEPHRINE***	***Initial* Rate**	***Maximum* Rate***
10 kg	Mix **6 mg** (i.e., 0.6 X 10) in 100 ml	1 drop/minute (= 1 μg/min)	10 drops/min (= 10 μg/min)
20 kg	Mix **12 mg** (i.e., 0.6 X 20) in 100 ml	1 drop/minute (= 2 μg/min)	10 drops/min (= 20 μg/min)
30 kg	Mix **18 mg** (i.e., 0.6 X 30) in 100 ml	1 drop/minute (= 3 μg/min)	10 drops/min (= 30 μg/min)
Adult Dose	1 mg in 250 ml D5W	15-30 drops/minute (= 1-2 μg/min)	*Titrate upward*

* Higher doses may be used if asystole persists and/or the patient fails to respond.

> **Note**- The beauty of preparing pediatric IV infusions using the above parameters (i.e., *mixing* ***0.6 mg*** of the drug *X* ***body weight*** in **kg**- *in* ***100 ml*** of dliluent)- is that the number on the infusion pump (which indicates the number of ***ml/hr*** infused)- will be *identical* to the number of ***drops/minute*** !!! Because of the small quantities of drug required for pediatric IV infusions- it is essential to use an *infusion pump* to ensure accuracy.

Atropine

As emphasized in the beginning of this section- ***Atropine*** should be considered a *second-line* drug (and no more than a *third-line* treatment measure) for management of pediatric bradyarrhythmias. The treatment of choice should always entail focused efforts to ensure that ventilation and oxygenation are adequate. IF despite these efforts pharmacologic therapy *is* still needed for treatment of pediatric bradycardia/asystole- the drug of choice should be ***Epinephrine*** (and not Atropine).

> The point to emphasize is that Atropine should probably *not* be used to treat pediatric bradycardia- until *after* Epinephrine has been tried *and* adequate oxygenation/ventilation has been assured.

- *IV Dosing of Atropine*- Give **0.02 mg/kg**. May repeat this dose every 5 minutes (if needed)- up to a ***total* dose** of **1.0 mg** in a child- or up to **2.0 mg** in an adolescent (AHA PALS Text- Pg 6-9).

  Do *not* give less than 0.1 mg in a single dose (regardless of the child's body weight). The *maximal* recommended dose of Atropine for use in pediatric resuscitation is 0.5 mg for a child (or 1.0 mg in an adolescent).

Weight of Patient	Single IV Dose of *Atropine*
10 kg	0.2 mg
20 kg	0.4 mg
30 kg	0.6 mg
Adult Dose	0.5- 1.0 mg

Dopamine

The pharmacologic effects of ***Dopamine*** are *dose-dependent.* As is the case for adults, infusion of *Epinephrine* may be preferable to Dopamine when there is marked circulatory instability- and/or when hypotension persists *despite* higher infusion rates of Dopamine.

- *At LOW infusion rates* (i.e., **5-10 µg/kg/minute**)- dilates renal and mesenteric blood vessels (so urine output may increase)- but heart rate and BP will usually *not* be affected (i.e., predominant *dopaminergic* effect).

- *At MODERATE infusion rates* (i.e., **10-20 µg/kg/minute**)- increases cardiac output- usually with only a modest effect on peripheral vascular resistance and BP (i.e., *beta-adrenergic* effect prevails).

- *At HIGH infusion rates* (i.e., **>20 µg/kg/minute**)- results in intense peripheral vasoconstriction (as *alpha-adrenergic* effect takes over)- producing a significant increase in peripheral vascular resistance and BP.

> **Note**- Pediatric definitions of dose-related effects with Dopamine infusion differ slightly from those of adults. In general, infusion of Dopamine is begun at a relatively *higher* infusion rate (of **10 µg/kg/minute**) in pediatric patients (AHA PALS Text- Pg 6-13).

IV Infusion Dose of Dopamine

The recommended range for ***IV Infusion of Dopamine*** in pediatric patients is *between* **10-20 µg/kg/minute**. Preparation for IV infusion may be accomplished as follows:

- Mix [6 mg X body weight (kg)] of drug in 100 ml of **diluent** (D5W, NS, or Ringer's lactate). At this concentration:

  - 1 drop/minute = 1.0 µg/kg/minute
  - 10 drops/minute = **10 µg/kg/minute** (= usual *initial* rate of infusion)
  - 20 drops/minute = 20 µg/kg/minute (= *maximum* rate of infusion)

Weight of Patient	**How to Mix *Dopamine***	***Initial* Rate**	***Maximum* Rate**
10 kg	Mix **60 mg** (i.e., 6 X 10) in 100 ml	10 drops/minute (= 100 µg/min)	20 drops/min (= 200 µg/min)
20 kg	Mix **120 mg** (i.e., 6 X 20) in 100 ml	10 drops/minute (= 200 µg/min)	20 drops/min (= 400 µg/min)
30 kg	Mix **180 mg** (i.e., 6 X 30) in 100 ml	10 drops/minute (= 300 µg/min)	20 drops/min (= 600 µg/min)
Adult Dose	200 mg in 250 ml D5W	30 drops/minute (= 400 µg/min)	*Titrate upward*

> **Note**- The beauty of preparing pediatric IV infusions using the above parameters (i.e., *mixing* ***6 mg*** of the drug *X* ***body weight*** in **kg**- *in* ***100 ml*** of dliluent)- is that the number on the infusion pump (which indicates the number of ***ml/hr*** infused)- will be *identical* to the number of ***drops/minute*** (*as well as* to the number of ***µg/kg/minute***) !!! Because of the small quantities of drug required for pediatric IV infusions- it is essential to use an *infusion pump* to ensure accuracy.

Lidocaine

Because malignant ventricular arrhythmias are much less commonly seen in association with pediatric cardiopulmonary arrest- *Lidocaine will not be needed in most pediatric codes.*

- ***Bolus Dose**- for **IV** or **IO** administration* = **1.0 mg/kg**. Thus, a **10 kg** child should receive a **10 mg** bolus dose of Lidocaine- a 20 kg child should receive 20 kg- and so on.

IV Infusion Dose of Lidocaine

The recommended range for ***IV Infusion of Lidocaine*** in pediatric patients is *between* **20-50 µg/kg/minute**. Preparation for IV infusion may be accomplished as follows:

- Mix 120 mg of Lidocaine in 100 ml of D5W (= **1,200 µg/ml** as the *concentration* of drug). At this concentration:

  - 1 drop/kg/minute = 20 µg/kg/minute (*Initial* rate)
  - 2.5 drops/kg/minute = 50 µg/kg/minute (*Maximum* rate).

Weight of Patient	**How to Mix *Lidocaine***	***Initial* Rate**	***Maximum* Rate**
10 kg	120 mg in 100 ml D5W	10 drops/min (= 20 µg/kg/min X 10 kg = 200 µg/min = 0.2 mg/min)	25 drops/min (= 0.5 mg/min)
20 kg	120 mg in 100 ml D5W	20 drops/min (= 400 µg/min = 0.4 mg/min)	50 drops/min (= 1.0 mg/min)
30 kg	120 mg in 100 ml D5W	30 drops/min (= 600 µg/min = 0.6 mg/min)	75 drops/min (= 1.5 mg/min)
Adult Dose	1,000 mg in 250 ml D5W	≈30 drops/min = 2 mg/min	4 mg/min

Note- The beauty of preparing pediatric IV infusions using the above parameters is that the number on the infusion pump (which indicates the number of ***ml/hr*** infused)- will be *identical* to the number of ***drops/minute*** !!! Because of the small quantities of drug required for pediatric IV infusions- it is essential to use an *infusion pump* to ensure accuracy.

Adenosine

As noted at the beginning of this section, the most common tachyarrhythmia to produce hemodynamic instability in *infants* is ***PSVT***- which often attains heart rates in excess of 200-250 beats/minute in this age group.

Because of its rapid rate- PSVT may *not* be well tolerated when it occurs in infants or small children. If allowed to persist, infants in particular face a great risk of developing congestive heart failure and/or shock. The *younger* the infant, the *faster* the ventricular rate (especially if >180 beats/minute), and the *longer the duration* of the tachycardia (especially if over 24 hours)- the more likely (*and the sooner*) that heart failure will develop. Clinically then, if the infant does not readily respond to a ***vagal* maneuver** (i.e., application of an *ice pack* to the face for ≈15 seconds) or pharmacologic therapy (i.e., ***Adenosine***)- *and/or* at *any* time develops signs of hemodynamic compromise- *then* ***emergency cardioversion*** *may be needed.*

In most cases, pharmacologic therapy *can* be used and will be effective for PSVT (so that emergency cardioversion will *not* be needed). ***Adenosine*** has become the drug of choice in this situation for pediatric patients. Adenosine is extremely effective and appears much *less* likely to produce adverse hemodynamic effects in infants or young children than Verapamil. Even if adverse effects do occur, the exceedingly short half-life of Adenosine (of *less* than 10 seconds) tends to limit their duration.

Note- Although ***Verapamil*** has been a drug of choice for treatment of PSVT in adults, the drug should be used with extreme caution (if at all) in younger children- especially if they are acutely ill. This is because excessive heart rate slowing, decreased contractility, and profound hypotension (from vasodilatation and negative inotropy) can all occur and produce potentially disastrous consequences in such patients.

- ***IV Dosing of Adenosine*** - Give **0.1 mg/kg** for the *initial* dose. Double this amount (i.e., to **0.2 mg/kg**) if there is no effect. The *maximal* recommended dose of Adenosine for use in pediatric resuscitation is 12 mg.

  As is the case for adults- remember the importance of *rapid* administration of Adenosine (giving the drug *as fast as possible* over 1-3 seconds)- so as to prevent deterioration of drug in the IV tubing. To further facilitate absorption- follow each IV bolus with a fluid flush.

Weight of Patient	Initial IV Dose of *Adenosine*	2nd (*and Subsequent*) Doses
10 kg	1 mg	2 mg
20 kg	2 mg	4 mg
30 kg	3 mg	6 mg
Adult Dose	6 mg	12 mg

Sodium Bicarbonate

Respiratory failure is the most common cause of cardiac arrest in children. As a result, the most important treatment priority in pediatric resuscitation is to improve ventilation- *NOT to administer Sodium Bicarbonate.* Next to oxygen, Einephrine is the drug of choice for treatment of cardiopulmonary arrest in children. ***Sodium Bicarbonate*** should be considered *only* if the arrest is prolonged- or if the patient was *known* to have a severe preexisting/underlying metabolic acidosis.

- ***IV (or IO) Dose***- Give **1 mEq/kg** (where 50 ml of 8.4% solution = 50 mEq).

Weight of Patient	**IV (or IO) Dose of SODIUM BICARBONATE**
10 kg	10 mEq (1/5 ampule)
20 kg	20 mEq (2/5 ampule)
30 kg	30 mEq (3/5 ampule)
Adult Dose	50-100 mEq (1-2 ampules)

Defibrillation/Cardioversion

VT and V Fib are extremely uncommon terminal events in pediatric arrests. As a result, defibrillation and synchronized cardioversion will only *rarely* be needed during pediatric resuscitation.

- ***Defibrillation Dose***- **2 J**(joules)**/kg** for the *initial* attempt. If unsuccessful- *double* the dose (to **4 J/kg**)- and repeat X 2 (shcoking in *rapid* succession).

- ***Synchronized Cardioversion Dose***- **0.5 J**(joules)**/kg** initially. Increase this amount as needed for subsequent cardioversion attempts.

Weight of Patient	***1st Defib* (2nd - 3rd Shock)**	***Cardioversion***
10 kg	20J (then 40J- 40J)	5 J
20 kg	40J (then 80J- 80J)	10 J
30 kg	60J (then 120J- 120J)	15 J
Adult Dose	200J (then 300J- 360J)	*Variable* (≈50-200 J)

CHAPTER 3

Key Clinical Issues in ACLS/Airway

Section 3A: *KEY Clinical Issues in ACLS*

Clinical Issue #1:

- *What if you can't establish IV access?*
  - *Which drugs can be given by the **E**ndo**T**racheal (**ET**) route?*
    - *What dose of drug is recommended when administering by the ET route?*

Answer- On occasion, IV access may be difficult (if not impossible) to achieve. In this situation, administration of drug by the ***E**ndo**T**racheal (ET) route* provides a suitable alternative for three of the most commonly used medications in cardiopulmonary resuscitation: *Atropine, Lidocaine, Epinephrine.* In addition, *oxygen* (which *is* a drug!)- as well as *Narcan* and *Valium*- can also be given by the ET route. This leaves the emergency care provider at least three *mnemonics* to choose from to facilitate recall of these drugs:

A- L- E	A- L- O- E	N- A- V- E- L
- ***A*** *tropine*	- ***A*** *tropine*	- ***N*** *arcan*
- ***L*** *idocaine*	- ***L*** *idocaine*	- ***A*** *tropine*
- ***E*** *pinephrine*	- ***O*** *xygen*	- ***V*** *alium*
	- ***E*** *pinephrine*	- ***E*** *pinephrine*
		- ***L*** *idocaine*

Practically speaking- the emergency care provider should use *whatever* drug access site is established first. In most cases this will be a peripheral IV line (that hopefully will be with a large bore catheter placed in a proximal site such as the anticubital or external jugular vein). As soon as a skilled operator adept at central line placement arrives on the scene- insertion of a central venous catheter (into either the internal jugular or subclavian vein) may be attempted- especially if the patient is *not* responding to treatment. In the event that IV access is unavailable but the patient *is* intubated- medication should be administered (*without* delay) by the ET route. Once effective IV access is established- medication can then be *readministered* (if/as needed) by the IV route.

- **Dosing Considerations-** Because absorption of drug is *not* as reliable by the ET route as by IV administration- a *larger* dose (i.e., ≈ **2** to **2.5 times** the IV dose) is recommended when the ***ET route*** is used (AHA Text- Pg 1-11).

Clinical Issue #2:

- *What if the rhythm is **Refractory V Fib** ?*

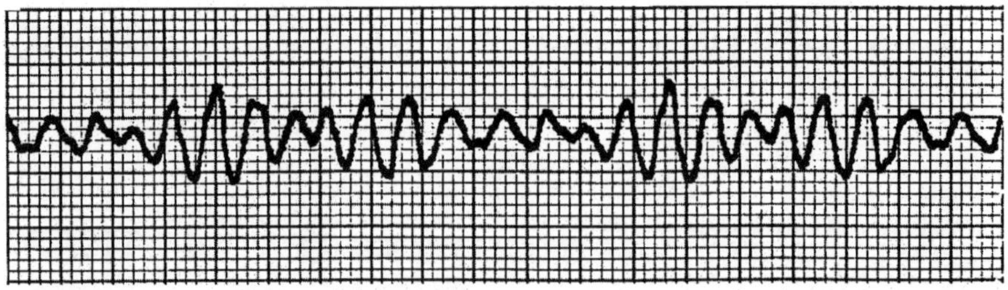

Answer- Persistence of V Fib *despite* administration of appropriate *initial* interventions defines the condition as *"refractory."* This situation is clear indication for special treatment considerations.

In clinical practice the term ***Refractory V Fib*** is usually applied after failure to respond to initial attempts at *basic CPR- intubation- ventilation- defibrillation* (4 or more times)- and one or more doses of *Epinephrine.* Appropriate treatment measures now include:

- Use of *more* Epinephrine. Consideration *might* be given at this time to use of ***HDE*** (if this is not already being done).
- A trial of ***Antifibrillatory Therapy.*** AHA Guidelines recommend ***Lidocaine*** as the initial antifibrillatory agent of choice. The drug may be given in a *single* dose (of **1.5 mg/kg**) to patients in cardiac arrest.
- A search for a *potentially reversible* cause(s) of the cardiac arrest (i.e., consideraton of the *"D" = Differential Diagnosis* of the *2° Survey*). Important causes of refractory cardiac arrest to consider include *electrolyte* abnormality- *acid-base* disturbance- *hypovolemia- hypothermia-* drug *overdose-* and/or development of a *complication* of CPR.
- *If Lidocaine fails-* Consideration of ***Bretylium*** (as a 2nd-line antifibrillatory agent). Give 5 mg/kg (or a single **500 mg IV** bolus) initially- and repeat in 5 minutes (giving ≈10 mg/kg for this 2nd IV bolus) if the V Fib persists.
- Consideration of ***Magnesium Sulfate-*** in a dose of **1-2 gm IV** (which may be repeated)- especially for patients who are likely to be hypomagnesemic.
- Continued repeat *countershock* (as needed and appropriate). Perform CPR for at least 30-60 seconds after each drug administration before reattempting countershock.
- Possible empiric trial of an ***IV ß-Blocker-*** especially if increased sympathetic tone is likely to be associated with (or responsible for) the arrest.
- Consideration of ***Sodium Bicarbonate*** (realizing that *true* indications for use of this drug in the setting of cardiac arrest have become quite *limited*).

(See also pages 37-43.)

Clinical Issue #3:

- *What energy level is "optimal" for defibrillation?*

Answer- AHA Guidelines currently recommend selection of **200 joules** as the *initial* energy level for defibrillation of adults. However, 200 joules is *not* necessarily the *"optimal"* energy level for defibrillation of every patient in cardiac arrest (AHA Text- Pg 4-6). This is particularly true for certain patients who inherently have low ***T**rans**T**horacic **R**esistance (**TTR**)* values. Such individuals may receive an excessive amount of *current* when standard energies (i.e., 200 joules) are routinely used for defibrillation- an effect that may result in structural myocardial damage, and/or actual failure to defibrillate. In contrast, patients with *high* TTR values may not receive enough current- *despite* selection of a *seemingly* adequate energy level for defibrillation. Complicating the issue further is the clinical reality that body size and weight are *not* reliable indicators of TTR! *Even emaciated elderly subjects may sometimes have unexpectedly high TTR values* (See pages 174-178).

Future use of ***current-based* defibrillators** that are able to *instantaneously* measure TTR (and *adjust* current delivery accordingly) should help to resolve the problem of determining *optimal* energy needs for specific patients (AHA Text- Pg 4-7). Until such time that these devices become generally available- use of **200 joules** should continue as the standard *initial* energy level recommended for defibrillation of adults.

Clinical Issue #4:

- *What if V Fib recurs later on in the code?*
  - *What energy level should be used for repeat defibrillation?*

Answer- If V Fib *recurs* at a later point in the code (i.e., in a patient who has already been defibrillated *out of* V Fib)- AHA Guidelines advise that *"shocks should be reinitiated at the energy level that previously resulted in successful defibrillation"* (AHA Text- Pg 4-6). While fully acknowledging this recommendation, we nevertheless prefer to *drop back* to **200 joules** in most cases because:

i) Defibrillation is *not* benign. Use of excessive energy can clearly produce conduction system damage- and even asystole.

ii) Just because a patient fails to respond to 200 joules at an earlier point in the code does *not* necessarily mean that they won't respond to this same energy at a *later* point in the code (i.e, *after* oxygenation, administration of Epinephrine and antiarrhythmic medication, correction of electrolyte and acid-base abnormalities, etc.).

The approach we suggest to this issue is simple: If the patient fails to respond to repeat defibrillation at the lowered energy level (i.e., of 200 joules)- *increase* the energy level (to 360 joules)- *and defibrillate again.* Little time should be lost by this approach- and it should allow defibrillation to be accomplished at the *lowest* possible energy level.

Bottom Line- Selection of an energy level of *either* **200** *or* **360 joules** is probably appropriate for the initial attempt at *repeat* defibrillation. If the lower energy level is selected but is unsuccessful- the next repeat attempt should be with 360 joules.

Alternatively, one might begin repeat defibrillation at an intermediate energy level (i.e., of 300 joules)- increasing this to 360 joules if V Fib persists *(See also pages 172-173).*

Clinical Issue #5:

- *What is the rationale for using **H**igh-**D**ose **E**pinephrine (**HDE**)?*
    - *Is it likely that increased use of HDE will have a significant impact in saving lives?*

Answer- Although Epinephrine exerts both *alpha-* and *beta-adrenergic* effect- the more important action of the drug (*by far!*) in the setting of cardiac arrest is its ***alpha-adrenergic*** (= *vasoconstrictor*) ***effect***. As a result of alpha-adrenergic induced vasoconstriction- aortic *diastolic* pressure is increased. This enhances the gradient for coronary perfusion, and helps to maintain blood flow to the heart during cardiac arrest. Blood flow to the brain is also increased by the action of Epinephrine as a result of preferential shunting of blood from the external to the internal carotid artery.

The clinical reality is that the "optimal" dose of Epinephrine for use during cardiac arrest remains unknown. The finding that has become clear is that the alpha-adrenergic action of Epinephrine is essential for increasing *Coronary Perfusion Pressure (CPP)* in the arrested heart- and that much *higher* doses of the drug (i.e., ***HDE***) may be needed in some patients to achieve CPP values that are adequate for resuscitation. Unfortunately, studies to date have failed to demonstrate improved long-term survival with the use of higher doses of drug. Practically speaking, such results should *not* be unexpected- since *realistic* chances for survival are likely to be exceedingly small *regardless* of the dose of Epinephrine used- *IF* the victim of out-of-hospital cardiac arrest fails to respond to initial attempts at defibrillation and initial dosing with SDE.

AHA Guidelines suggest the following approach for the dosing of Epinephrine during cardiac arrest:

- Begin with ***SDE*** (i.e, **1 mg IV** of the 1:10,000 soln.). SDE is most likely to work when the rhythm is V Fib (instead of asystole) and the duration of the arrest is short.
- *If SDE is unsuccessful*- either continue with SDE for subsequent dosing (giving the drug every 3-5 minutes as needed)- and/or *increase* the dose of Epinephrine according to one of several ***HDE alternatives*** (AHA Text- Pg 1-16):

    - Administration of **2-5 mg** IV boluses- *OR* -
    - *escalating* **1- 3- 5 mg** IV boluses- *OR* -
    - dosing at **0.1 mg/kg** as an IV bolus.

Bottom Line- The "optimal" dose of Epinephrine is simply not known. Regardless of one's belief about whether or not higher doses (i.e., HDE) might be more effective in some situations- the recommended approach in cardiac arrest is to begin with **SDE** (i.e., **1 mg IV**). After this first dose, one may *either* continue with SDE dosing- *or* increase the dose as suggested above.

AHA Guidelines acknowledge the uncertainty that exists regarding the *optimal* dosing of Epinephrine by stating- *"Use of higher doses of Epinephrine (**HDE**) can NEITHER be recommended NOR discouraged* (AHA Text- Pg 7-4).

(See also pages 123-127.)

Clinical Issue #6:

- At what point should a code be stopped?

- What is the maximal number of times that a patient can be defibrillated?

Answer- There is no "maximal number" of times that a patient can be defibrillated. As long as the patient remains in V Fib- a *potentially* treatable rhythm is present that *may* respond to defibrillation . . . .

Having said this, as V Fib persists ***beyond* 20-30 minutes** *despite* appropriate BLS/ACLS- *realistic* chances for converting the patient *out of* this rhythm (and achieving long-term survival with *intact* neurologic function) become increasingly small. Consideration might therefore be given to *stopping* resuscitative efforts after this period of time. This premise relates *both* to arrests that occur in the hospital- as well as to those that occur in the field. Although transport to an emergency facility is still required in many communities before allowing EMS personnel in the field to cease resuscitative efforts- increased awareness of the dismal prognosis of these patients may eventually alter this practice. Practically speaking- the chances for *meaningful* long-term survival (i.e., *with* intact neurologic function) from out-of-hospital cardiac arrest are exceedingly small- *IF* adequately performed BLS and ACLS measures (including repeated defibrillation by trained EMS personnel) fail to restore a spontaneous pulse in the field.

> ***Exceptions*** to the above rule (i.e., when you definitely *would* want to continue full resuscitative efforts for **more** than 20-30 minutes) include:
>
> 1) *Resuscitation of children*
> 2) *Hypothermia*
> 3) *Drowning*
> 4) The patient who goes *in* and *out* of V Fib multiple times
>
> For each of these situations- a *realistic* possibility may exist for converting the patient out of V Fib (and restoring normal function)- *despite* the extended period that the patient was in arrest.

Clinical Issue #7:

- What if you are uncertain about the rhythm?

*- How should you approach the patient with a **W**ide-**C**omplex **T**achycardia (**WCT**) of **Uncertain Etiology**?*

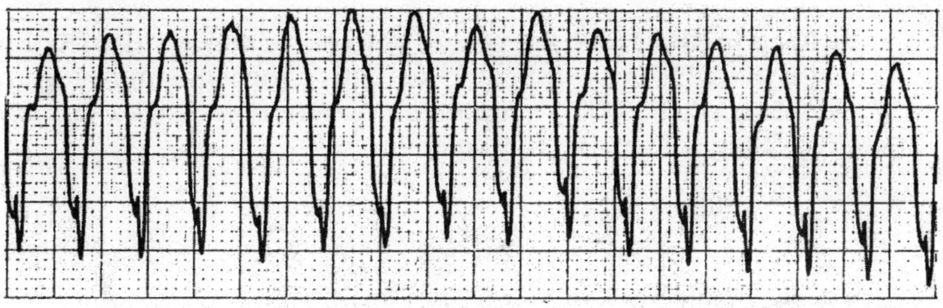

Answer- An extremely important clinical entity in emergency cardiac care regards the evaluation and management of the patient with a ***WCT*** (***W****ide-****C****omplex* ***T****achycardia*) of ***Uncertain Etiology.*** Clinically- we define this entity as the presence of a tachycardia in which the QRS complex is *wide* (i.e., ≥0.12 second)- and *normal* atrial activity is absent (or at least *not* immediately evident). In most cases, the ventricular rhythm will be regular (or at least *almost* regular)- although we emphasize that VT need *not* necessarily be a regular rhythm. Marked irregularity of the ventricular response (i.e., the presence of an *irregularly* irregular rhythm in which R-R intervals *continually* change from beat to beat)- suggests A Fib, in which QRS widening is likely to result from *preexisting* bundle branch block. Less marked irregularity of a WCT rhythm could represent *either* VT- *or* SVT (with aberrant conduction or bundle branch block).

The rhythm on the previous page is an example of a regular WCT. The rate of this rhythm is about 230 beats/minute, and there is no evidence of atrial activity. Clinically- the approach we suggest when confronted with a rhythm of this nature consists of the following:

- *FIRST- Determine the patient's* ***hemodynamic status.*** This is *by far* the most important action to accomplish. If the patient is hemodynamically unstable- *specific diagnosis of the tachyarrhythmia no longer matters.* This is because synchronized cardioversion now becomes *immediately* indicated *regardless* of what the rhythm happens to be.

- *IF the patient IS hemodynamically STABLE-* there may then be time to try to determine the etiology of the arrhythmia. This may be done by obtaining a 12-lead ECG, comparing it to prior 12-lead tracings or rhythm strips on the patient, and/or considering use of vagal maneuvers *if/as* appropriate. Remember that ***sustained VT*** is statistically far more likely to be the cause of a WCT than *SUPRAventricular* tachycardia with either aberrant conduction or preexisting bundle branch block. This is especially true if the WCT occurs in an *older* patient who has *underlying* heart disease.

- *IF doubt remains* (about the diagnosis)- ***Assume VT- and treat the patient accordingly!*** This dictum holds true *regardless* of how stable the patient looks (and *regardless* of the patient's blood pressure).

- *Avoid* use of Verapamil/Diltiazem in the treatment of WCT (unless you are *100% certain* of a *SUPRAventricular* etiology).

- *Regarding specific treatment-* AHA Guidelines recommend trying ***Lidocaine*** first (on the assumption that the rhythm is most probably VT). This may be followed with ***Adenosine*** (if Lidocaine is unsuccessful)- and then ***Procainamide***- and/or ***Magnesium*** (if deficiency of this cation is suspected)- and/or ***Bretylium.*** If hemodynamic decompensation occurs at *any* time during the process- prepare for *immediate* ***synchronized cardioversion.*** Cardioversion may also be appropriate when the patient fails to respond to medical therapy (AHA Text- Pg 1-33).

> Keep in mind that Adenosine is likely to convert the rhythm *only* if the WCT is *supraventricular* with a mechanism of *reentry* (i.e., primarily PSVT). We therefore prefer *not* to use this drug if we strongly suspect VT as the etiology.

(See also pages 65 and 85-88.)

Clinical Issue #8:

- *How to determine* ***hemodynamic stability*** *in a patient with tachycardia? In a patient with bradycardia?*

Answer- The most important parameter to assess in a patient with ***tachycardia*** is whether the rhythm is *hemodynamically* "significant". Specifically, the question to address is whether the rhythm is causing the patient problems (i.e., producing *signs* or *symptoms* of concern) as a *direct result* of the rate:

- ***Signs of Concern***- include hypotension (i.e., systolic BP ≤80-90 mm Hg), shock, heart failure/pulmonary edema, and/or Acute MI.
- ***Symptoms of Concern***- include chest pain, shortness of breath, and/or decreased mental status.

The definition of *hemodynamic stability* is equally applicable for *SUPRAventricular* tachyarrhythmias- as it is for VT. Thus, a patient with tachycardia who is hypotensive, having chest pain, and mentally confused is probably in need of immediate cardioversion- *regardless* of whether the rhythm is VT or SVT. Additional points to keep in mind are:

i) that immediate cardioversion will usually *not* be needed when the heart rate of the tachycardia is *less than* 150 beats/minute.

ii) that some patients with sustained VT may be hemodynamically stable- and that they may *remain* in VT for surprisingly long periods of time (of minutes, hours- *and even days!*).

iii) that bedside clinical evaluation (i.e., *"You have to be there"*) is usually the best way to determine the need for specific treatment. Thus, a patient in VT may not necessarily need immediate cardioversion *despite* a blood pressure reading of 70 systolic- *IF* they are otherwise alert, comfortable, and asymptomatic.

iv) that a patient does *not* necessarily need to be alert in order to be hemodynamically "stable"- as many *other* factors may account for persistent lack of consciousness in the setting of cardiac arrest (i.e., severe metabolic insult, residual effects from drug overdose, post-ictal state, etc.). Thus *despite* continued unresponsiveness- a patient in a *sustained* tachycardia may remain *hemodynamically* stable as long as the rhythm is associated with evidence of good perfusion (i.e., good peripheral pulses and an adequate systolic blood pressure).

> Regarding the Patient with ***Bradycardia***- virtually *identical* parameters are used to assess hemodynamic significance as for *tachycardia* (i.e, the presence of associated hypotension, chest pain, shortness of breath, altered mental function, development of heart failure, etc.).

(See also pages 49-50 and 90.)

Clinical Issue #9:

- *What if the rhythm is* **SVT** ? (i.e., *How would you approach such a patient?*)
  - *What is the differential diagnosis of a* **regular SVT** ?
    - *Is it clinically useful to obtain a 12-lead ECG on such patients?* If so- *why?*

Lead II

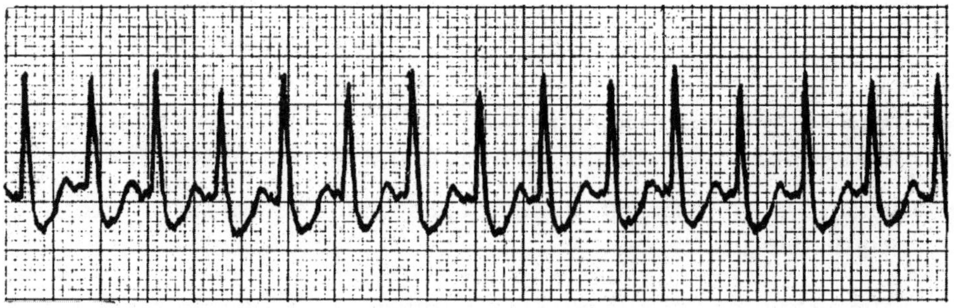

(See also pages 50-53, 56-58, 63, and 165-169.)

Answer- The rhythm shown above appears to be a ***regular* SVT** (***S****upra****V****entricular* ***T****achycardia*) at a heart rate of about **220 beats/minute**. There is no clear evidence of atrial activity. The clinical approach we suggest is as follows:

- *FIRST- Determine the patient's* **hemodynamic status**. This initial step is *equally* important when the rhythm is SVT- as it is when the rhythm is VT. This is because- *IF* the patient is acutely unstable, then *immediate* synchronized cardioversion is indicated *regardless* of what the rhythm happens to be.

- *IF the patient is hemodynamically STABLE*- there is time to try to determine the etiology of the tachyarrhythmia. The *first* step in this process is to **verify that the rhythm is *truly* supraventricular**. *It is all too easy to get fooled-* because on occasion, a portion of the QRS complex may lie on the baseline. When this occurs- the QRS complex may look to be narrower than it really is. Thus, although the QRS complex in this particular case *appears* to be narrow- one can *not* be certain of this from inspection of the *single* monitoring lead shown above (i.e., it is hard to be sure in this tracing where the QRS complex ends- and the ST segment begins). Our clinical approach would clearly be different if the QRS complex was wide instead of narrow (which would make the rhythm a WCT of *uncertain* etiology).

Bottom Line- If at all possible, it helps to obtain a ***12-lead* ECG** on the patient *during* the tachycardia. Doing so at the *earliest* feasible moment (i.e., assuming that the patient is hemodynamically stable)- may provide invaluable information:

- it confirms that the QRS complex is *truly* narrow in all 12 leads (or that the QRS is wide)
- it may reveal evidence of atrial activity that was not initially seen in the lead being monitored
- it may provide additional information that helps in the diagnostic process.

- *IF you confirm SVT and the patient is STABLE*- one should now proceed with ***differential diagnosis***. Optimal treatment depends on determining the etiology of the SVT. Practically speaking- there are 3 clinical entities to consider in the differential diagnosis of a ***regular SVT***. They are:

  i) *Sinus Tachycardia*
  ii) *Atrial Flutter*
  iii) *PSVT*.

  Regularity of the rhythm rules out A Fib (although care should be taken in determining regularity- because *rapid* A Fib may *almost* look regular). Distinction between the 3 entities listed above can often be made from clues on the 12-lead ECG, by comparison of the tachycardia with prior tracings on the patient, and/or by use of a vagal maneuver (*See below*). All of these measures may help to reveal the nature of atrial activity (and/or the *lack* thereof).

> We emphasize the importance of determining ***heart rate*** in the diagnostic process:
>
> - ***Sinus Tachycardia***- rarely exceeds 150-160 beats/minute in a supine (i.e., hospitalized) adult. A rate of 220 beats/minute (as is present in this case) is clearly too fast to be sinus tachycardia.
>
> - ***Atrial Flutter***- almost always presents with a ventricular response that is close to 150 beats/minute (in the *untreated* patient). This is because the atrial rate of untreated flutter is almost always close to 300/minute (250-350 range)- and the AV node most commonly allows 2:1 AV conduction (i.e., $300 \div 2 \approx 150$ beats/minute).
>
> *By the process of elimination*- the rhythm in this case is most likely to be ***PSVT*** (since a rate of 220 beats/minute is highly unlikely for either sinus tachycardia or A Flutter).

- *Consider a **vagal maneuver***- as either a diagnostic and/or therapeutic trial. Application of a vagal maneuver will either abruptly convert PSVT to normal sinus rhythm- or have no effect at all. In contrast, if applied to a patient in sinus tachycardia, A Fib, or A Flutter- a vagal maneuver is likely to transiently *slow* the ventricular response (and hopefully allow detection of the underlying atrial mechanism).

- *Begin drug therapy (based on your best guess of the etiology of the rhythm)*. AHA Guidelines recommend ***Adenosine*** as the drug of 1st choice for the treatment of PSVT (AHA Text- Pg 1-33). If Adenosine is ineffective, consideration might then be given to the use of *Verapamil/Diltiazem.*

  AHA Guidelines also recommend Adenosine as the drug of 1st choice for treatment of SVT when the etiology is uncertain (AHA Text- Pg 1-33). Even if the drug fails to convert the rhythm- it is likely to *transiently* slow the rate enough to allow correct diagnosis (i.e., *"chemical Valsalva"*).

  The optimal treatment approach will differ slightly for other forms of SVT. Rate-slowing drugs (i.e., Verapamil/Diltiazem, Digoxin, or beta-blockers) are often used first with rapid A Fib/Flutter. Conversion of these rhythms can then be achieved by correction of the underlying/precipitating disorder, addition of other antiarrhythmic agents (i.e., Quinidine, Procainamide, etc.), and/or synchronized cardiversion (if needed). A point to emphasize is that treatment of A Fib/Flutter may *not* necessarily be needed in the acute care setting if the ventricular response is not very rapid and the patient is hemodyanamically stable.

The last diagnostic entity in the list- *sinus tachycardia*- should generally *not* be treated with drugs. Instead, the treatment of choice for sinus tachycardia should always be aimed at identifying and correcting the underlying cause of this disorder.

Clinical Issue #10:

- *What if the rhythm of your patient is that shown below? How would you approach such a patient?*

- *How is treatment of this rhythm different from treatment of known VT?*

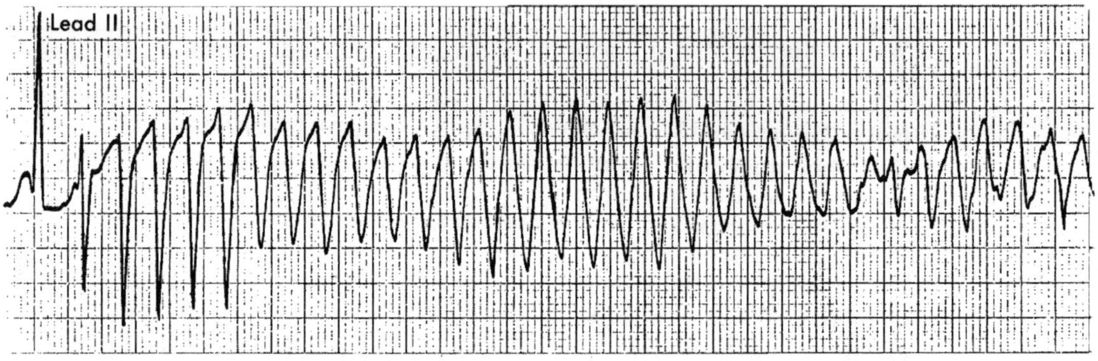

Answer- The rhythm shown above is ***Torsade de Pointes*** (i.e., *"twisting of the points"*). This term was selected to reflect the *alternating polarity* (i.e., from positive to negative) of the QRS complex with respect to the ECG baseline. Diagnostically- *Torsade* is differentiated from "typical" (i.e., monophasic) VT by marked variation in QRS morphology *during* the tachycardia. Torsade is often asssociated with preexisting ***QT prolongation***. Early recognition of this rhythm is extremely important- because treatment differs greatly from that of "conventional" VT. The clinical approach we suggest to Torsade is as follows:

- *FIRST*- Determine the patient's hemodynamic status. ***Cardiovert*** (or ***defibrillate***) the patient if actutely unstable. Although often responsive to electrical therapy, Torsade has the disturbing tendency to *repeatedly* recur- often until the underlying *cause* of the rhythm can be found and corrected.

- *As soon as possible*- Identify and treat the underlying cause of the rhythm. Common precipitating causes of *Torsade* to consider include overdose with tricyclic antidepressants or phenothiaziness, hypokalemia/hypomagnesemia, and/or use of drugs that lengthen the QT (such as Quinidine or Procainamide). Be sure to *avoid* use of IV Procainamide when treating a patient with Torsade!

- Give ***Magnesium Sulfate***- in a dose of **1-2 gm IV** (over 1-2 minutes)- which may be repeated one or more times. AHA Guidelines indicate that *higher* doses of Magnesium (i.e., of up to 5-10 gm) have been used with success in the treatment of some patients with Torsade (AHA Text- Pg 1-39).

- If Magnesium is ineffective- consider ***overdrive pacing*** (if available) as the next treatment of choice.

Clinical Issue #11:

- *When should you* ***Cardiovert*** *a patient?*

  - *Why is it safer to cardiovert than to use unsynchronized countershock?*

Answer- The advantage of ***Synchronized*** **Cardioversion** is that the electrical discharge is programmed to occur on the upstroke of the R wave (i.e., at a point *away* from the "vulnerable period"). This greatly reduces the chance that the electrical impulse will occur at a time that precipitates deterioration of the rhythm to V Fib. In contrast with defibrillation, delivery of the electrical impulse is completely *unsynchronized-* and therefore equally likely to occur at any point in the cardiac cycle.

The principal indication for use of *synchronized* cardioversion is in the treatment of ***tachyarrhythmias*** (including *both* VT and *SUPRAventricular* rhythms) that are either hemodynamically *unstable-* and/or which fail to respond to other measures. Clinically, cardioversion is needed *emergently* only if the patient is (or becomes) acutely unstable. If the patient with tachycardia is *not* acutely unstable, an initial trial of medical therapy is often preferred. Cardioversion may still be needed *later* in some of these patients (i.e., if medical therapy fails to control the rhythm)- but in such cases it can usually be performed under less urgent conditions (i.e., there should at least be time to *sedate* the patient and call anesthesia to the bedside).

> Practically speaking, it is highly *unlikely* that synchronized cardioversion will be needed on an *emergent* basis- IF the heart rate of the tachyarrhythmia is *less* than **150 beats/minute** (AHA Text- Pg 1-33).

A point to keep in mind is that synchronization may sometimes be problematic in certain patients with VT- *especially* when the QRS complex is broad or bizarre in shape *and/or* the rate is excessively rapid. In such cases, it may be difficult for the *machine* to distinguish between T waves and the QRS complex. If *for any reason* the process is *delayed* and the patient is acutely unstable- *forget about cardioversion,* and go immediately to *unsynchronized* shock (= defibrillation)!

(See also pages 53-55 and 179-183.)

Clinical Issue #12:

- *What initial* ***energy level*** *is recommended for* ***cardioversion*** *of the various arrhythmias?*

  - *How do A Fib and A Flutter differ in their response to synchronized cardioversion?*

    - *What should you do if cardioversion of an arrhythmia inadvertently precipitates V Fib?*

Answer- AHA Guidelines recommend use of the following ***Standard Sequence of Energy Levels*** for synchronized cardioversion of the various tachyarrhythmias (AHA Text- Pg 1-35):

- *1st Attempt*- **100 joules**
  - *IF unsuccessful*- increase energy to **200 joules-** - then to **300-** and finally to **360 joules**.

Several ***exceptions*** exist to the above general recommendations (i.e., when a different energy selection might be preferable for cardioversion of certain arrhythmias). These exceptions include:

- ***Polymorphic VT*** (i.e., VT with an *irregular* morphology and rate)- which often requires a *higher* energy level for successful cardioversion. AHA Guidelines therefore suggest *starting* with **200 joules**- which may need to be increased if the rhythm persists.
- ***Atrial Flutter***- which often responds to *lower* energy levels (probably because it is a very *organized* arrhythmia with rapid but very regular atrial activity). AHA Guidelines therefore allow for selection of **50 joules** as the *initial* energy level for attempts at converting A Flutter.
- ***Atrial Fibrillation***- which in our experience is also often a relatively difficult rhythm to successfully cardiovert when lower energy levels are used. *We* therefore prefer to *start* with **200 joules** for our *initial* attempt at cardioverting A Fib- and to increase this to 360 joules if a second attempt is needed. Other associated clinical factors (i.e., left atrial size, duration of time that the patient has been in A Fib, persistence of a precipitating cause, etc.)- often determine whether or not the patient with A Fib will respond to cardioversion.

> An interesting clinical point to emphasize is that although the measures used to treat A Fib and A Flutter are similar- the *response* to treatment is often quite different. Thus, similar medications are recommended to *slow* the rate (i.e., Digoxin, Verapamil/Diltiazem, beta-blockers)- and *convert* the rhythm (i.e., Quinidine, Procainamide, etc.)- but rapid A Fib is clearly more likely to respond to this therapy. Despite even high doses of rate-slowing agents, the ventricular response of A Flutter often remains unacceptably rapid.
>
> In contrast- A Flutter is generally much more responsive to synchronized cardioversion (which often works at surprisingly low energy levels).

Despite the most approrpiate of precautions- synchronized cardioversion may occasionally precipitate deterioration of a tachycardia to V Fib. The *KEY* to effective management is to *anticipate* this possibility. Should it occur- simply *turn off the SYNCH mode*- and *immediately* defibrillate the patient. The chances are excellent that prompt defibrillation of inadvertently precipitated V Fib will restore the rhythm to sinus.

Finally- we note that cardioversion should be *avoided* (if at all possible) in patients who are known (or suspected) to have Digoxin *toxicity*. Practically speaking- the procedure is usually safe if performed on a patient who is taking Digoxin but whose level is clearly *within* the therapeutic range.

Clinical Issue #13:

- *When should you use the* ***Precordial Thump*** ? What is the drawback of the thump?
- *What about the* ***Cough*** ?

Answer- The ***Precordial Thump*** is a sharp, quick blow delivered to the mid-portion of the sternum. The potential problem with the thump is the complete lack of control over when in the cardiac cycle the energy will be delivered. As a result, the rhythm could be aggravated if the thump is *inadvertently* delivered during the "vulnerable" period.

AHA Guidelines currently view the thump as an *optional* (**Class IIb**) action that should be considered for treatment of pulseless VT/V Fib in *witnessed* arrest- *only* when no defibrillator is available. When a defibrillator *is* available- "it makes sense to go *directly* to that therapy, and *not* waste even a minimum of time with the thump" (AHA Text- Pg 1-15). Use of synchronized cardioversion is far preferable to the thump for treatment of VT *with* a pulse.

To perform ***Cough Version*** the patient is instructed to *"Cough hard- and keep coughing"*- as soon as the arrhythmia is noted. The mechanism for why *Cough CPR* works is uncertain. It *may* be due to improved coronary perfusion (from the increase in intrathoracic pressure generated by the cough)- activation of the autonomic nervous system- *and/or* conversion of mechanical energy from the cough into an electrical depolarization impulse (albeit one of only a few joules). Despite the uncertainty about its mechanism, what *has* become clear- *is that the cough is usually a benign procedure that may effectively convert sustained VT to sinus rhythm in a surprising number of cases.*

> **Bottom Line-** Consider the use of ***Cough Version*** (advising forceful, repetitive coughing) to *conscious* patients in sustained VT. This procedure may work, and it is unlikely to exacerbate the arrhythmia. In contrast- *avoid* use of the ***Thump*** for sustained VT *with* a pulse (because of the substantially increased risk that the thump might precipitate deterioration to V Fib).

(See also pages 169-171.)

Clinical Issue #14:

- *What if the rhythm is a* ***Bradycardia*** ? (i.e., *How to approach a patient when the rate is too slow?*)

Answer- The term ***"Bradycardia"*** encompasses a diverse group of cardiac rhythms that are unified by the finding of a slow ventricular rate (i.e., of *less* than 60 beats/minute). The principal clinical entities included within this definition are sinus bradycardia (often with sinus arrhythmia)- A Fib with a *slow* ventricular response- the AV blocks- escape rhythms (AV nodal and idioventricular)- and asystole.

Clinically- the approach we suggest when confronted with a rhythm of this nature consists of the following:

- *FIRST*- Determine if the patient has a pulse. If the patient is *pulseless*- then by definition, the rhythm is ***PEA*** (*Pulseless Electrical Activity*)- and a different set of priorities must be addressed. These include:

  i) Performing CPR (since PEA is a *non-perfusing* rhythm)
  ii) Searching for (and trying to correct) the cause of the PEA
  iii) Administration of *Epinephrine* and/or *Atropine*
  iv) Consideration of a fluid challenge.

- *If a pulse IS present* - then determine the patient's hemodynamic status. Specifically, determine if the bradycardia is causing serious signs or symptoms as a *direct result* of the reduction in heart rate. Based on this information (and the *severity* of symptoms)- interventions to consider include:

  - ***Atropine***- in a dose of **0.5-1 mg IV**. Atropine may be repeated (every 1-5 minutes) up to a *total* dose of ≈**3 mg** (0.04 mg/kg)- *as needed* according to the clinical situation.

  - ***TCP*** (*TransCutaneous Pacing*)- which *is* appropriate as the *first* intervention when the bradycardia is severe and/or the clinical condition is unstable. Pacing is also *preferable* to Atropine when the rhythm being treated is advanced AV block with ventricular escape (i.e., with a wide QRS complex).

  - Use of a ***Pressor Agent***. This may be IV infusion of *either* ***Dopamine*** or ***Epinephrine***- depending on the *severity* of symptoms.

> **Note-** Pacing should *not* be delayed while waiting to achieve IV access (or for Atropine to take effect). *When bradycardia is severe-* apply ***TCP*** as soon as it becomes available. Use of a ***pressor agent*** is generally best reserved for treatment of *Atropine-resistant* bradycardia when TCP is unavailable (or ineffective).

(See also pages 89-91 and 104-110.)

Clinical Issue #15:

- *How to approach the patient with* ***Hypotension*** ?
  - *What are the elements of the* ***"Cardiovascular Triad"*** ?

Answer- The causes of ***Shock*** are many. *All* shock states share the common denominator of *"inadequate cellular perfusion and inadequate oxygen delivery for existing metabolic demands"* (AHA Text- Pg 1-40). Having stated this, the actual clinical presentation of a patient in shock may vary greatly- depending on the *specific cause* of the shock state (i.e., sepsis, spinal shock, cardiogenic shock)- and depending on which *compensatory mechanisms* have been called into play in an effort to correct the problem. Common clinical manifestations of shock include *impaired mentation* and *reduced urine output* (from hypoperfusion of the brain and kidneys)- as well as compensatory changes of *tachycardia* and *peripheral vasoconstriction* (in an effort to increase cardiac output and shunt blood centrally). The resulting reduction in peripheral blood flow may produce the clinical finding of *cool, mottled* extremities.

AHA Guidelines emphasize the importance of the ***Cardiovascular Triad*** for formulating a practical clinical approach to the patient who is hypotensive- but *not* in full cardiac arrest (AHA Text- Pg 1-40). According to this concept- *all* forms of ***Hypotension*** can be categorized as resulting from one (*or more*) of the following problems:

i) A *problem* with ***Rate*** (i.e., rate *too fast* or rate *too slow*)- with management decisions based on the Algorithms for treatment of ***Tachycardia*** and ***Bradycardia***.

ii) A *problem* with the ***"Pump"***- as seen in Acute MI with cardiogenic shock, or other predisposing cause of ventricular dysfunction/pulmonary edema.

iii) A *problem* with ***Volume***- as seen with *hypovolemia* from blood loss, dehydration, or other cause of volume depletion- and/or a *relative* reduction in intravascular volume (as may occur with excessive vasodilatation).

> In addition to the 3 elements of the *Triad* described above (i.e., *rate*- the *pump*- and *volume*)- AHA Guidelines also describe a ***4th element*** that relates to *problems* resulting from an alteration in ***vascular resistance.*** This last element may *secondarily* produce a problem with volume (i.e., from excessive *vasodilatation* as noted above)- and/or a secondary problem with the "pump" (i.e., if *vasoconstriction* produces an increase in afterload that ultimately leads to a fall in cardiac output).

It should be emphasized that management decisions depend on identifying and addressing the specific element(s) of the *Cardiovascular Triad* that are causing the patient's hypotension. Empiric trial with a ***fluid challenge*** (i.e., rapid IV administration of ≈**150-500 ml** of normal saline) is often appropriate as an *initial* step- followed as needed by use of a pressor agent (i.e., ***Dopamine*** for less severe hypotension- and ***Norepinephrine*** when systolic pressure is <70 mm Hg).

Clinical Issue #16:

- *What if the monitor shows a **"flat line"** rhythm?* How can you be sure that this rhythm truly represents asystole?
    - In addition to asystole- *what other entities should be considered in the differential diagnosis of a flat line rhythm?*
        - *Should a flat line rhythm ever be shocked?*

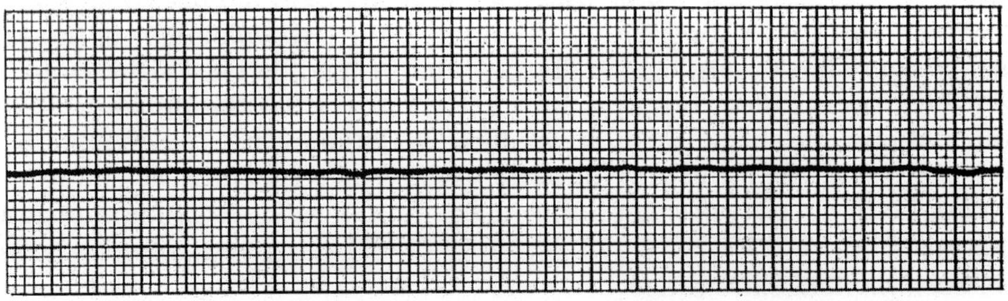

Answer- The diagnosis of ***Asystole*** is made from the electrocardiographic finding of a *truly **flat*** **line** (i.e., a line that is flat in ***all*** leads)- in a patient who is *pulseless.*

- ***Fine V Fib*** may occasionally ***"masquerade"*** as asystole (i.e., if the predominant vector of the fibrillation rhythm happens to be *isoelectric* to the single monitoring lead being looked at).

> **Note-** Rotating quick look paddles by 90° (or for the monitored patient, viewing the rhythm in additional leads)- will quickly resolve the issue of whether electrical activity is present or not.

Practically speaking, the phenomenon of fine V Fib *masquerading* as asystole is *not* commonly seen. As a result, recognition of a flat line rhythm in a single lead does *not* justify routine defibrillation (in the desperate hope that shocking the flat line may convert the rhythm). Clinically- *it is probably far better to take an extra moment to view additional leads* (and determine *with certainty* the etiology of the rhythm)- *than to "blindly" shock a flat line rhythm based on the finding of a single lead.* AHA Guidelines acknowledge that shocking asystole *can* make the rhythm worse (i.e., by "stunning" the heart/producing *profound* parasympathetic discharge)- and that this may reduce even more the chance for return of spontaneous cardiac activity (AHA Text- Pg 4-7).

- In addition to asystole and fine V Fib, the *differential diagnosis* of a ***flat line* rhythm** should also include the possibility of *loose leads* (or leads *not* connected to the patient or the monitor)- *no power-* and/or *signal gain turned down too low* to produce a rhythm on the monitor (AHA Text- Pg 1-14).

(See also pages 99-101.)

Clinical Issue #17:

- *What if in treating SVT with IV Verapamil/Diltiazem the patient develops excessive bradycardia or asystole?*
- *What is the treatment approach for* ***Calcium Channel Blocker Toxicity*** ?

Answer- The calcium channel blockers *Verapamil* and *Diltiazem* have negative inotropic and chronotropic efffects- as well as direct vasodilatory properties. As a result, patients who receive an excessive amount of these drugs may develop significant ***bradyarrhythmias*** (including progressively severe sinus bradycardia, AV block- and even asystole). ***Hypotension*** often occurs from the reduction in heart rate- *and/or* from vasodilatation- *and/or* from impaired myocardial contractility. In addition, mental status changes may sometimes be seen (i.e., from CNS hypoperfusion)- which in severe cases can lead to lethargy, seizures, and even coma.

AHA Guidelines suggest the following approach for treatment of patients who develop ***Calcium Channel Blocker Toxicity*** (AHA Text- Pg 10-23):

- Provision of supplemental oxygen.
- Glucose determination (since hyperglycemia has been associated with calcium channel blocker toxicity).
- Administration of a ***Fluid Challenge*** (as *initial* treatment of hypotension)- rapidly infusing ≈**500-1,000 ml** of normal saline.
- Use of ***Calcium Chloride***- in a dose of **500-1,000 mg** (i.e., 5-10 ml) given by *slow* IV infusion (over 5-10 minutes).
- Use of ***Epinephrine*** by IV infusion- beginning at a rate of ≈**2 µg/minute** (and increasing this dose as needed). Because Epinephrine may *sensitize* the vasculature to Calcium's effects- AHA Guidelines advise *repetition* of **Calcium** after giving Epinephrine (up to a *total* dose of 2-4 gm of Calcium).
- Use of ***Glucagon***- in a dose of **1-5 mg IV** (if bradycardia/asystole persists).
- Use of ***Pacing*** (if bradycardia/asystole persists).
- Use of ***Atropine*** (although Atropine is generally *not* a very effective drug for treatment of bradycardia caused by calcium channel blocker toxicity).

> **Note-** Although it should seem intuitively obvious to treat *Calcium Channel Blocker Toxicity* with **Calcium Chloride**- use of this drug is often *overlooked* in this situation. *Don't forget Calcium Chloride.*

Clinical Issue #18:

- *When is **Pacing** indicated for bradycardia?*
    - *What is meant by the term **"anticipatory pacing readiness"** ?*
        - *When might "pacing readiness" be more appropriate than actual initiation of pacing?*

Answer- The major indication for pacing with bradycardia occurs when the patient is felt to be symptomatic as a *direct result* of the reduction in heart rate. However, even when heart rate is significantly slowed pacing may *not* necessarily be needed- IF the patient is otherwise unaffected (i.e., normotensive, and asymptomatic). Despite this, it would still seem prudent to *anticipate* the *possibility* that the bradycardia might suddenly *become* hemodynamically significant (perhaps *without* warning)- especially when the clinical setting is that of a cardiopulmonary emergency. AHA Guidelines therefore allow that "in conscious patients with *hemodynamically stable* bradycardia it may be *reasonable* to attach electrodes to the patient - and leave the pacemaker in ***Standby Mode*** "- ready to turn on at *any* moment- IF the patient's condition were to deteriorate at *any* time during the treatment process (AHA Text- Pg 5-3).

> The advantages of ***anticipatory pacing readiness*** (i.e., use of TCP in the *Standby Mode*)- are that it may obviate the need for transvenous pacing (which is an invasive procedure)- and/or *minimize* the time needed to implement TCP if hemodynamic decompensation suddenly occurs. *Pacing readiness* is especially appropriate for patients with bradyarrhythmias that are likely to either resolve on their own or with treatment (i.e., *drug-induced* bradycardia). It is also appropriate for treatment of *new* 2° or 3° AV block- and/or *new* bifascicular block- that occurs in the setting of Acute MI in a *hemodynamically stable* patient (AHA Text- Pg 5-2).

If the decision is made to use TCP in the *Standby Mode*- it may be advisable to verify that mechanical capture is possible, and that the patient will be able to tolerate pacing in the event it is needed (AHA Text- Pg 1-32 and Pg 5-5).

(See also pages 184-187.)

<u>Section 3B:</u> *Airway Management and Ventilation*

The importance of controlling the airway in patients presenting with cardiac and/or respiratory emergencies cannot be overemphasized. For outcome to be favorable, spontaneously breathing patients should be provided with supplemental oxygen- those who are not adequately ventilating must be assisted- and patients in respiratory arrest must be intubated and oxygenated. This chapter discusses the modalities and techniques used to accomplish these tasks.

Opening the Airway

The first priority in managing the patient with respiratory difficulty is to ensure patency of the airway. The two maneuvers recommended for doing this are the chin-lift and jaw-thrust.

In the unconscious supine patient, the musculature that normally supports the tongue and epiglottis relaxes. As a result, one or both of these structures may fall back and occlude the airway (Figure 3B-1). This accounts for the fact that the most common cause of airway obstruction in the unconscious patient is soft tissue in origin.

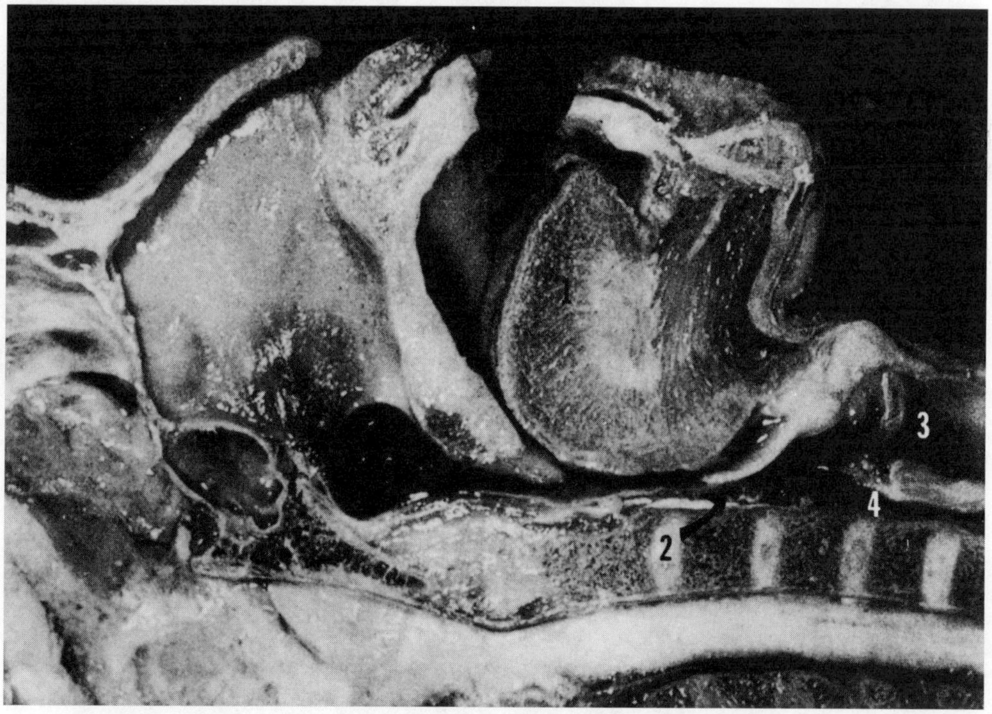

Figure 3B-1- Cross-section of the head demonstrating how the tongue and epiglottis occlude the airway in the supine position when the musculature is relaxed (1) tongue; (2) epiglottis; (3) trachea; (4) esophagus.

The degree of airway obstruction may be aggravated in the patient who is making spontaneous attempts to breathe. Inspiratory efforts create a negative pressure that frequently draws the tongue and epiglottis back even more into the throat, further compromising the airway. Because the tongue and epiglottis are attached to the lower jaw- procedures aimed at displacing the mandible forward will lift these structures off the posterior pharynx and open the airway. This is the way in which the chin-lift and jaw-thrust maneuvers work.

The Head-Tilt/Chin-Lift

The head-tilt/chin-lift maneuver is the recommended method of choice for opening the airway because it is easier to learn and more effective than the jaw-thrust. The technique is performed by placing the palm of one hand on the patient's forehead and the fingers of the other hand under the patient's chin. The fingers are positioned on the bony structure of the chin so as to avoid compression of soft tissues which might compromise the airway. With the hand on the forehead acting as a stabilizing force, the head is tilted backward by gently pulling the chin in a cephalad direction (Figure 3B-2).

As the head is tilted back, the mouth will almost always open. When this occurs- *resist* the urge to force the mouth closed. Instead, concentrate on using the fingers under the chin to assist in supporting the head-tilt position.

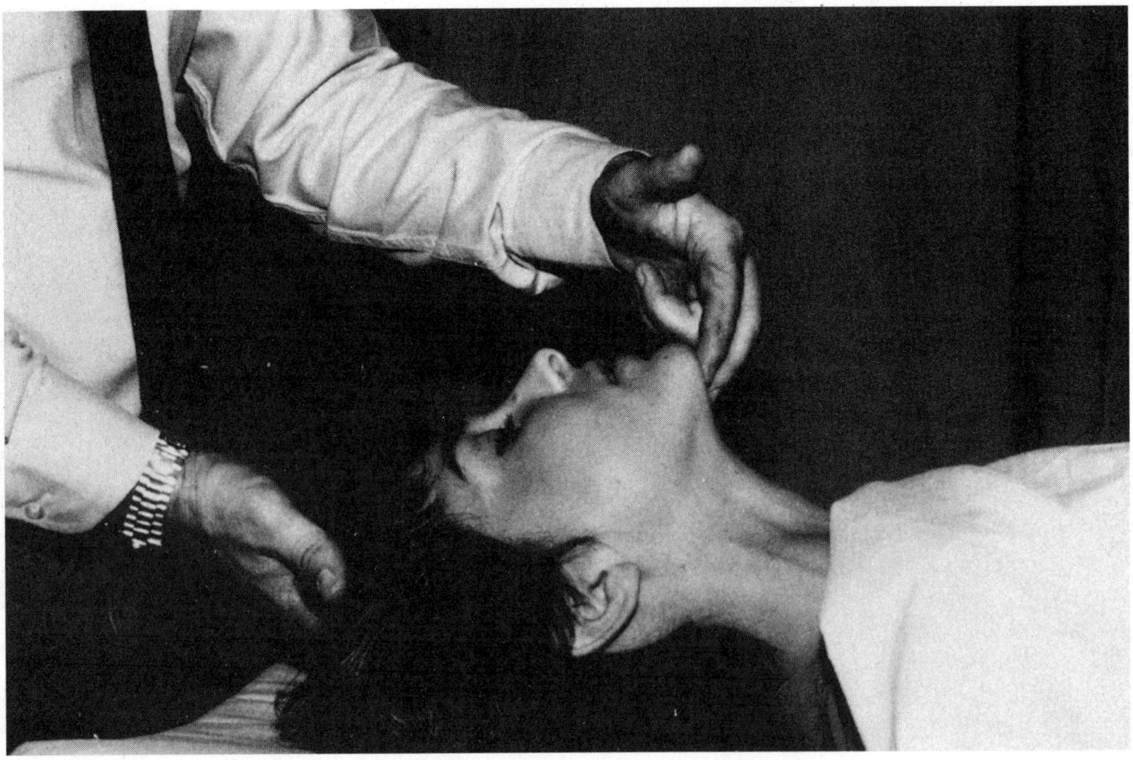

Figure 3B-2 - Head tilt / chin lift.

The Jaw-Thrust

Although slightly more difficult to perform than is the head-tilt/chin-lift maneuver- the jaw-thrust is the procedure of choice when the possibility of cervical spine injury exists. This maneuver allows the rescuer to support the head and open the airway *without* flexing or extending the cervical spine. One hand is placed on each side of the patient's head, and the index and/or middle fingers are used to displace the mandible anteriorly. This lifts the tongue off the hypopharynx (Figure 3B-3).

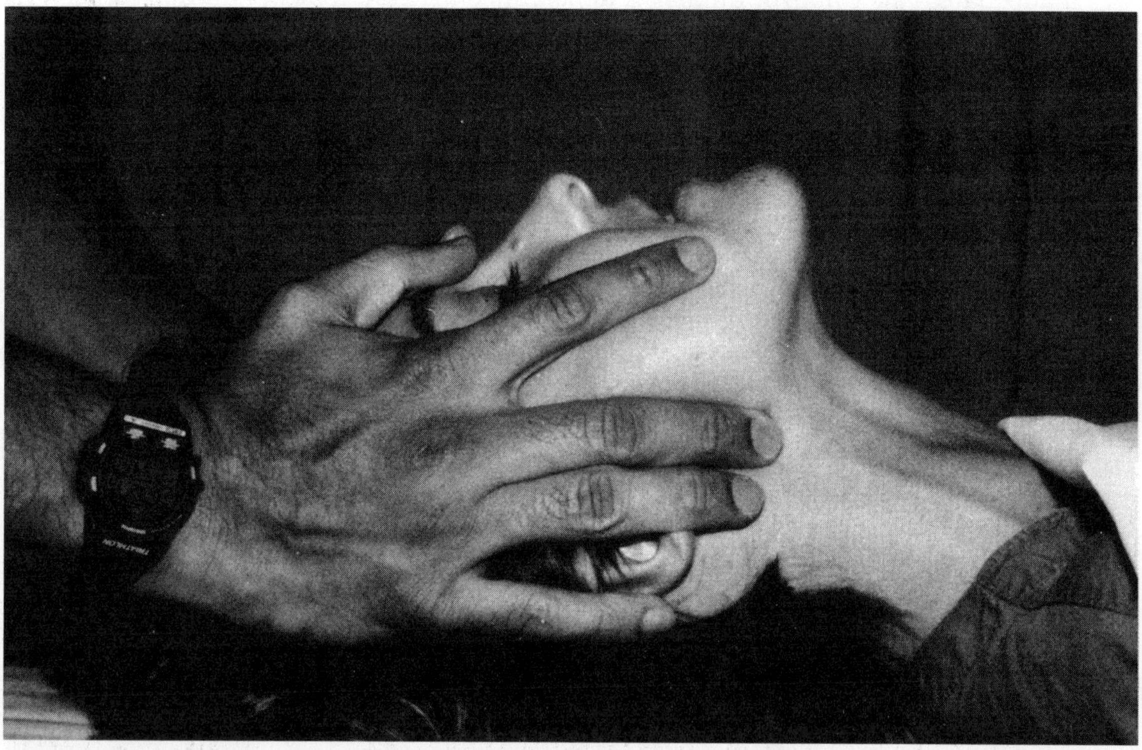

Figure 3B-3 - Jaw thrust.

The Head-Tilt/Neck-Lift

Although the head-tilt/neck-lift technique used to be the most commonly taught method for opening the airway- *it is no longer recommended.* Tilting the head back and lifting the neck is an *indirect* method of opening the airway. It is much less effective than the other two procedures that displace the mandible forward. The head-tilt/neck lift technique also poses the greatest risk when cervical spine injury is a possibility.

Assessing the Adequacy of Respiration

To provide optimal airway management, the emergency care provider must first be able to assess the adequacy of respiration. It is important to remember that there are two components of respiration: ventilation and oxygenation. Understanding the role that each component plays in respiration is essential. Simply stated, ***ventilation*** is the process of delivering gas to the patient's lungs; ***oxygenation*** is the process of getting oxygen into the blood. *Ventilations* can be spontaneous, assisted, or controlled. In each case a patient's lungs must receive an adequate volume of gas (tidal volume) over a defined time interval (minute ventilation) in order for good gas exchange to occur. *Oxygenation* is the process of delivering oxygen to lungs so that it can be transported to the tissues. In cases where the heart and/or lungs are not functioning properly- increased levels of oxygen must be administered to ensure adequate oxygen delivery to the lungs.

The parameters used to monitor the adequacy of respiration include skin color, breath sounds, tidal volume, respiratory rate, the work of breathing, and end-tidal carbon dioxide.

Evaluating the patient's ***skin color*** will sometimes provide the first clue that the patient is hypoxic. For example, the presence of *cyanosis* suggests that oxygenation is inadequate. Pallor and/or an ashen appearance indicate that in addition to poor ventilation, cardiac output may also be diminished.

All lung fields should be auscultated for ***breath sounds***. The finding of good, symmetric breath sounds suggests that the airway is patent and that air movement is adequate. On the other hand, asymmetric or abnormal breath sounds indicates that there may be a problem in the airway. This may be due to *obstruction* (from foreign body, soft tissue, or mucous plugging); cardiopulmonary disease (such as bronchospasm, pneumonia, or congestive heart failure); or improper tube placement (such as right mainstem intubation or tracheal intubation with the esophageal obturator).

Respiratory rate should be counted. In our experience, failure to do so is the most frequently overlooked part of the physical exam of an acutely ill patient. We emphasize the importance of *counting*- because of the ease with which one may overestimate or underestimate the frequency of respiration by casual inspection.

A conscious effort should also be made on the part of the observer to assess the ***work of breathing***. This may be done at the bedside by looking for:

i) tachypnea
ii) suprasternal and substernal retractions
iii) use of accessory chest and abdominal muscles.

> **Note**- In addition to the above mentioned respiratory changes that are associated with increase in the work of breathing- ***cardiac* changes** (i.e., in pulse rate or blood pressure) may also be evident.

The next two parameters to monitor are ***tidal volume*** and ***respiratory rate***. The product of these two parameters make up the ***minute ventilation***. Most adults breathe in a quantity of about 500 ml of air at an average rate of 12 times each minute. This results in a minute ventilation of 6 L/minute (500 ml X 12 = 6,000 ml). Because of the *inverse* relationship between tidal volume and respiratory rate- alterations in one of these parameters may be at least partially compensated by corrective alterations in the other. For example, minute ventilation may remain adequate despite a decrease in tidal volume- provided that the patient *hyperventilates* (and therefore increases respiratory rate proportionately).

> **Note**- The AHA recommendation for ventilation of adults is to deliver a tidal volume of between 10-15 ml/kg- at a respiratory rate of 12-15 times/minute (AHA Text-Pg. 2-1).
>
> Accurate assessment of tidal volume requires the use of a spirometer. In the absence of such equipment (or in an emergency setting)- one may surmise that the tidal volume is *probably* adequate if breath sounds are full and equal in the presence of good, symmetric chest excursion.

End-Tidal CO_2 ($ETCO_2$) Monitoring Devices

Capnography (the measure of end-tidal volume carbon dioxide concentrations in expired air) has long been used as a noninvasive method for evaluating the efficacy of respiratory function. Capnography equipment used to be cumbersome and far too impractical for use in the prehospital setting. Recent development of inexpensive, disposable, and easy-to-use adult and pediatric end-tidal CO_2 ($ETCO_2$) monitoring devices (Nellcor, Pleasanton, Ca.) has rekindled interest in this area. In addition, lightweight portable multiparameter noninvasive monitors that are able to simultaneously monitor blood pressure, oximetry, ECG and $ETCO_2$ are now available.

There are three types of $ETCO_2$ monitors- colormetric, mainstream and sidestream:

- The ***Nellcor* ETCO₂ device** is a colormetric monitor that readily attaches *in-line* between the endotracheal tube and the ventilatory support unit. The patient is given six or more breaths to prime the chemical indicator in the device (which will now register an accurate reading of the percentage of CO_2 in expired air). Color coding of the chemical indicator in the device facilitates recognition of baseline CO_2 concentration and of changes in $ETCO_2$ as they occur.

- The ***mainstream* method** requires that an infrared adapter and sensor be placed in the ventilation circuit. The sensor determines the amount of exhaled CO_2 by analyzing the exhaled gas as it passes through the circuit.

- The ***sidestream* method** requires a small adapter to be placed on the end of the endotracheal tube. A small vacuum tube is connected to the adapter and then to the capnograph. The capnograph pump then extracts about 200 ml/min from the adapter, and analyzes the gases withdrawn from the ET tube. The disadvantage of this method is that the patient and ventilatory system must be able to compensate for the 200 ml of gas being extracted by the capnograph.

Clinical Applications of Capnography

Capnography may be useful to the emergency care provider in a number of clinical settings. $ETCO_2$ monitoring is achieving increasing recognition as a noninvasive method for assessing the efficacy of ongoing cardiopulmonary resuscitation. In general, the prognosis for victims of cardiac arrest with persistently low $ETCO_2$ readings is extremely poor- especially when values are below 10 mm Hg. While other factors obviously play an important role in determining the likelihood of survival from cardiac arrest- the finding of a low $ETCO_2$ reading during resuscitation is useful clinically because it suggests the need for some *additional* intervention if there is to be a reasonable chance for survival.

$ETCO_2$ monitoring is now considered a standard of care for confirming proper endotracheal tube placement, especially when intubation has been performed by paramedics in the field. Auscultation of the chest for the presence of adequate air movement and symmetric breath sounds is *not* nearly as reliable an indicator as used to be thought. Moreover, auscultation of the chest may be quite difficult from the back of a moving ambulance or in a noisy aircraft.

> **Note**- $ETCO_2$ readings should significantly increase if the endotracheal tube has been correctly placed. Persistently low readings suggest esophageal intubation, inadequate CPR, and/or nonviability of the patient.
>
> In a similar manner- $ETCO_2$ monitoring can be used in the prehospital setting to confirm proper EOA (or EGTA) placement.

Cardiac changes associated with respiratory distress may be very different for adults compared to pediatric patients. In general, adults develop sinus tachycardia with respiratory distress. As a result of hypoxia, ventricular ectopy may develop- sometimes progressing to ventricular tachycardia and/or cardiac arrest from ventricular fibrillation. In contrast, heart rate almost always *decreases* in pediatric patients who become hypoxemic. If uncorrected, heart rate continues to drop- leading to severe bradycardia and ultimately cardiac arrest from asystole. Fortunately, appropriate treatment with prompt correction of hypoxemia will usually reverse cardiac changes in both children and adults.

> ***KEY***- The above parameters must be frequently assessed while caring for patients in cardiac and/or respiratory distress. Unless frequent *serial* examinations are performed- changes in hemodynamic or ventilatory status can be ever so easily overlooked.

Monitoring the Adequacy of Oxygenation

In addition to assessing the adequacy of ventilation- the *efficacy* of ventilation (i.e., the adequacy of *oxygenation*) should also be assessed if at all possible. This can be done using pulse oximetry, transcutaneous oximetry (TcO_2), and arterial blood gas (ABG) analysis.

Oximetry

Pulse oximetry provides continuous measurement of ***oxygen saturation*** or **SaO_2** (Figure 3B-4). SaO_2 readings in the range of 96% to 100% generally correspond to high PaO_2 concentrations (i.e., >80 mm Hg). It is important to emphasize that oxygen saturation is related to PaO_2 by the oxyhemoglobin dissociation curve- and that the slope of this

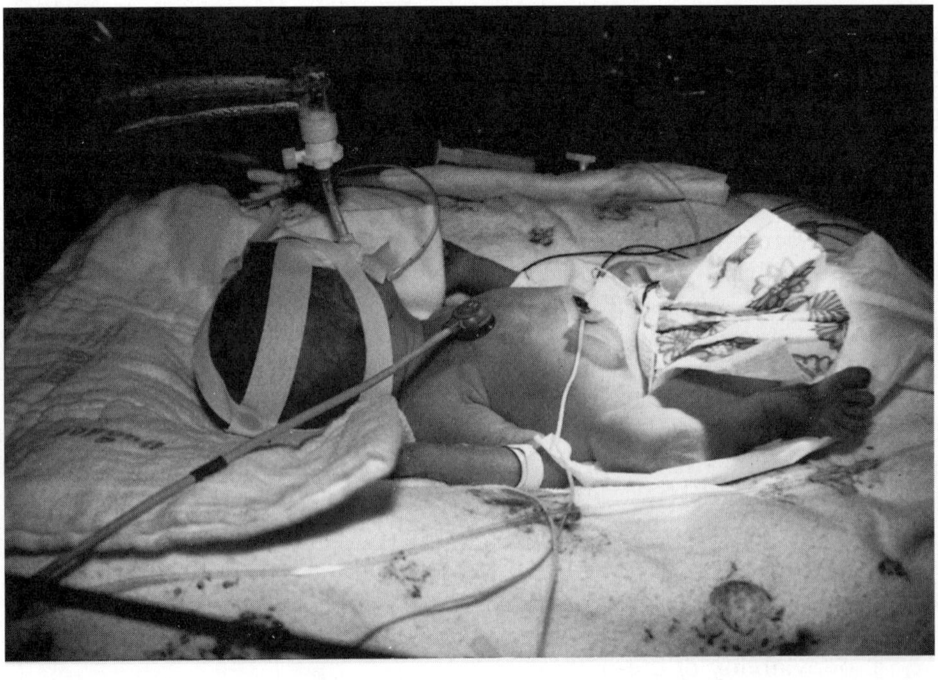

Figure 3B-4 - Application of a transcutaneous sensor to the chest of this infant for monitoring.

curve changes significantly when SaO_2 drops below 95%- and especially sharply when it drops into the range between 90% to 92%. A *seemingly* small decrease in SaO_2 (i.e., from the 96-97% range)- down to the 91-92% range may therefore correspond to a deceptively large drop in PaO_2 (to a value as low as 60 mm Hg!). Clinically, this means that oximetry can *not* be used as a substitute for ABG readings once SaO_2 readings drop much below the 96% range. However, when used as a tool to *continuously* monitor oxygen saturation, oximetry may be used as a *noninvasive* alternative to drawing repetitive ABGs.

Note- There are a number of other potential drawbacks to pulse oximetry that should be mentioned. These are that this measurement becomes inaccurate with hypothermia (especially <35 C), hypotension (<50 mm Hg), severe vascular disease, vasopressor therapy, anemia, hyperbilirubinemia, and with abnormal hemoglobin (as may be seen when there are increased concentrations of carboxyhemoglobin or methemoglobin). As a result- use of oximetry may have significant limitations in evaluating certain hemodynamically unstable patients (including some victims of cardiac arrest).

Transcutaneous Oximetry

Transcutaneous oximetry is frequently used in neonatal intensive care units, as well as in some cases where pulse oximetry is not applicable. Rather than measuring oxygen saturation- transcutaneous sensors monitor the *partial pressure* of oxygen in the arterial blood. Because they are applied to the patient's chest or abdomen (instead of to an extremity area)- transcutaneous sensors more accurately reflect arterial *oxygenation* when peripheral perfusion is poor. Transcutaneous oxygen sensors must be pre-calibrated prior to collecting data. They are heated (which may be uncomfortable to the patient), and require frequent site changes.

In emergency situations, pulse oximetry and $ETCO_2$ determinations offer several advantages over transcutaneous oximetry. Pulse oximeters are much easier to use. The device is simply attached to an ear lobe, toe, or finger- and sensing can begin within seconds (Figure 3B-5). An $ETCO_2$ device is advantageous because it can be placed on a BVM, endotracheal tube or tracheostomy tube.

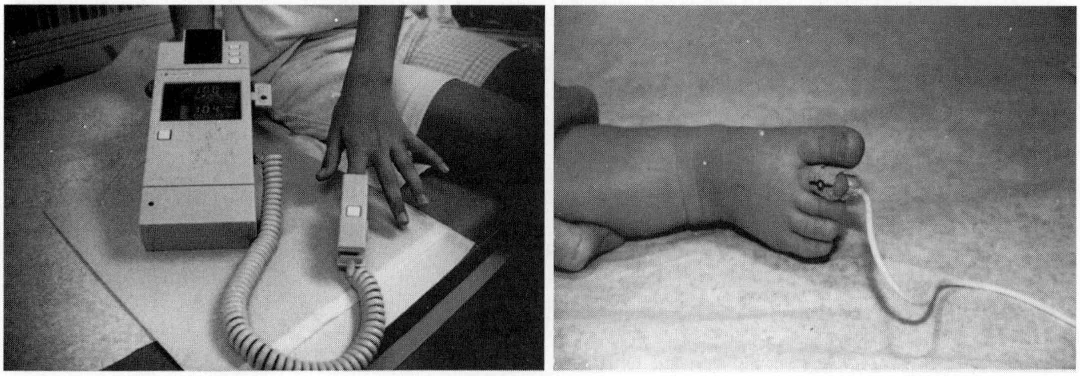

A B

Figure 3B-5- A) Application of a clip-on pulse oximeter to the finger; B) Application of a wrap around pulse oximeter to the toe.

Arterial Blood Gas Analysis

Serial arterial blood gas (ABG) analysis would seem to be the ideal evaluative method for assessing the adequacy of oxygenation. Unfortunately, a number of practical problems are associated with the use of ABG studies in an emergency setting.

Drawing ABGs is an invasive procedure that carries with it the risk of any of the complications that may arise from puncture of an arterial vessel. Finding the artery in a hypotensive or pulseless patient is often an extremely difficult task. Performing an Allen test in the upper extremity to verify collateral circulation (i.e., the presence of an ulnar artery pulse) may not always be possible. Using the femoral artery is not without problems either- because pulsations detected in the groin area during external chest compression do *not* necessarily identify this vessel. Because of the lack of valves in the central venous system- *retrograde* transmission of pulsations in the femoral vein may occur during CPR (and give the false impression that the femoral vein is the femoral artery).

As discussed in previous sections- ABGs obtained during cardiopulmonary resuscitation do *not* necessarily reflect the true state of acid-base balance on a cellular level. This is because of the marked discrepancy that rapidly develops during cardiac arrest between *arterial* pH (as measured by ABGs)- and the pH of mixed *venous* blood. A marked discrepancy is also seen between arterial $PaCO_2$- and the $PaCO_2$ of mixed venous blood. Readings from mixed *venous* blood (rather than ABGs) much more accurately reflect events at the cellular level during cardiac arrest.

> **Note**- PaO_2 readings obtained during cardiac arrest are often surprisingly high. It is well to remember that such readings result from the exceedingly slow passage of blood through the lungs- which allows more than adequate time for full saturation. Such readings do *not* necessarily reflect satisfactory peripheral oxygenation.

A final limitation of ABGs as a reflection of the adequacy of oxygenation is that they cannot be analyzed in the field. Even if ABG samples could be drawn in the prehospital setting- the delay in delivery to the hospital laboratory for analysis would render the results meaningless.

In selected settings (such as the prehospital setting)- an attractive alternative to ABG studies may be the combined use of pulse oximetry to monitor oxygenation, and $ETCO_2$ monitoring to appraise ventilation. Both are effective, inexpensive modalities that are extremely convenient for estimating the adequacy of oxygenation and assessing ventilation.

Adjuncts for Improving Oxygenation

In the conscious, spontaneously breathing patient, one of the main priorities is to provide supplemental oxygen. Although many devices are available for accomplishing this objective- we address only the four most commonly used modalities.

The Nasal Cannula

The nasal cannula is a piece of tubing with two ports designed to deliver supplemental oxygen through the nares. It is easily applied by slipping the tubing over the ears and sliding the prongs into the nares (Figure 3B-6).

The advantage of the nasal cannula is that it is well tolerated by most individuals. This device is particularly valuable in patients with chronic obstructive pulmonary disease (COPD)- for whom low concentrations of oxygen (24% to 28%) are often desirable. On the other hand, when higher concentrations of oxygen are needed- a nonrebreathing oxygen mask and/or Venturi mask is preferable.

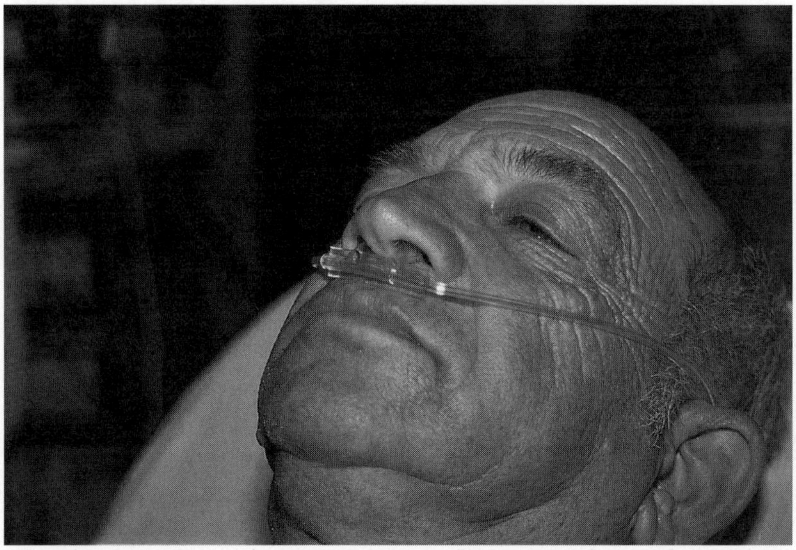

Figure 3B-6- Nasal cannula

> **Note**- In normal persons, respiratory drive depends on arterial carbon dioxide (CO_2) concentration. In contrast, hypercarbia loses its value as a stimulus for respiration in patients with COPD. Such individuals come to depend on *hypoxemia* for their respiratory drive. For this reason, administration of high concentrations of oxygen to such patients may be potentially dangerous: by correcting hypoxemia, ventilation may be suppressed to the point of causing respiratory arrest! The FiO_2 of supplemental oxygen should therefore be kept at *low* levels (i.e., 2 L/minute- or less) for *spontaneously* breathing patients with COPD.

The problem with use of the nasal cannula is that the actual amount of inspired oxygen varies greatly, depending on *both* tidal volume and whether the patient predominantly breathes through their nose or mouth. Under normal circumstances, most adults breathe primarily through their nose. In contrast, adults tend to change this pattern with respiratory distress- and *breathe through their mouth.* The value of a nasal cannula is dramatically reduced if it is used in a patient who is breathing primarily through their mouth.

> **Note-** Simply observing the patient will often suggest whether they are breathing primarily through their nose or mouth. In general, it is extremely difficult for adults to breathe through the nose if one's mouth is open. *Verify this statement by trying it out on yourself!* It may therefore be preferable to provide supplemental oxygen by *mask* (rather than nasal cannula)- for those individuals with respiratory distress whose mouths remain open.

The Oxygen Mask

The oxygen mask is a plastic device with a number of small vents on each side which allow for inspiration and expiration of ambient air. There is also a port for delivery of supplemental oxygen on the lower portion of the mask. Five to 10 L of oxygen may be administered, providing an FiO_2 of up to 50%.

The principal drawback of this device is the tremendous variability in actual inspired oxygen concentration. This is because the amount of air entrained from the outside (that mixes with the supplemental oxygen) is dependent on the patient's inspiratory flow rate. Because of the variability in delivered FiO_2 with the oxygen mask- a non-rebreather or Venturi mask is usually preferable when high and/or precisely determined concentrations of oxygen are required.

The Non-Rebreathing Oxygen Mask

The non-rebreathing oxygen mask is far superior to the basic plastic oxygen mask described above. Because this device can consistently deliver an FiO_2 of up to 90%- it is the adjunct of choice when high concentrations of oxygen are needed.

Several modifications account for the superiority of this device (Figure 3B-7). The first is that a flutter (one-way) valve has been added to one or both sides of the non-rebreather mask. This allows exhaled air to escape, but prevents ambient air from being inspired. In contrast, the open (air) holes on each side of the basic mask allow passage of both inspired

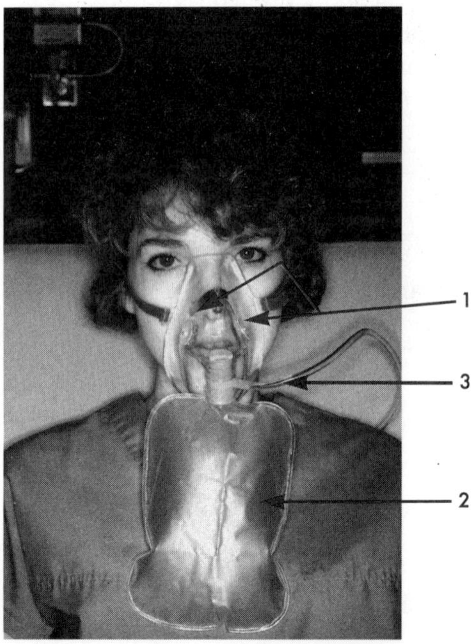

Figure 3B-7- Nonrebreathing oxygen mask. This mask differs from the standard oxygen mask because it has flutter (one-way) valves (1) and an oxygen reservoir (2). Also shown is oxygen tubing (3) through which supplemental oxygen is directed into the reservoir.

and expired air. The other major difference between these two devices is that the basic mask directs the supplemental oxygen into the mask- while the non-rebreathing mask directs it into a reservoir bag. A one-way valve prevents exhaled air from entering this reservoir- so that the patient entrains 100% oxygen from the reservoir on inhalation. In contrast, the concentration of inspired oxygen from the basic mask is much less than 100% because supplemental oxygen has mixed with ambient air.

Note- The reservoir bag should remain completely filled when using the nonrebreathing oxygen mask, so that ample supplemental oxygen is available for each breath. In order to ensure that this occurs- high flow rates (of ≈10-15 L/minute) must be used. In addition, the mask must fit snugly on the face to prevent ambient air from seeping in around the mask and mixing with oxygen inhaled from the reservoir bag.

The Venturi Mask

The Venturi mask (Figure 3B-8) is similar in concept to the basic oxygen mask, but features one important modification: it allows relatively *fixed* concentrations of supplemental oxygen to be inspired. Oxygen concentrations of 24%, 28%, 35%, and 40% can be delivered- using either 4 or 8 L/min flow rates. The advantage of this mask is much greater control of the oxygen concentration administered to the patient. Consistent oxygen delivery has made the Venturi mask the favored device for providing precise FiO_2 rates to patients with COPD.

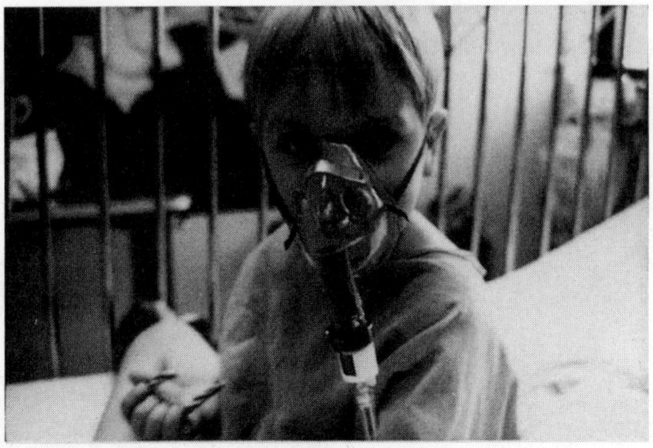

Figure 3B-8- Venturi mask. The Venturi mask allows delivery of a *fixed* oxygen concentration of 24%, 34% or 40%.

Airway Adjuncts

In the semiconscious or unconscious patient, invasive measures may be needed to maintain patency of the airway for ventilation. The three devices used are the oral, nasopharyngeal airway and the endotracheal tube.

The Oral Pharyngeal Airway

The oral pharyngeal airway is a semicurved, tubular device (Figure 3B-9). When properly positioned, the proximal end of the airway rests on the teeth, and the distal tip lies between the base of the tongue and the back of the throat. This prevents the tongue from occluding the airway, and allows ventilation to occur through the lumen of the tube. The oral pharyngeal airway is only indicated for patients who are *unconscious* and have *no gag* reflex.

Note- Appropriate sizing of the oral pharyngeal airway may be estimated at the bedside or in the field by aligning the tube on the side of the patient's face. Choose an airway that extends from the tragus to the corner of the mouth (Figure 3B-10).

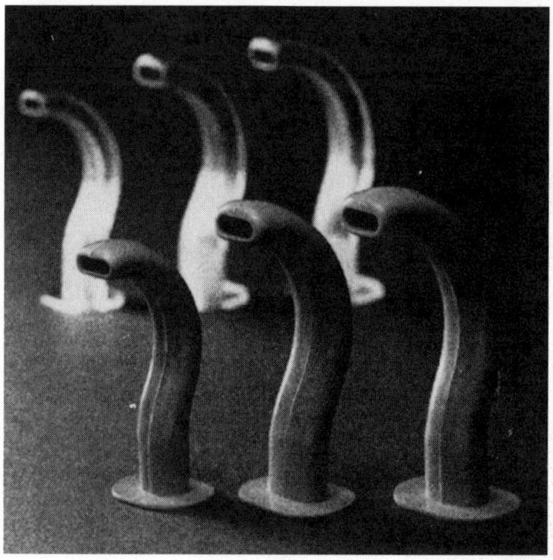

Figure 3B-9- Examples of oral pharyngeal airways.

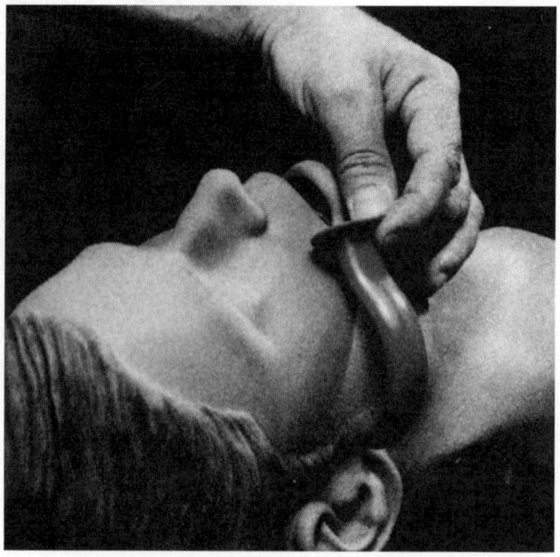

Figure 3B-10- Sizing the oral pharyngeal airway.

Technique for Insertion:

There are two ways to position the oral pharyngeal airway. The quickest method is to insert the device *upside down* into the mouth (Figure 3B-11A). As soon as the distal end reaches the hard palate, the airway is gently rotated 180 degrees- and then slipped *behind* the tongue into the posterior pharynx (Figures 3B-11B and 3B-11C).

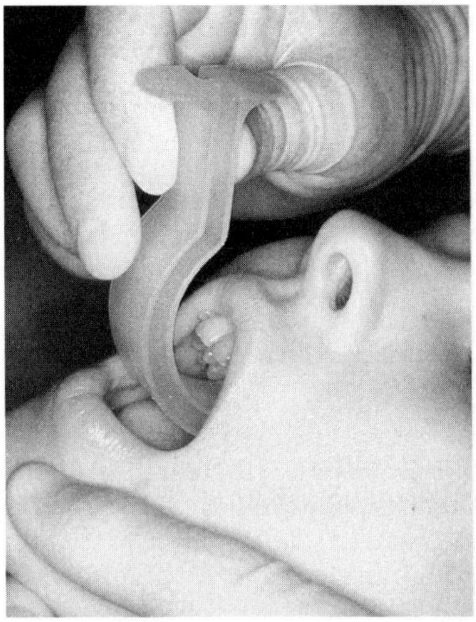

Figure 3B-11A- Insertion of the oral pharyngeal airway. The device is inserted upside down into the mouth

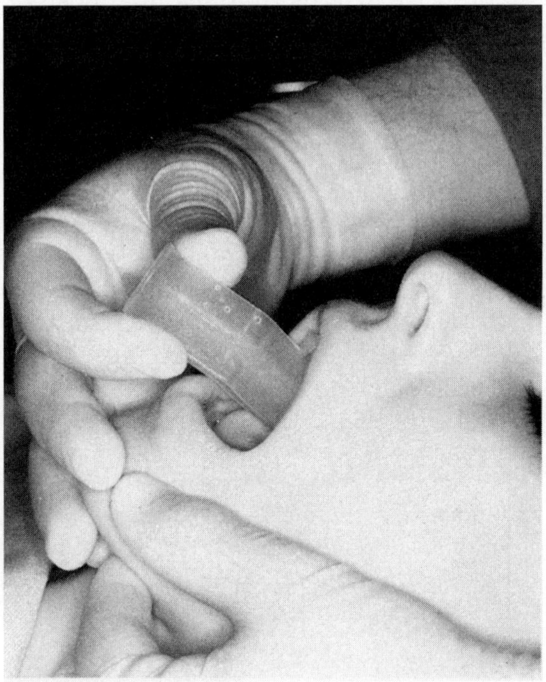

Figure 3B-11B- then rotated 180 degrees.

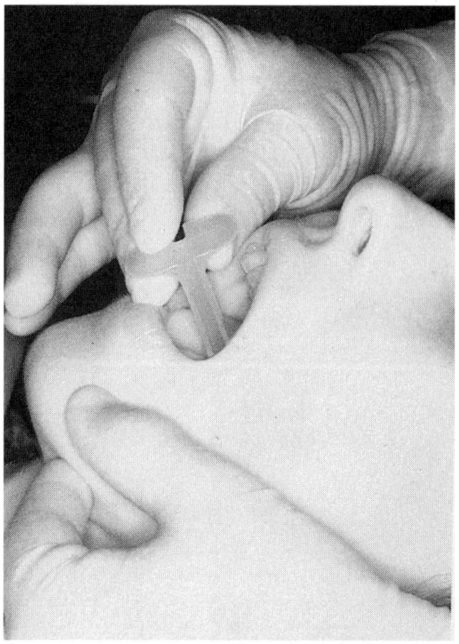

Figure 3B-11C- then slide into its final position. The distal tip should be at the back of the tongue, and the proximal end resting on the lips.

The second technique for insertion of the oral pharyngeal airway requires a tongue blade. The tongue is depressed and the airway is inserted *right side up* into the oral pharynx. With either technique- the flange of the tube should sit comfortably on the lips once the device has been properly inserted into it's final position (Figure 3B-12).

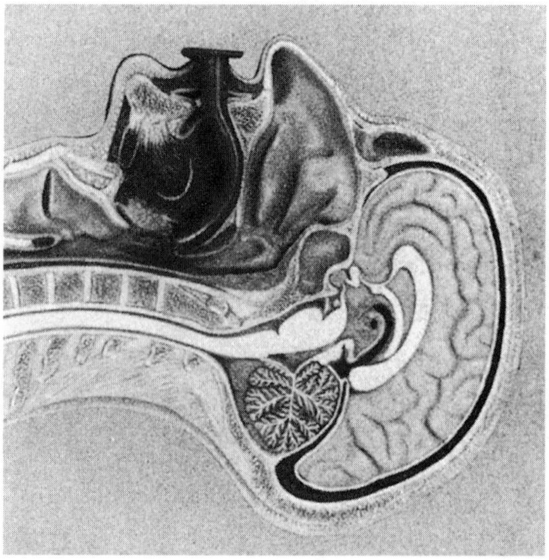

Figure 3B-12- Correct final position of an oral pharyngeal airway.

Special Considerations Regarding Oral Airway Insertion:

- Although the second technique for insertion of the oral airway may seem intuitively easier (i.e., *direct* visualization with the use of a tongue blade)- one must be sure to insert the airway *deep* enough so as to come to rest *behind* the tongue. Unless careful attention is focused on accomplishing this directive, it may be all too easy to stop short- in which case the device may actually *cause* airway obstruction (by pressing on the tongue and pushing it back to occlude the airway).

- If the oral airway repeatedly comes out of the mouth- it is likely to be *improperly* seated (and compressing the tongue into the posterior pharynx). This may further obstruct the airway. *Don't continue to force the airway in.* Instead- *remove it entirely.* Then try to insert it again.

- Although the lumen of the oral airway is adequate for ventilating the patient- it should *not* be used for suctioning because the lumen is not large enough to allow passage of the suction catheter (Figure 3B-13). The suction catheter is instead inserted *adjacent* to the airway. Suction is then performed in the usual manner (Figure 3B-14).

- The oral pharyngeal airway should be used only in *unconscious* patients. Insertion of this device in a conscious or semiconscious patient is likely to activate the gag reflex (when the back of the tongue or posterior pharyngeal wall is touched)- and thus precipitate vomiting. Alert patients (or semiconscious patients with an intact gag reflex)- are therefore *not* suitable candidates for insertion of an oral pharyngeal airway.

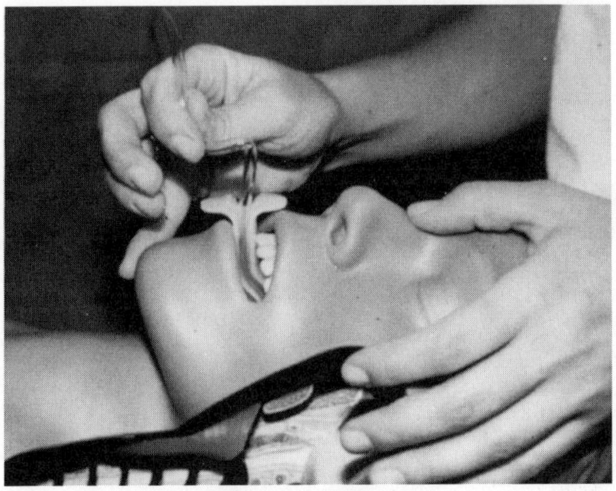

Figure 3B-13

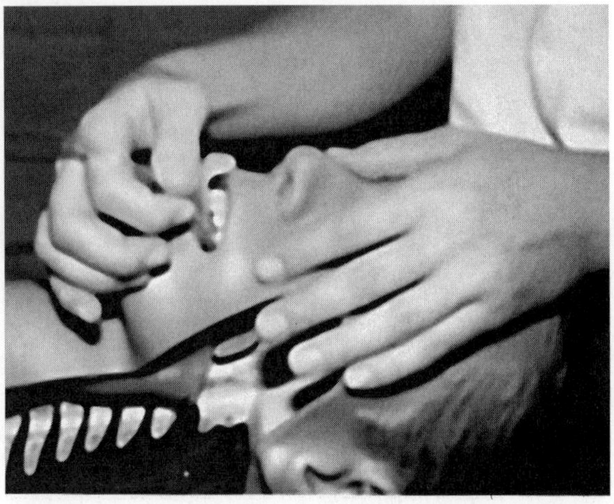

Figure 3B-14

Figure 3B-13- Although the lumen of the oral airway is adequate for *ventilation*, it is *not* large enough to allow passage of a suction catheter. In the above illustration, attempted passage results in kinking of the suction catheter.

Figure 3B-14- The correct way to suction a patient with an oral airway in place is to insert the suction catheter into the mouth adjacent to (but not through) the oral airway.

The Nasopharyngeal Airway (Nasal Trumpet)

The nasopharyngeal airway is an extremely compliant rubber tube that measures approximately 15 cm in length (Figure 3B-15). The tube is designed so that its distal tip sits in the posterior pharynx, while the proximal tip rests on the external nares. The lumen of this device permits the passage of air into the lower respiratory tract.

> **Note**- The principal advantage of the nasal pharyngeal airway is that it is usually well tolerated in the patient who retains a sensitive gag reflex. This makes it the airway adjunct of choice for the conscious or semiconscious patient who experiences respiratory difficulty.

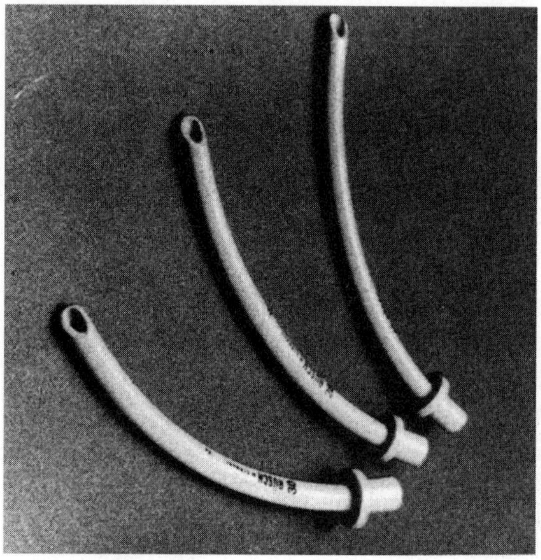

Figure 3B-15- Examples of nasopharyngeal airways.

Technique for Insertion:

The tube should be lubricated with 2% lidocaine gel *prior* to insertion. The purpose of the lidocaine is twofold: it anesthetizes the nasal mucosa in the posterior pharynx (so as to minimize sensitivity of the gag reflex), and lubricates the tube to facilitate insertion.

The nasopharyngeal airway is then advanced into the nares by placing the bevel against the septum of the nose (Figure 3B-16A)- and gently sliding the tube *backward* in line with the base of the ears (Figure 3B-16B). In this way, the tube passes *parallel* to the floor of the nasal cavity (Figure 3B-16C). When completely inserted- the distal end is seated in the posterior pharynx (Figure 3B-16D).

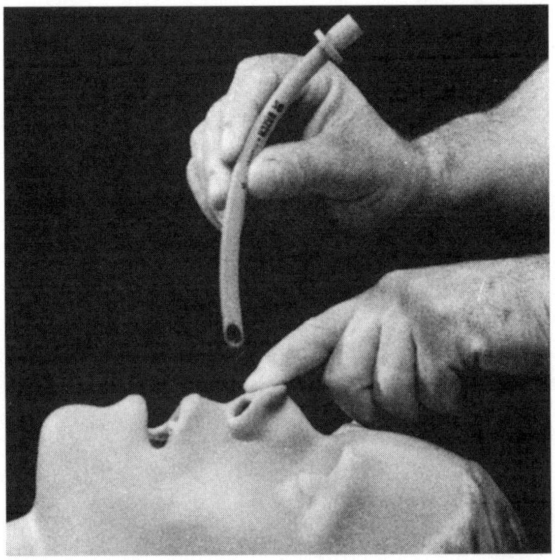

Figure 3B-16A

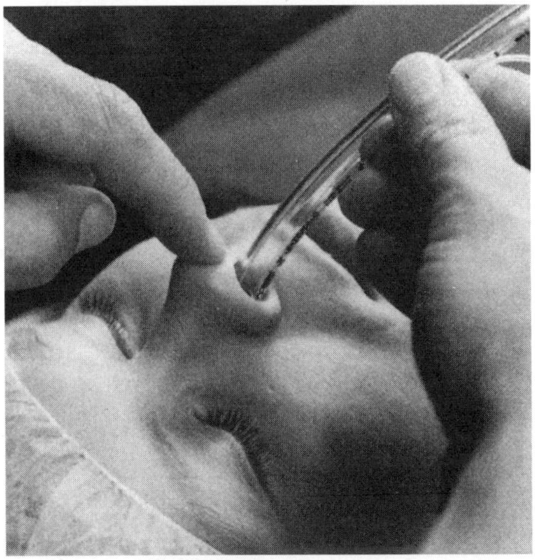

Figure 3B-16B

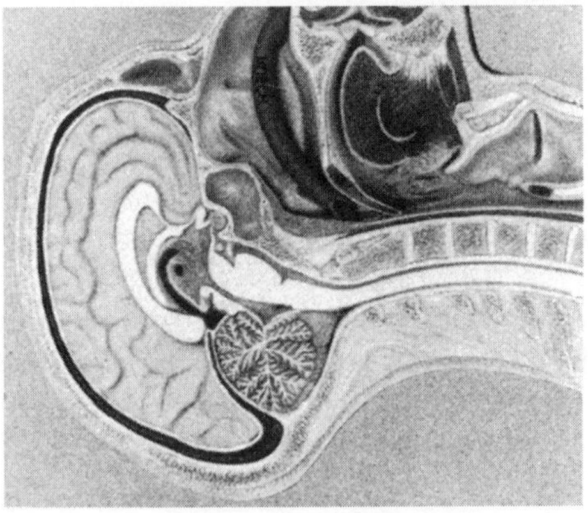

Figure 3B-16C

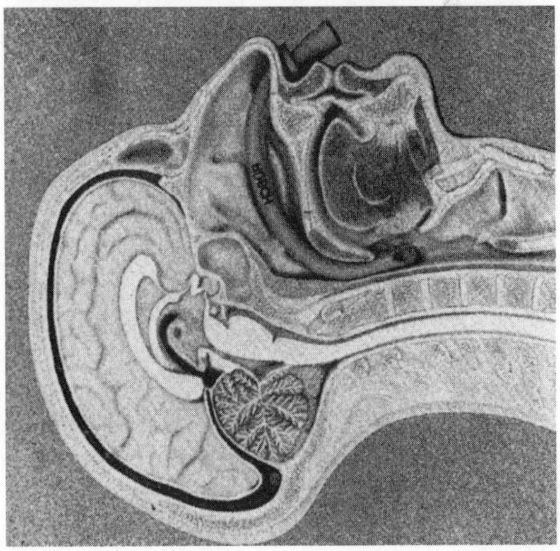

Figure 3B-16D

Figure 3B-16A- Proper bevel position of the nasopharyngeal airway during insertion. In this illustration the bevel is placed against the septum as the airway is inserted into the right nares.

Figure 3B-16B- Carefully slide the nasopharyngeal tube into the nasal cavity, as demonstrated in this photo, which is illustrating the same technique using a ET tube.

Figure 3B-16C- Passage of the nasopharyngeal airway parallel to the floor of the nasal cavity.

Figure 3B-16D- Correct position the nasopharyngeal airway after insertion.

Special Considerations:

- In most cases, proper insertion of the nasal trumpet will result in correct position of the distal end in the posterior pharynx. On occasion, however- the tube may either be too short or too long. Be alert to the fact that if this happens- *adequate ventilation may not be achieved.*

- While most conscious or semiconscious patients are able to tolerate this device- the gag reflex of certain particuarly sensitive individuals may still be activated.

- Forceful introduction of the airway into the nasal passage should be avoided (since this may cause abrasions or lacerate the nasal mucosa- and therefore produce significant bleeding).

Suction

Immediate accessibility to properly functioning suction equipment is equally important as availability of other airway adjuncts. Such equipment is needed to remove secretions and particulate matter that could otherwise be aspirated or compromise the airway. Suction units should be portable, durable, and capable of generating at least 300 mm Hg of negative pressure. When suctioning the oral pharynx- a large-bore catheter and tube should be used in order to ensure that all large particulate matter will be evacuated. Smaller catheters are generally adequate for nasopharyngeal and/or endotracheal suction.

Suction Technique:

Adequate ventilation does *not* occur during suctioning. As a result, patients should always be hyperoxygenated *before* beginning suctioning. The suction procedure itself should never be carried out for more than 15 seconds at a time to minimize the chance of hypoxemia.

Suction of the oral pharynx is performed by inserting the catheter in the patient's mouth, and *intermittently* applying negative pressure. The *KEY* to endotracheal suctioning is *not* to apply negative pressure during insertion of the catheter down the endotracheal tube. Suction is applied intermittently- and *only* while slowly withdrawing the catheter.

Artificial Ventilation

Assisted Ventilations

Regardless of whether a patient is intubated or not, ventilations should be administered in the same manner. In either situation- the *KEY* to ventilation will reside with delivering each breath *slowly* and evenly over a 1 to 2 second time period. Ventilating in this manner reduces airway pressure in the mouth, and therefore decreases the likelihood that gastric insufflation will occur in the patient with an unprotected airway. It also enhances the opening of alveoli in the lung, which results in increased alveolar extraction of oxygen. This method of ventilation mimics our own intrinsic respiratory pattern- and therefore optimizes the ability of the lungs to function properly. In contrast, delivering breaths rapidly would be counterproductive, and would lessen the chance that adequate air will reach the lungs for optimal gas exchange.

> ***KEY***- It should be emphasized that if resistance is encountered at *any* time during ventilation- *do not continue.* Instead, assess the patient *immediately* for the possibility of airway obstruction. Although some patients clearly require higher airway pressures for adequate ventilation (because of restrictive disease or reduced compliance)- it is essential to first *rule out* airway obstruction *before* you proceed with more forceful ventilation.

Ventilation During CPR

Ventilating a patient during CPR is a special skill in itself that requires continuous monitoring and close attention to detail to ensure proper performance. Incorrect ventilation (i.e., application of either excessive or inadequate inspiratory pressure) may result in hypoxemia, increased intracranial pressure, or gastric insufflation- especially in patients who are not intubated. It may also result in accompanying tachycardia or bradycardia.

As is the case for assisted ventilation- when performing CPR, ventilations must also be administered *slowly* and smoothly (i.e., over a 1 to 2 second time period). Only by doing so can one avoid generation of turbulent air flow and ensure even distribution to all lung fields. In addition, the parameters of respiration should ideally remain constant. Thus, each ventilation should be administered at the same speed and pressure to result in as constant a minute ventilation as possible.

CPR is *not* a benign procedure. In addition to fracturing ribs or the sternum- CPR may cause cardiac or pulmonary parenchymal changes (contusions), liver laceration, and/or pneumothorax or hemothorax. Unfortunately, some of these complications are *not* amenable to immediate treatment. Resuscitative efforts (including external chest compression) need to continue if a patient remains pulseless- *regardless* of whether there are cardiac contusions or fractured ribs. In contrast, other potential complications of CPR (such as tension pneumothorax or cardiac tamponade) mandate immediate recognition and treatment if resuscitation is to have any chance for success.

Practically speaking- the goal of achieving optimal ventilation during CPR is a task much easier wished for than accomplished. Pulmonary parenchymal changes are a common (expected) accompaniment of even perfectly performed CPR. This unfortunate clinical reality is made abundantly clear from inspection of Figure 3B-17- which illustrates the typical appearance of the lungs after a relatively short period (*less* than 15 minutes) of

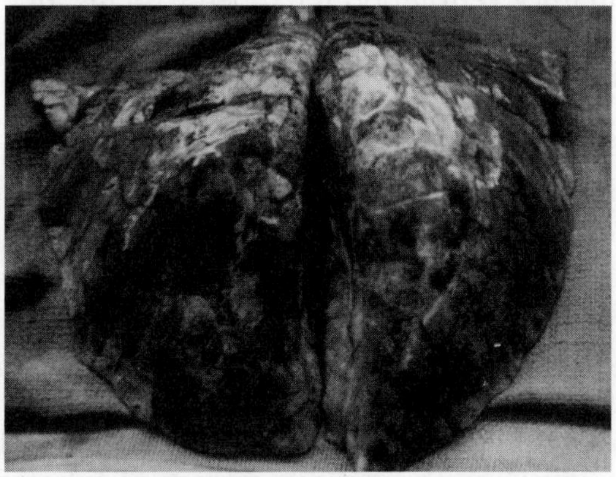

Figure 3B-17- Example of typical pulmonary contusions that occurred during external chest compressions. The darkened areas are areas of contusions and hemorrhage.

CPR. Note that numerous areas of pulmonary contusion, hemorrhage, and atelectasis are already evident. As a result of these anatomic alterations- pathophysiologic changes are produced which lead to increased pulmonary vascular resistance with impaired pulmonary flow and suboptimal oxygenation. Parenchymal damage (and associated pathophysiologic changes) would probably be even more significant in those patients with underlying pulmonary disease who undergo CPR. As might be expected, lung compliance is dramatically reduced by this process- and *continues* to decrease (i.e., the lungs become stiffer) the longer resuscitation is in progress. Accordingly, ventilation during CPR becomes progressively more difficult and less effective.

Clearly, the first step toward reducing the deleterious pathophysiologic changes produced in the pulmonary parenchyma by CPR is to minimize the duration of the resuscitative process. Attention to a number of other factors may also be helpful. For example, undue emphasis is often placed on strict interposition of ventilation after every fifth compression during basic life support. Practically speaking- blood flow is *not* decreased when a portion of the ventilatory cycle overlaps with the next chest compression. In fact, blood flow to the arrested heart may actually *increase* by simultaneous occurrence of ventilation and compression. While we are definitely *not* suggesting to disregard AHA recommendations for basic life support (to administer ventilations during the pause after each fifth chest compression)- we *are* emphasizing the tremendous importance of being sure that ventilation is not unduly hurried.

KEY- Ventilation must be delivered *slowly* and smoothly (to ensure as even distribution of air to all lung fields as possible).

For those patients who *remain* in cardiac arrest- intubation should be accomplished as expeditiously as possible. Subsequent ventilation (which is usually accomplished by compression of a bag-valve device) should continue to be smooth with a slow and even delivery- keeping respiratory parameters as constant as possible (while still maintaining the flexibility to adapt to alterations in lung compliance as the resuscitative process goes on).

Ventilatory Adjuncts

The devices described below are used to assist ventilation of patients in respiratory distress or to provide mandatory ventilation for those who are not breathing at all.

The Pocket Mask (Mouth-to-Mask)

The pocket mask is very similar to the mask used in conjunction with the bag-valve devices (Figure 3B-18). The major difference is that the mouth-to-mask unit has an additional port where supplemental oxygen can be administered, providing inspired oxygen concentrations of 50% when the flow rate is 10 L/minute. The port used for attachment of the reservoir bag with the bag-valve device is the port through which the rescuer ventilates the patient with the pocket mask.

The most attractive feature of the pocket mask is that it allows the rescuer to perform mouth-to-mouth ventilation *without* the need for direct contact with the mouth of the victim. Addition of a disposable, inexpensive exhalation (one-way) valve further ensures the safety of the rescuer (by diverting the victim's stream of exhaled air)- and should alleviate concerns about contracting an infectious disease (such as AIDS or tuberculosis). As noted earlier, tidal volumes attainable by ventilation with the pocket mask are superior to those achieved from ventilation with a BVM unit.

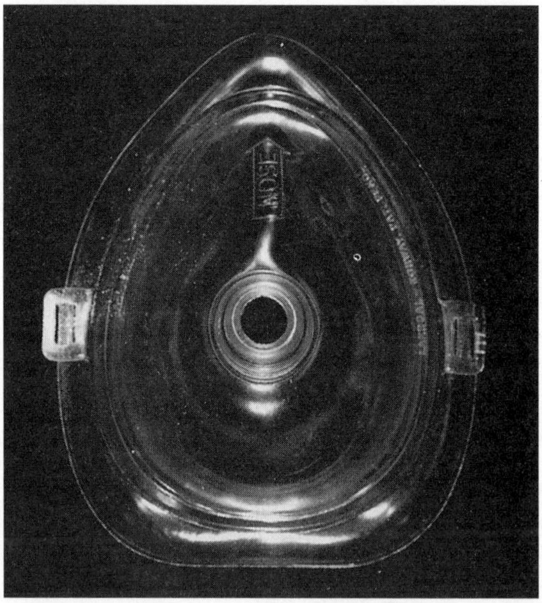

Figure 3B-18- Pocket Mask

Technique for Use:

When using the pocket mask, the rescuer positions himself/herself above the head of the patient. The mask is placed on the patient's face and secured through a coordinated interplay of the fingers of both hands. The thumbs stabilize the mask over the bridge of the nose, while the index fingers hold the mask in place over the chin. The three remaining fingers of each hand are positioned under the chin, and act in concert to maintain the the head tilt which keeps the airway patent (Figure 3B-19).

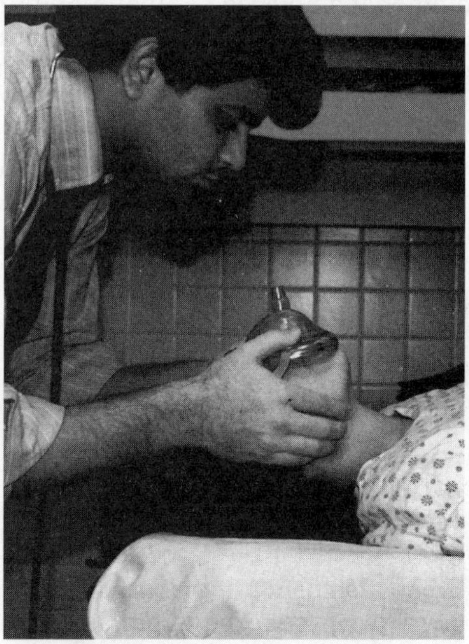

Figure 3B-19- Proper application of the pocket mask. The rescuer is at the head of the patient in good position for ventilation.

Self-Inflating Reservoir Bags

The self-inflating resuscitation bag (bag-valve mask or BVM) is a unit consisting of a bag and an adapter that can be attached to a mask or endotracheal tube (Figure 3B-20). This is the most common device for delivering assisted ventilations in emergency situations.

The ideal BVM unit should have the following characteristics:

i) A clear mask
ii) A self-inflating, easy-to-grip bag
iii) A system for delivery of supplemental oxygen
iv) An oxygen reservoir
v) No pop-off valve.

The reason for the clear mask is that it allows the emergency care provider to see if regurgitation has occurred. The bags of most BVM units are made of smooth rubber that becomes especially slippery when wet. An easy-to-grip bag would facilitate handling the unit when ventilating the patient.

A system for delivery of supplemental oxygen is important. An FiO_2 of up to 40% may be provided by attaching a high-flow source of supplemental oxygen to the bag. With the additional attachment of an oxygen reservoir and a flow rate of 10 to 15 L/minute- an FiO_2 of up to 90% may be delivered.

Pop-off valves are not desirable for BVM units used to manage the airways of patients in cardiac arrest because of the dramatic decrease in lung compliance that occurs in this setting. As we have already mentioned, much higher than usual airway pressures are often needed to ventilate such patients. Pop-off valves could be self-defeating, as they might prevent generation of sufficient peak airway pressure to overcome this increase in airway resistance.

BVM units are the most commonly employed ventilatory adjunct in emergency situations. Nevertheless, significant drawbacks are associated with their use. These include fluctuations in peak airway pressure, tidal volume, and ventilatory rate; variability in delivered oxygen concentrations when a reservoir is not used; and face mask leaks.

Contrary to popular belief, tidal volumes generated with BVM units in the unprotected airway are far less than those generated by mouth-to-mouth or mouth-to-mask ventilation. This is *not* true for intubated patients- since leakage of air through (around) the face mask is no longer a problem, and both of the rescuer's hands are now free to squeeze the bag.

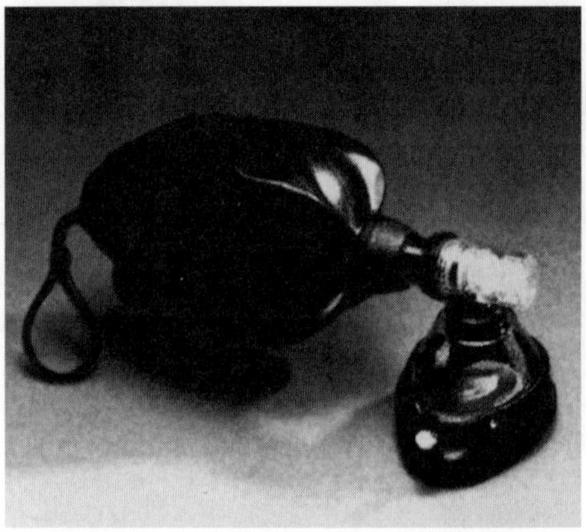

Figure 3B-20- Example of a self-inflating bag-valve mask (BVM).

Technique for Using Bag-Valve Mask:

The most difficult part about ventilating a patient who is not intubated using a BVM device is that one rescuer must simultaneously perform three tasks (Figure 3B-21A). A patent airway and tight face seal must be maintained with one hand- while the other hand is used to ventilate the patient. Unless each of these tasks is performed correctly, inadequate ventilation is likely to result.

Insertion of an oral or nasopharyngeal tube may assist in maintaining patency of the airway. The mask of the BVM unit is then applied to the patient's face and secured by positioning the index finger on the portion that covers the chin- while the thumb holds the upper part of the mask *firmly* against the bridge of the nose (pushing down to ensure a good face seal). The remaining three fingers are placed on the base of the mandible and support the head in the tilt position (by careful upward pressure). Once the fingers are correctly in place, their action is similar to that when squeezing a rubber ball. The other hand is used to squeeze the bag (Figure 3B-21B).

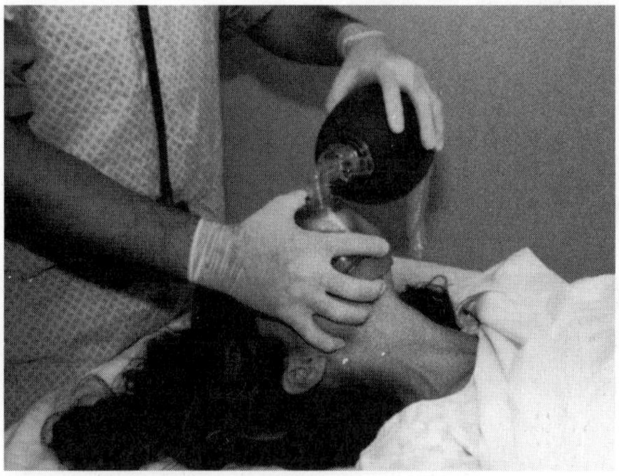

Figure 3B-21A- Use of BVM by a single rescuer. This task requires the simultaneous accomplishment of three tasks: maintaining a patient airway and face seal with one hand, while ventilating the patient with the other hand.

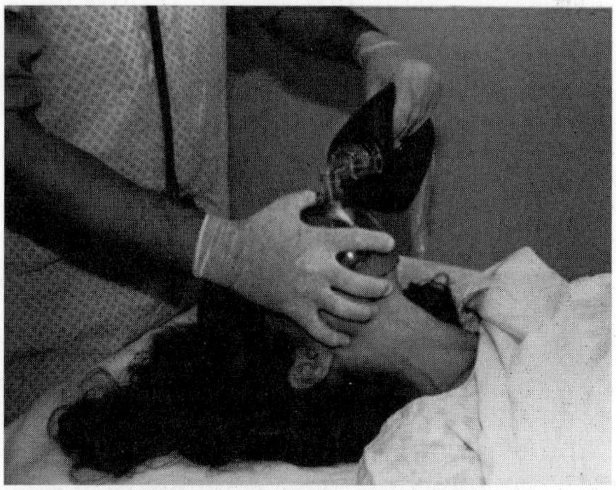

Figure 3B-21B- Follow-up to Fig. 3B-21A, illustrating actual ventilation as the single rescuer squeezes the bag.

To prevent high peak airway pressures and decrease the likelihood of gastric distention in the patient with an unprotected airway- the bag must be squeezed slowly. Use of a second rescuer is extremely helpful in this regard, since it allows one rescuer to concentrate on securing a good face seal with the use of both hands- while the second rescuer may also use both hands to squeeze the bag (Figure 3B-21C). When proper ventilation is being administered, the chest will be observed to rise and fall with each insufflation of the bag.

> **Note**- An additional advantage of the BVM unit is that it provides the rescuer with a sense of the compliance of the patient's lungs.

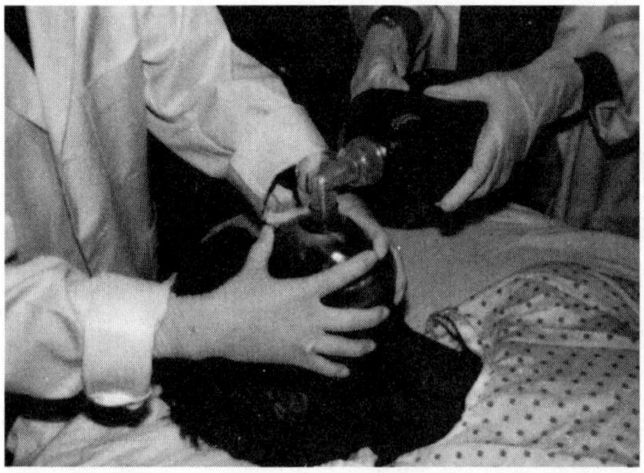

Figure 3B-21C- Addition of a second rescuer greatly facilitates proper ventilation with a BVM (unit). One rescuer concentrates on maintaining a patent airway and tight face seal, while the second rescuer is able to use both hands to deliver ventilations.

Flow-Inflation Reservoir Bag

The flow-inflation reservoir (anesthesia) bag (Mapelson-D bag) requires even more skill to operate than does a BVM. It consists of an anesthesia bag, a piece of plastic tubing (that is approximately 1 foot long), an exhaust valve, and a standard endotracheal tube connector (Figure 3B-22). The latter is usually attached to the oxygen source and an endotracheal tube. Advantages of this bag over the standard BVM are that you can apply CPAP (continuous positive airway pressure) and PEEP (positive end-expiratory pressure). In addition, ventilation with 100% oxygen is guaranteed. In contrast, one is never entirely sure of the concentration of oxygen delivered with the BVM (because of the variability in the amount of entrained room air).

In general, Mapelson-D bags are used much less commonly than BVM units. This device should be operated only by individuals highly trained in its use. In the hands of an inexperienced provider, the risk of barotrauma (and tension pneumothorax) is great.

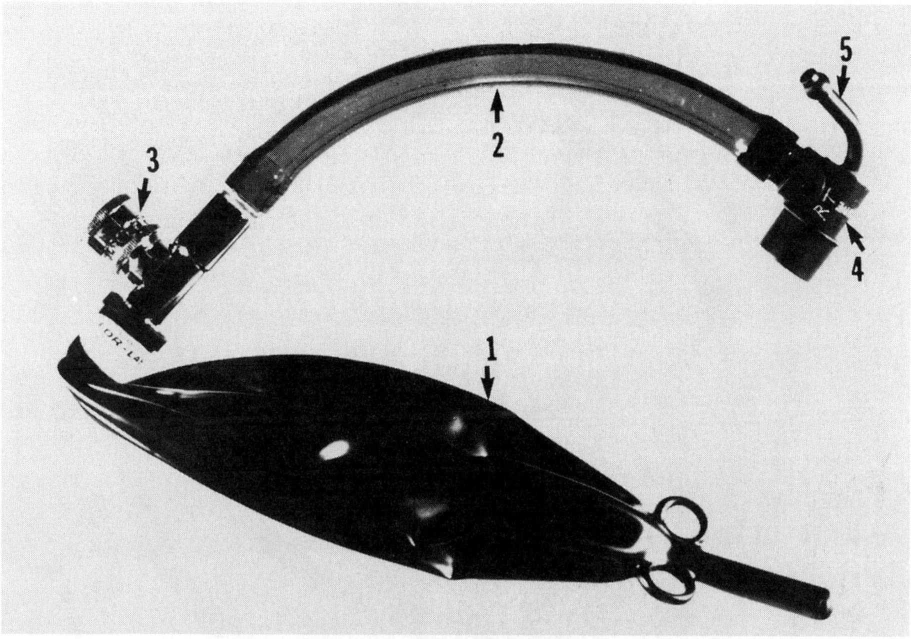

Figure 3B-22- Flow-inflation reservoir bag: (1) anesthesia bag; (2) plastic tubing; (3) exhaust valve; (4) standard ET tube connector; (5) connector for oxygen supply tubing.

Oxygen-Powered Breathing (O_2PBD)

The oxygen-powered breathing device has been used to ventilate the victim in respiratory arrest and provide supplemental oxygen to spontaneously breathing patients. When used in the former setting, the O_2PBD functions as a manually cycled, pressure-limited ventilator (Figure 3B-23). Activation of the unit by the rescuer provides spontaneous flow rates of up to 120 L/minute. Ventilation is terminated either by release of the activation button, or when peak airway pressure attains 40 mm Hg (54 cm H_2O).

Concerns about the use of this device relate to the high inspiratory flow rates it generates (and turbulent flow it produces) when manually operated- as well as the potential for producing gastric insufflation in the patient with an unprotected airway. Recent modifications in newer models (and manufacture of conversion kits for older models) have improved the safety of the O_2PBD by allowing reduction of flow rates to 40 L/minute. Nevertheless, the device must still be used with extreme caution in adults (especially in patients who are not intubated)- and it is not recommended for use in children.

The O_2PBD may be most useful when employed as a demand valve for spontaneously breathing patients. In this capacity, generation of as little as 1 cm H_2O negative airway pressure activates a flutter valve within the unit that allows the patient to inhale 100% oxygen. This aspect of the device is extremely advantageous in providing spontaneously breathing patients supplemental oxygen without requiring large volumes of stored oxygen.

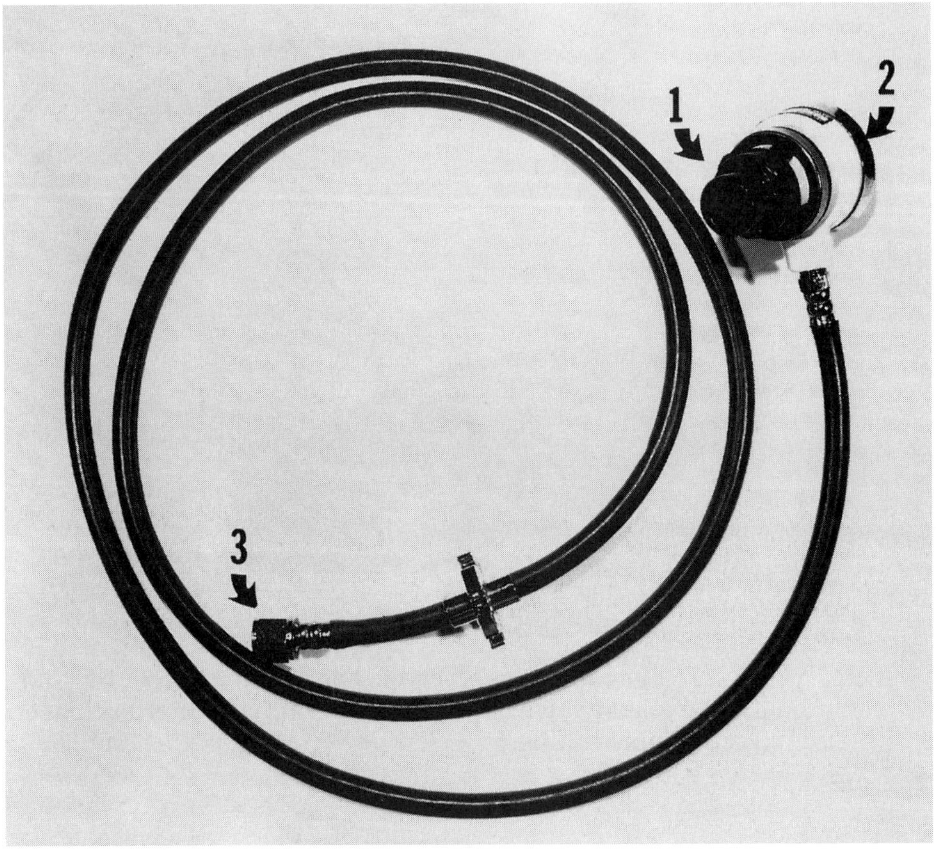

Figure 3B-23- Oxygen-powered breathing device: (1) 15/22mm connector for attaching the endotracheal tube; (2) flow regulator; (3) oxygen source connector.

Advanced Airway Management Techniques

Esophageal Obturator Airways

The principle of the esophageal obturator is to occlude the esophagus so that gastric insufflation is prevented and the ventilatory efforts of the rescuer can be directed into the trachea. Two types of obturators are currently available: the **esophageal obturator airway (EOA)** and the **esophageal *gastric* tube airway (EGTA)**. Although similar in appearance, important differences exist between the two types of obturators in the method of ventilation.

The ***EOA*** is the original esophageal obturator airway. This device was first described in 1968. It consists of a tube approximately 37 cm in length with a blind tip on its distal end. Inflation of a cuff just above this tip occludes the esophagus. When properly inserted, the cuff should lie slightly below the level of the carina of the trachea (Figure 3B-24).

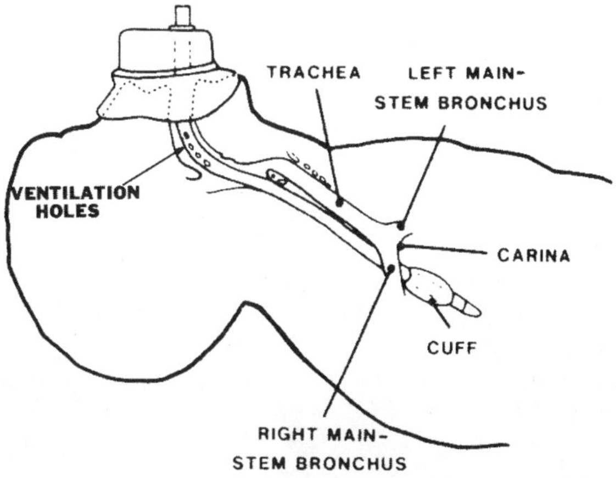

Figure 3B-24- Correct positioning of esophageal obturator airway (EOA) after insertion. The cuff of the EOA lies just below the carina. (Reproduced with permission. *Textbook of Advanced Cardiac Life Support,* 1994 Copyright American Heart Association.)

The proximal end of the tube is open and fits snugly into a specially designed face mask. Small ventilation holes are present in the upper third of the tube. When the EOA is correctly positioned, the holes lie at the level of the posterior pharynx. It is through these small holes that ventilation occurs.

The ***EGTA*** was developed in 1977. It improved on the design of the EOA by adding a route for decompression of the stomach (Figure 3B-25). This lessens the chance of regurgitation and aspiration. Instead of having a blind tip on the distal end of the obturator tube, an opening was made through which a nasogastric tube could be passed into the stomach. The small holes which had previously been used for ventilation with the EOA are no longer present with the EGTA tube. Instead, a second port has been added to the mask through which ventilation occurs in a similar fashion as with the bag-valve mask (Figure 3B-26).

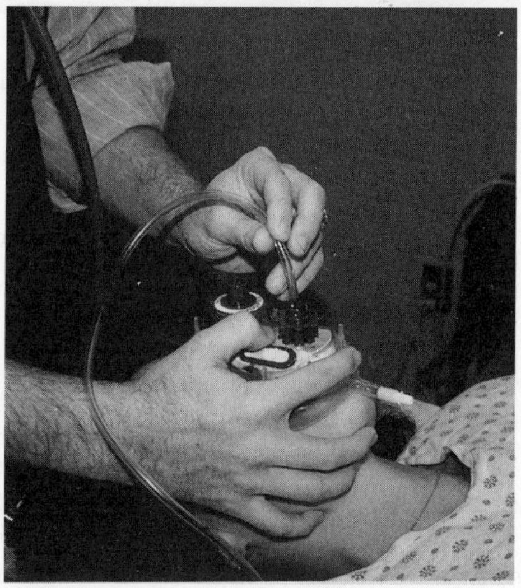

Figure 3B-25- Inserting a gastric tube through the lumen of the EGTA (tube) to decompress the stomach.

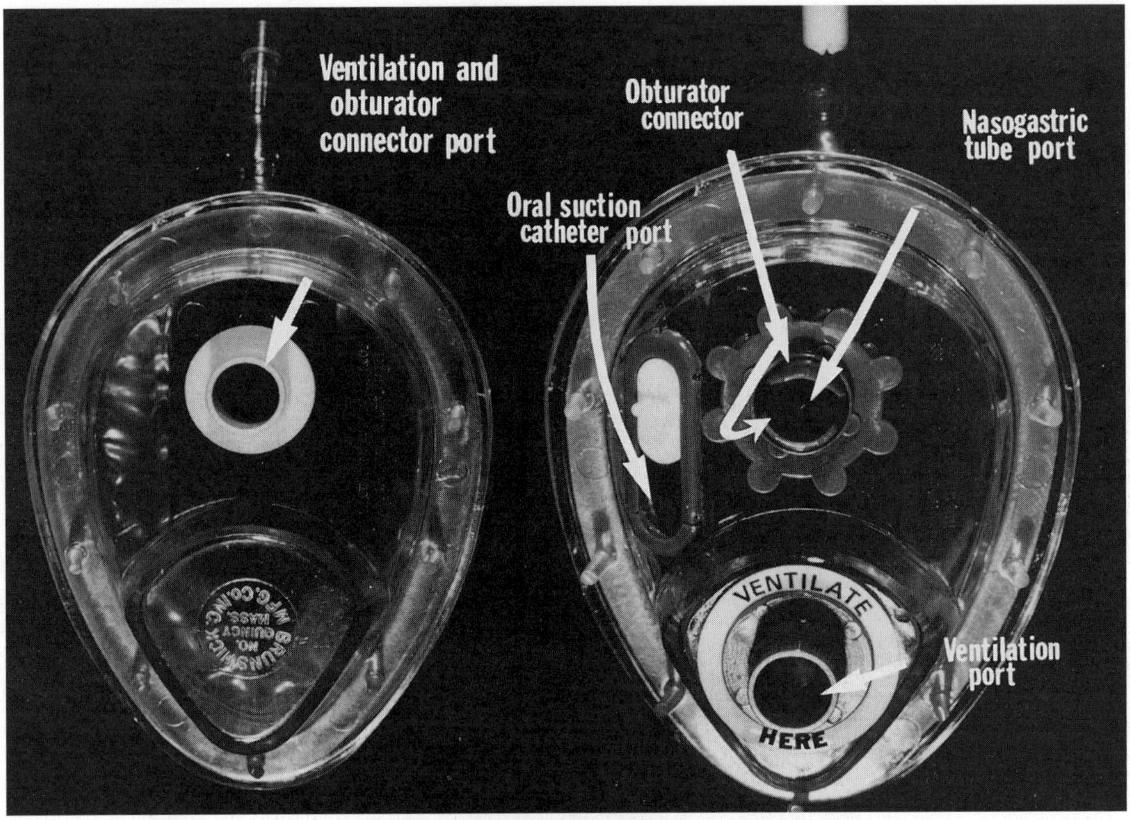

Figure 3B-26- Comparison of EOA (left) and EGTA (right) face mask. Ventilation with EOA is accomplished via the ventilation holes shown in Figure 3B-24. In contrast, ventilation with the EGTA is accomplished through a special ventilation port. In both cases, air is directed into the trachea by virtue of the fact that the esophagus is occluded.

Technique for Insertion:

The principle for insertion of the EOA and the EGTA is the same. The mandible is lifted forward by the rescuer's hand, as the patient's head is gently flexed to assist passage of the tube into the esophagus (Figures 3B-27A and 3B-27B). The EOA/EGTA is inserted into the oral pharynx and *blindly* advanced. It should follow the natural curvature of the pharynx and enter into the esophagus (Figure 3B-27C). At this point the mask should be seated on the face (Figure 3B-27D).

Never force advancement of the tube. If resistance is encountered along the way- simply withdraw the tube slightly and reposition the patient's head. Then try again to advance the tube.

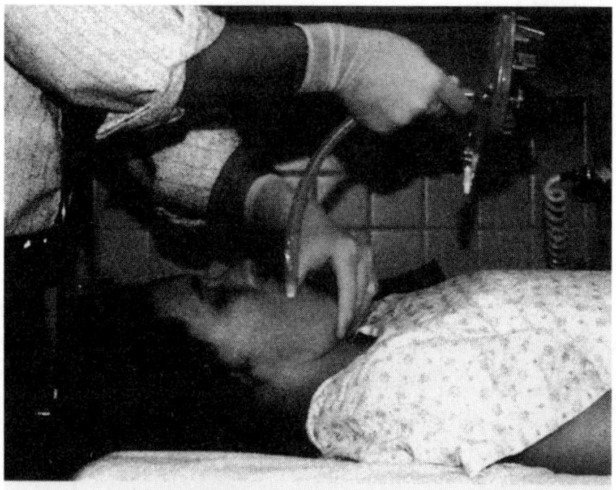

Figure 3B-27A- Position of the head (gently flexed forward) while inserting the obturator airway.

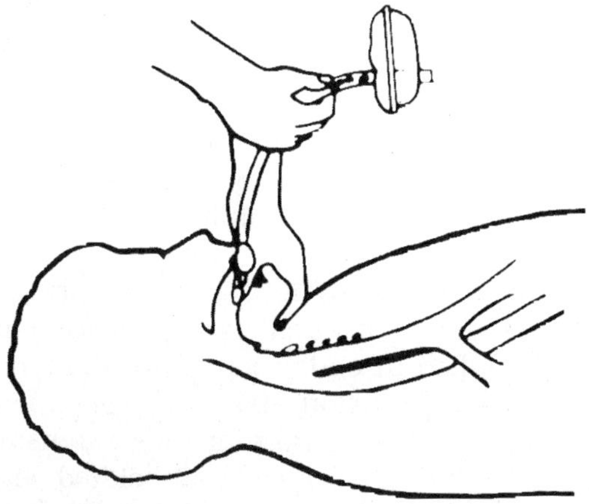

Figure 3B-27B- Schematic representation of Figure 3B-27A. (Reproduced with permission. *Textbook of Advanced Cardiac Life Support*, 1994 Copyright American Heart Association.)

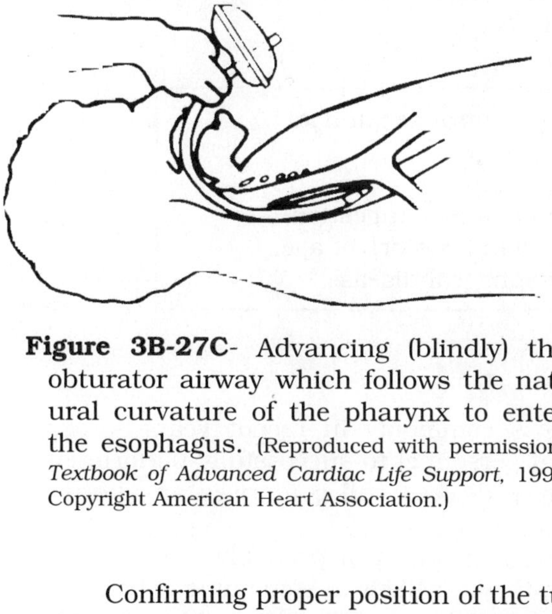

Figure 3B-27C- Advancing (blindly) the obturator airway which follows the natural curvature of the pharynx to enter the esophagus. (Reproduced with permission. *Textbook of Advanced Cardiac Life Support*, 1994 Copyright American Heart Association.)

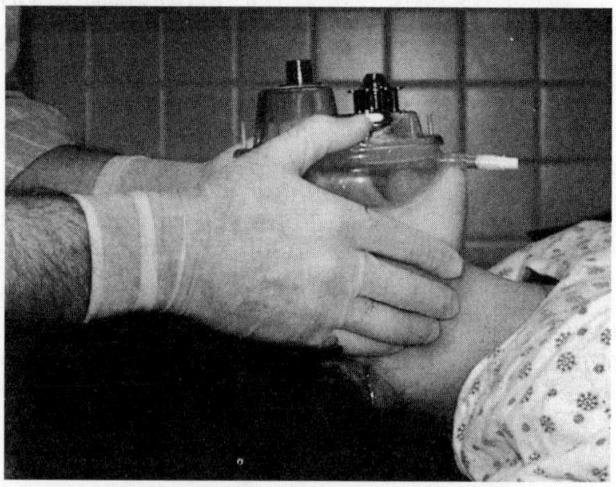

Figure 3B-27D- Final position of the obturator airway mask.

Confirming proper position of the tube is critical. If the trachea is inadvertently intubated and the cuff of the tube inflated with 20 to 30 ml of air, significant damage may occur to this structure. Several positive pressure ventilations should be delivered to test for tube position. Even though some of this air will enter the esophagus, enough should go into the trachea to produce a rise and fall of the chest wall if the tube is properly situated in the esophagus. The cuff may now be inflated with 20-30 ml of air. Further confirmation of proper tube placement can be obtained by auscultating over the apices and lateral lung fields for good bilateral breath sounds, and observing for symmetric chest excursion.

Another way to confirm proper tube placement is by $ETCO_2$ monitoring. Extremely low $ETCO_2$ readings suggest that the obturator may have inadvertently intubated the trachea-whereas increasing $ETCO_2$ readings are consistent with proper tube placement.

Special Considerations:

As was the case for ventilating a patient with a BVM, obtaining a good face seal is essential for ensuring adequate ventilation with the EOA/EGTA. Realize that head positioning in preparation for EOA/EGTA insertion is the *opposite* of that for preparing to intubate endotracheally. That is- the neck is slightly extended back, and the chin is flexed forward. Doing so minimizes the chance of inadvertently entering the trachea when the tube is inserted.

The EOA/EGTA was initially advocated as an alternative method of endotracheal intubation. Its greatest application has been in the prehospital setting, where operators skilled in endotracheal intubation are not always available. Advantages of the EOA are that insertion may be accomplished rapidly (in *less* than 10 seconds) by trained individuals- and that neck extension is *not* needed for the procedure. However, significant problems have been associated with its use. These include:

i) Inadequate tidal volumes due to face mask leak.
ii) Inadvertent endotracheal intubation.
iii) Esophageal laceration and rupture.
iv) High incidence of gastric regurgitation on removal of the tube.

Because of these problems, endotracheal intubation is universally acknowledged as the procedure of choice for managing the unprotected airway.

Note- Use of the EOA/EGTA is *contraindicated* if:

i) The victim is conscious.
ii) There is suspicion of caustic ingestion.
iii) The victim is less than 16 years of age.
iv) There is known esophageal disease.

Additional Considerations:

The EOA/EGTA has been used much less commonly in recent years- probably because of the increased ability of paramedical personnel to successfully perform endotracheal intubation. Nevertheless, use of these devices still comprises an alternative method for securing an airway.

Practically speaking, most emergency care providers will probably never have the opportunity to insert an EOA/EGTA. However, they *are* likely at some time to be involved with the *removal* of this device- especially if they work in an emergency facility. It is therefore essential to at least gain familiarity with the technique for removal of the tube.

If the patient is still not breathing spontaneously on arrival in the emergency department- endotracheal intubation must be performed *before* the esophageal obturator is withdrawn in order to protect the airway. Because of the extremely high incidence of gastric regurgitation with removal of the EOA/ EGTA- the patient's head should be turned to the side, and suction must be readily available.

Hyperventilate the patient *prior* to any manipulation. The face mask of the obturator is then detached by squeezing the connector on the proximal end of the tube that protrudes through the mask (Figure 3B-28). To make room for the laryngoscope, the obturator tube is pushed to the *left* side of the mouth with the rescuer's index finger. Intubation can now be performed in the usual fashion. A beneficial result of the fact that the EOA/EGTA is still in place in the esophagus is that the rescuer is far less likely to mistakenly intubate this structure.

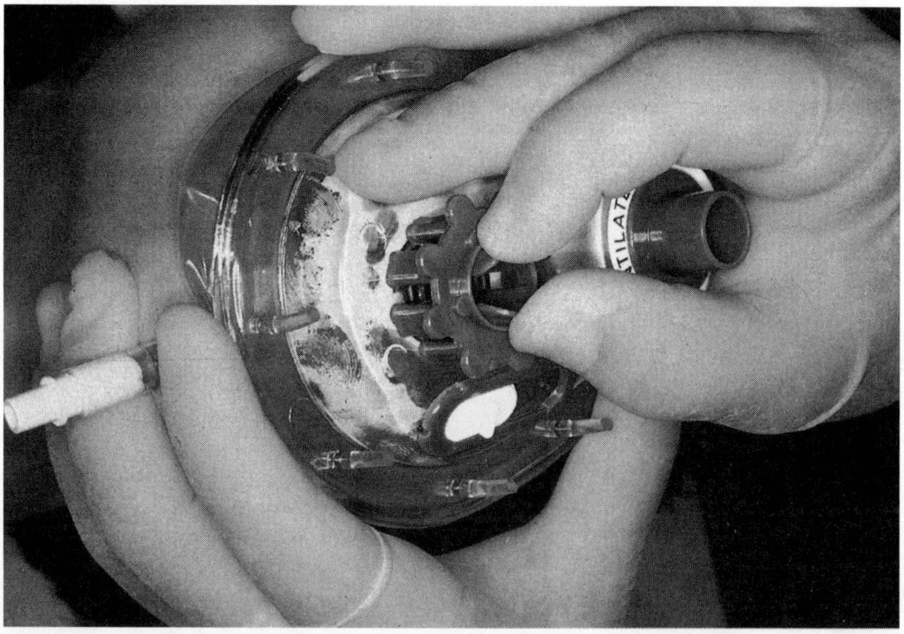

Figure 3B-28- Releasing the EGTA face mask. The prongs on the proximal tip of the obturator are squeezed together to release the mask.

Once correct placement of the endotracheal tube has been confirmed, the EOA/EGTA may be removed. This should be done by deflating the balloon, turning the patient on the side, and vigorously suctioning the oral pharynx at the same time that the tube is withdrawn.

Endotracheal Intubation

The most definitive means of managing the airway for the nonbreathing, unresponsive patient is with endotracheal intubation. The advantages of intubation are:

i) Prevention of aspiration.
ii) Reduced risk of inducing gastric insufflation.
iii) Allows for administration of high concentrations of inspired oxygen and positive pressure ventilation.
iv) Provides emergency access for drug administration (when IV access has not yet been obtained).
v) Provides access for suctioning of the tracheobronchial tree (with endotracheal or nasotracheal intubation).

Two types of laryngoscope blades may be used to perform this procedure: the **Miller** (i.e., ***straight***) **blade** and the **MacIntosh** (i.e., ***curved***) **blade.** The technique for visualization of the vocal cords will be similar *regardless* of which blade is used. The only difference in the procedure is in the placement of the tip. When using the ***curved* blade**, the tip is inserted *into* the vallecula. The soft tissue is then lifted- and the laryngeal opening is visualized (Figure 3B-29). In contrast, when the ***straight* blade** is used- the epiglottis itself is lifted to provide visualization (Figure 3B-30).

KEY- It *matters little* which blade is chosen for intubation. Far more important for the emergency care provider is to decide on his/her preference- and to become comfortable in the use of that one type of blade.

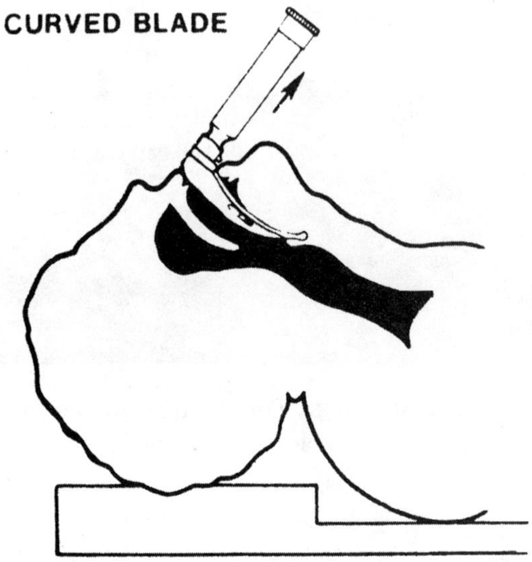

Figure 3B-29- Proper placement of the curved blade in the vallecula.
(Reproduced with permission. *Textbook of Advanced Cardiac Life Support,* 1994 Copyright American Heart Association.)

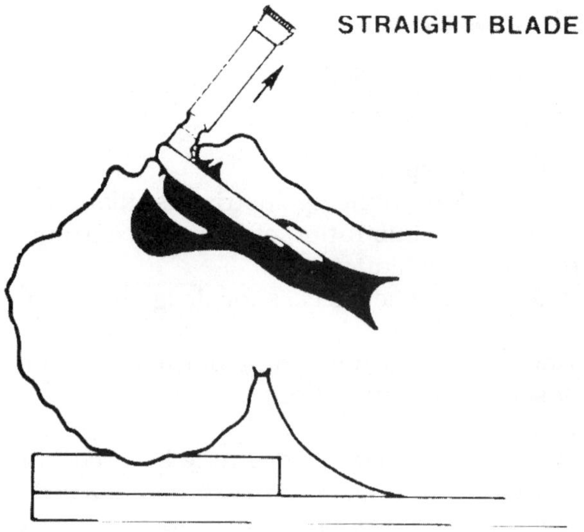

Figure 3B-30- Proper placement of the straight blade. The epiglottis is lifted with the distal tip of the blade to visualize the aperture of the trachea.
(Reproduced with permission. *Textbook of Advanced Cardiac Life Support,* 1994 Copyright American Heart Association.)

Special Features:

An advantage of the ***curved* blade** is its relatively large surface area compared to the straight blade. This facilitates manipulation of the tongue, and provides a larger space in the oral cavity for passage of the endotracheal tube. It may also be somewhat easier technically to use the curved blade. On the other hand, visualization of the larynx may *not* be quite as good because the presence of the epiglottis below the curved blade may partially block the operator's view. With the ***straight* blade**- the epiglottis is lifted up and out of the line of view. *Each blade has its advocates.* As emphasized above- the choice of which one to use is simply a matter of personal preference.

> **Note**- The size of the endotracheal tube most commonly used to intubate adults is 7.5 to 8 mm in diameter for females, and 8 to 8.5 mm for males.

Prior to Intubation

All equipment must be routinely checked at frequent intervals. The time to find out that a laryngoscope bulb has burned out is *not* after the blade has been inserted into the pharynx. Similarly, the time to find out that the cuff is defective is *not* after the patient has been intubated.

Pre-oxygenation should always precede attempts at intubation. At no time should a patient remain unventilated for more than 20 to 30 seconds. If intubation is not successful within this time frame- *withdraw* the tube. Reventilate the patient with 100% oxygen for 20 to 30 seconds. Then try again.

Positioning the Patient

It is commonly assumed that hyperextension of the head and neck will facilitate endotracheal intubation. In reality, hyperextension produces the *opposite* effect- because it causes the axes of the oropharynx and trachea to become misaligned (Figure 3B-31). One technique that may make intubation easier is to place a small pillow or towel under the patient's occiput so as to lift the head slightly *without* extending it. This posture is known as the ***sniffing position*** (Figure 3B-32). As can be seen from Figure 3B-33- a much more *direct* line for visualization of the vocal cords (due to alignment of the axes of the oropharynx and trachea) is now evident.

> **Note**- As an aid to conceptualizing the ***"sniffing position"***- pretend you are holding a wonderfully fragrant flower in front of you. Now imagine how you would position yourself to take a sniff. *Do so.* Now consider what you have done to achieve the position- *flexed your neck forward,* and *slightly extended it.*

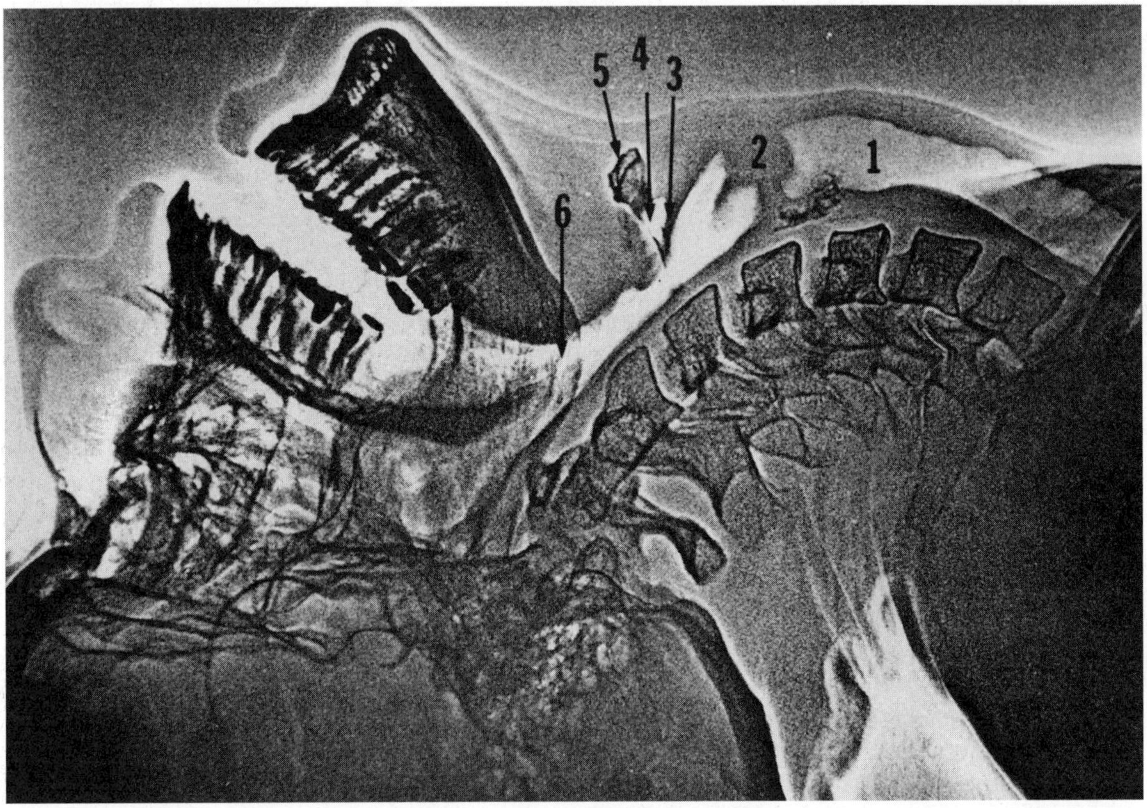

Figure 3B-31- Hyperextension of the neck. The axes at the oropharynx and trachea become misaligned with hyperextension making endotracheal intubation more difficult: (1) trachea; (2) vocal cord; (3) epiglottis; (4) vallecula; (5) hyoid cartilage; (6) oropharynx.

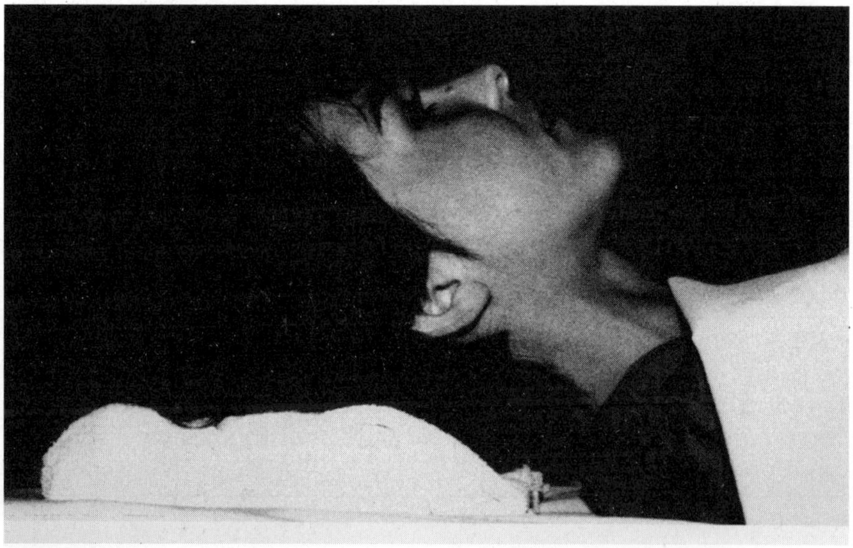

Figure 3B-32- Sniffing position. A pillow lifts the occiput without hyperextending the head.

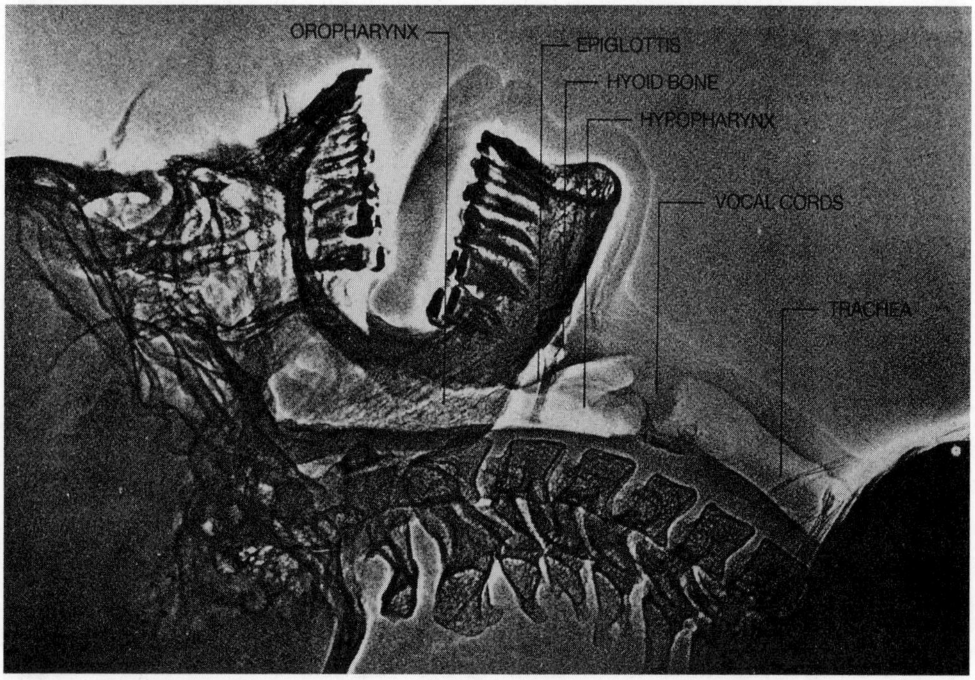

Figure 3B-33- X-ray demonstrating anatomic relationships in the sniffing position. Compared to Figure 3B-31, a much more direct line for visualization of the vocal cords is now evident.

Technique for Intubation:

The *KEY* priorities for endotracheal intubation are speed of insertion (to minimize the time of hypoxia) and proper technique. The two are *equally* important (and closely interrelated). Thus, attention to proper technique naturally improves speed, as operator familiarity and confidence increase (and the need for repetitive intubation attempts becomes less).

A common mistake is to rapidly insert the full length of the laryngoscope blade *without* attention to placement. This frequently puts the tip of the blade *beyond* the epiglottis and vallecula- making it extremely difficult for the operator to identify the anatomy. The operator is then forced to search for key structures on withdrawal of the blade. It is far simpler and more effective to insert the blade in a more controlled manner. This allows visualization of structures in their natural sequence *as the blade is advanced* through the airway.

> ***KEY***- Remember that the vallecula lies at the base of the tongue and is not nearly as deep in the throat as is commonly believed. It is therefore *not* necessary to insert the entire length of the laryngoscope blade into the patient's mouth for successful intubation.

After equipment has been checked and the patient properly positioned and pre-oxygenated, you are ready to begin the procedure. Insert the laryngoscope blade *carefully* into the patient's mouth, following the natural curvature of the tongue (Figure 3B-34). The hard palate and uvula are visualized as one tracks through the oral pharynx (Figure 3B-35). On arrival at the posterior pharynx, the tip of the blade is lifted. In most cases

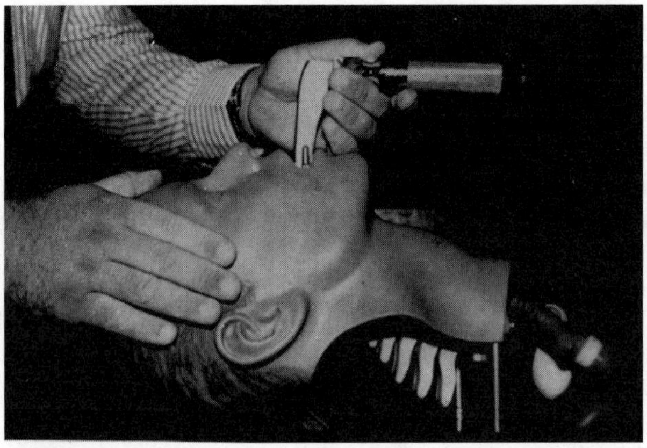

Figure 3B-34- Inserting the laryngoscope blade into the patients mouth, following the natural curvature of the tongue.

the epiglottis will now become readily visible (Figure 3B-36). If you are using the straight blade- the epiglottis itself is lifted to visualize the cords (Figure 3B-37). If the curved blade is used- the blade tip is inserted into the vallecula and then lifted a little higher to visualize the cords.

The teeth must *not* be used as a fulcrum to pry up the mandible when attempting to visualize the cords. Doing so makes it likely that a tooth will be fractured or dislodged. Instead, the operator should concentrate on lifting the laryngoscope handle *forward* and *anteriorly*- as if reaching to touch the point where the ceiling and wall meet (Figure 3B-38). In doing so, the principal movement is from the arm and elbow. Excessive wrist flexion does not help visualization, and it predisposes to trauma.

Once the epiglottis has been lifted and the laryngeal opening is in view, the following structures should be seen:

i) The arytenoid cartilages.
ii) The vocal cords.
iii) The glottic opening.

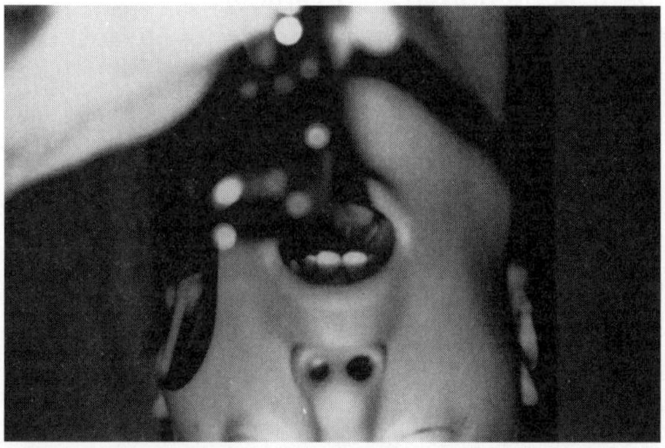

Figure 3B-35- Visualization of the hard palate and uvula as one tracks through the oral pharynx.

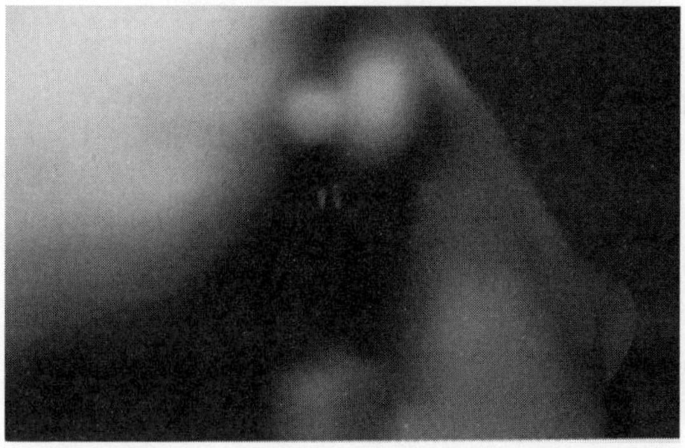

Figure 3B-37- Lifting the epiglottis with the straight blade to visualize the cords.

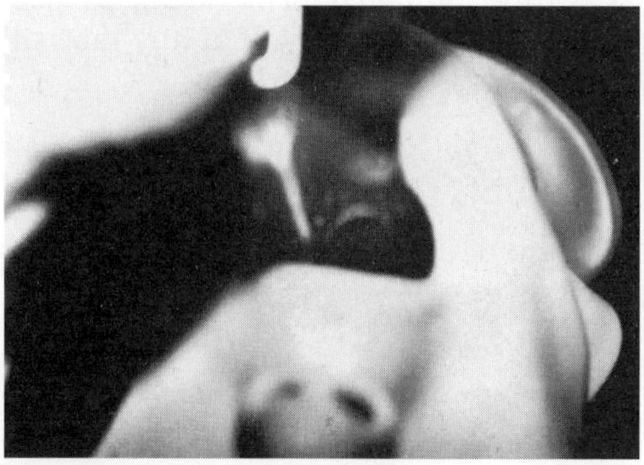

Figure 3B-36- Visualizing the epiglottis as the blade tip is lifted.

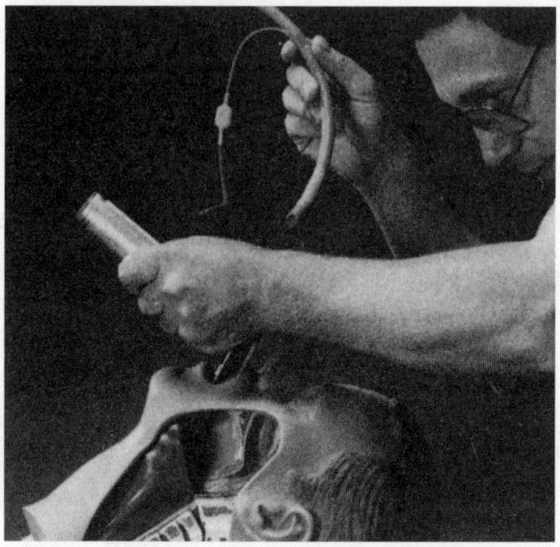

Figure 3B-38- Correct technique for insertion of the endotracheal tube, lifting the laryngoscope handle *forward* and *anteriorly* .

The arytenoid cartilages lie at the bottom of the rescuer's field of vision (Figure 3B-39). Behind them are found the white, glossy vocal cords, which are separated by the dark glottic opening. It is through this opening that the endotracheal tube is inserted. One should be extremely deliberate in watching the tube pass through this opening. Advance the endotracheal tube until the cuff just disappears from sight, which is approximately 2 cm beyond the cords (Figure 3B-40). Advancement beyond this point should be avoided because it may result in intubation of the right mainstem bronchus.

Once the tube is properly seated in the trachea it is held in position with the operator's *right* hand. Care must be taken not to dislodge the endotracheal tube or fracture any teeth while removing the laryngoscope. The cuff is now inflated with 5 to 10 ml of air. Correct position of the tube should be verified by auscultating the lung fields and epigastric areas as several ventilations are administered. One listens for the presence of good bilateral breath sounds and looks for symmetric chest excursion. Absent or diminished breath sounds on the left side of the chest suggest intubation of the right mainstem bronchus. This can usually be rectified by withdrawing the tube a short distance until breath sounds equalize. Should gurgling sounds be heard over the epigastrium with ventilations, the tube is in the esophagus. Immediately deflate the balloon and remove the tube. Final confirmation of proper tube placement is demonstrated radiographically.

Unfortunately, if at any time the cuff ruptures- the ET tube must be removed and the patient reintubated.

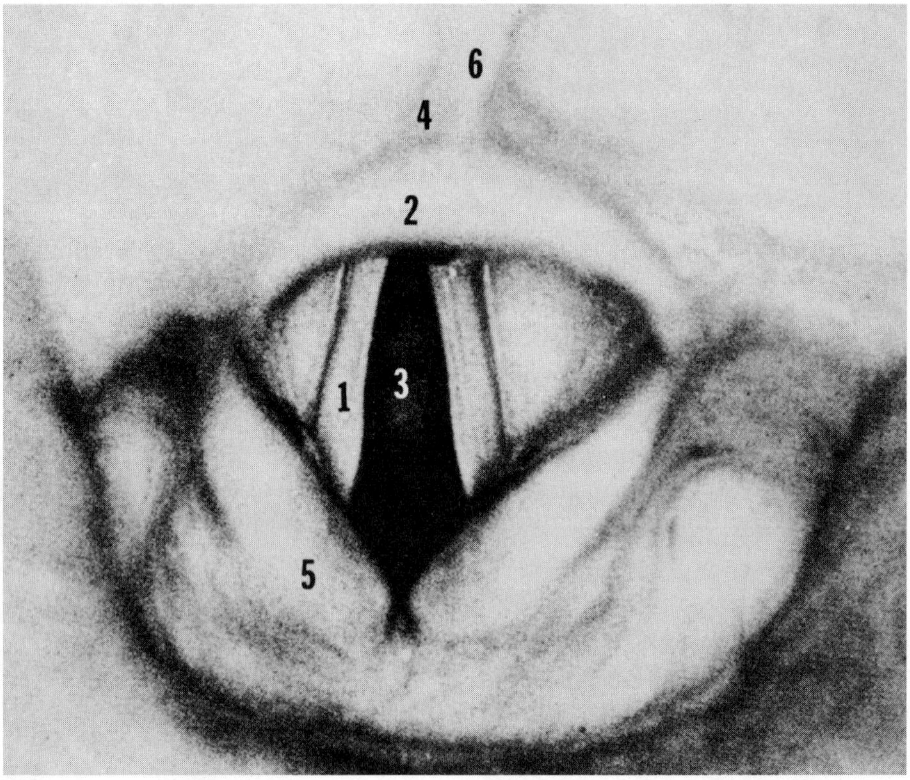

Figure 3B-39- Anatomy the area around the entrance to the trachea: (1) vocal cords; (2) epiglottis; (3) aperture of the cords; (4) vallecula; (5) arytenoid cartilage; (6) tongue.

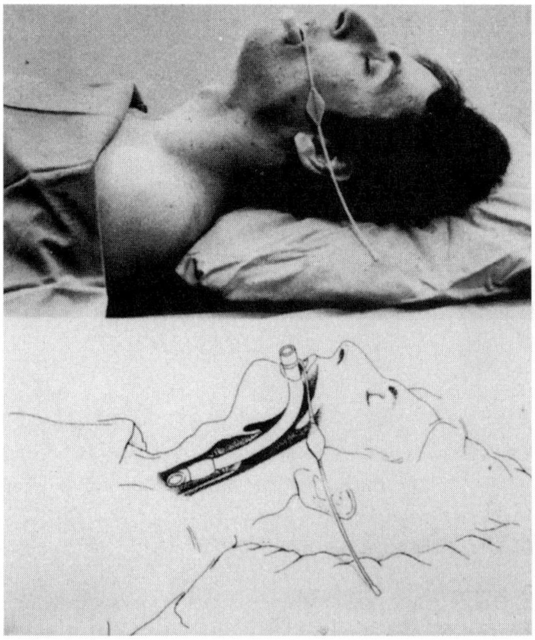

Figure 3B-40- Correct position of the endotracheal tube after insertion. The tube has been advanced through the cords until the cuff is approximately 1/2 to 1 inch past the vocal cords.

Use of a Stylet

Insertion of an endotracheal tube may sometimes be aided by the use of a ***stylet***. This malleable, firm wire is inserted into the endotracheal tube, with the distal end of the stylet lying at least 1 cm proximal to the distal end of the endotracheal tube. The reason for recessing the distal end of the stylet is to avoid traumatizing the airway. Molding the stylet so that the distal end of the endotracheal tube takes on a "hockey stick" appearance, and then guiding this curvature in an anterior direction usually facilitates entry through the cords.

The Sellick Maneuver

Another technique that may greatly assist the operator during endotracheal intubation is application of **cricoid pressure** (the ***Sellick* maneuver**). This technique serves the dual function of facilitating visualization of the glottis and preventing regurgitation of gastric contents until intubation can be completed. Unlike other tracheal cartilages which have a soft membranous posterior portion- the cricoid is a full cartilaginous ring. As a result, pressure on this structure can occlude the esophagus by compressing it against the vertebral bodies that lie below.

To perform the Sellick maneuver, one must first identify the *cricoid cartilage*. This is done by walking one's hands down in the midline from the thyroid cartilage (Adam's apple) into the depression below (the cricothyroid membrane)- and onto the next lying structure. This is the cricoid cartilage. Apply firm, *downward* pressure on the anterolateral aspects of this cartilage with the thumb and index finger of either hand (Figure 3B-41). Be sure to *maintain* this downward pressure until *after* the endotracheal tube has been inserted and the cuff is inflated (or else gastric regurgitation will occur)!

Proper hand placement is essential for the Sellick maneuver to work. Pressure must *never* be applied directly over the cricoid cartilage. Doing so will only compress the larynx and make intubation more difficult. Instead, the site for downward pressure application is along the *outer* edge (anterolateral aspect) of the cricoid cartilage.

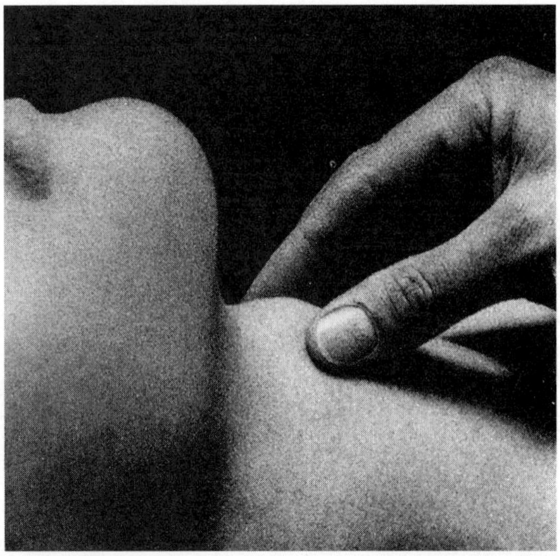

Figure 3B-41- Application of the Sellick manueuver. Firm *downward* pressure is applied to the anterolateral aspect to cricoid cartilage.

Special Considerations Regarding Intubation:

An interesting phenomenon to be aware of (and prepared for) is the development of ***hypotension*** immediately following the intubation of certain patients in acute respiratory distress. Considering the sequence of events leading up to emergency intubation, this phenomenon should not be unexpected:

- Endogenous catecholamines rise markedly in patients with acute air hunger as a natural result of the anxiety, fear, and severe stress they experience. Elevated catecholamines promote tachycardia and/or hypertension.

- Sedation will often be needed to facilitate intubation of acutely anxious patients with severe air hunger. This may cause hypotension by two mechanisms: i) the sedative drug shuts off the patient's endogenous catecholamine surge; and ii) many sedative drugs exert a direct vasodilatory effect on the arterial vasculature.

- Hypotension may be further aggravated by application of positive pressure ventilation after intubation which increases intrathoracic pressure (and leads to a reduction in venous return).

Blind Nasotracheal Intubation

The advantage of nasotracheal intubation is that it provides an alternative method for achieving definitive control of the airway in the spontaneously breathing patient who exhibits teeth clenching and/or who retains a sensitive gag reflex. A slightly smaller (6.5 to 7.5 mm in diameter) endotracheal tube is recommended for this procedure than for oral endotracheal intubation.

Technique for Insertion:

The technique for insertion is initially the same as that described for placement of a nasopharyngeal airway. The nasotracheal tube is lubricated with 2% lidocaine gel. It is inserted into the nares and advanced by placing the bevel against the septum of the nose- and then gently sliding the tube backward in line with the base of the ears (Figure 3B-42). In this way the tube passes *parallel* to the floor of the nasal cavity.

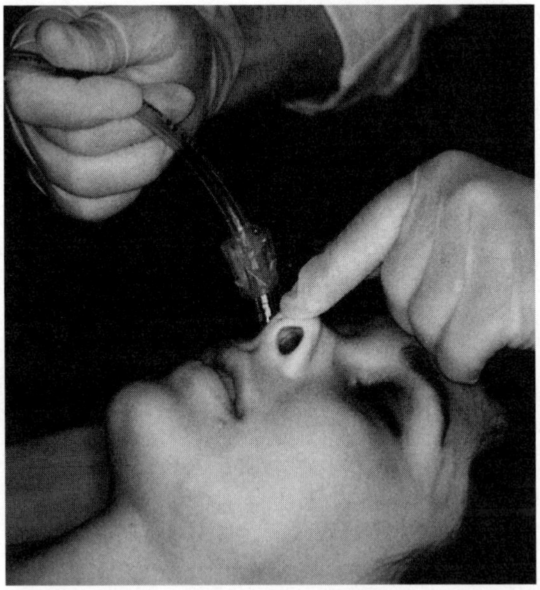

Figure 3B-42- Insertion of nasotracheal tube into the right nares.

In passing from the nasopharynx to the posterior pharynx, the tube must take a downward turn. Occasionally it may get hung up trying to negotiate this turn and abut against the posterior pharyngeal wall. Clinically, this should be suspected if resistance to further advancement is encountered or there is loss of air movement through the tube. Should this happen- immediately *withdraw* the tube a short distance. Reposition (slightly extend) the patient's head, and then reattempt to advance the tube. Do *not* try to force the tube forward- as this may result in mucosal injury and bleeding (or even in retropharyngeal perforation)!

At this point, direct your attention to listening (or feeling) for air movement through the tube (Figure 3B-43). As the distal end of the tube gets closer and closer to the laryngeal opening, the sound of air movement should become increasingly louder (Figure 3B-44). Continue to gently guide the tube toward the glottis. If at any time air movement ceases- withdraw the tube slightly, reposition the patient's head (if needed), and resume the process. When air movement sounds are at their loudest, hold the tube still. Try to *anticipate* the very next inspiratory effort of the patient. The moment this effort begins- attempt to advance the tube into the trachea. This often stimulates the patient's cough reflex. If the attempt is successful- inspiratory and expiratory air flow will be heard through the tube. If not- the esophagus may have been intubated. The tube should be immediately withdrawn, and another attempt made.

Once the patient has been intubated, final tube placement should be confirmed in the same manner as for oral endotracheal intubation.

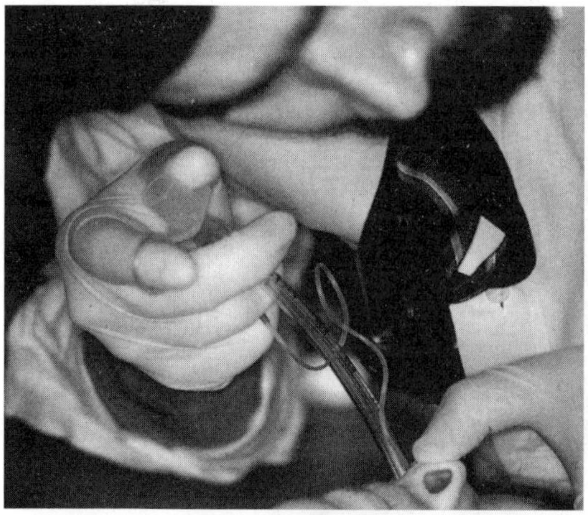

Figure 3B-43

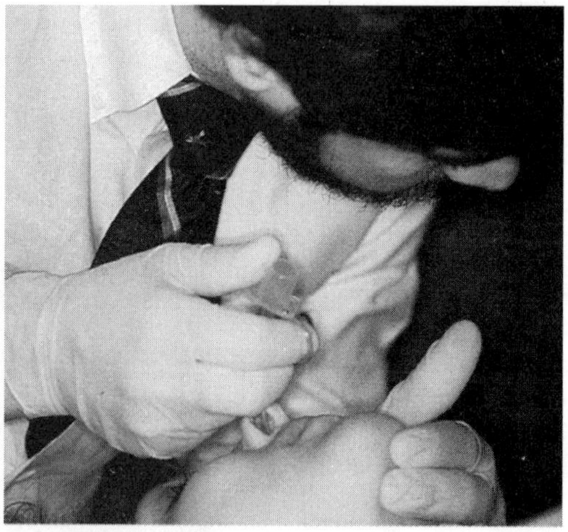

Figure 3B-44

Figure 3B-43- Listening for air movement as the tube is advanced.

Figure 3B-44- As the final position of the nasotracheal tube is approached, the sound of air movement becomes increasingly louder. Manipulation of the trigger at this point may facilitate tracheal intubation *(see Figure 3B-45).*

Special Considerations:

In recent years a device has been developed that greatly facilitates blind nasotracheal intubation (Endotrol, National Catheter Corporation, Brunswick, New York). By means of a *trigger* mechanism at the proximal end of the tube, controlled flexion of the distal end is now possible (Figure 3B-45). This allows the operator to direct the distal tip *anteriorly* (in the direction of the laryngeal opening) at the moment the tube is inserted into the trachea (Fig. 3B-44).

It is important to emphasize that since accurate placement with blind nasotracheal intubation is predicated on hearing (or feeling) air movement in the tube- the procedure *cannot* be performed in an apneic patient.

Note- At times the intubator may not desire having to place his/her face in the close proximity to the proximal end of the endotracheal tube (and to the patient's face) as shown in Figure 3B-44 in order to listen for air movement. This can be easily accomplished by use of a stethoscope (Figure 3B-46).

Simply remove the stethoscope head and place the distal end of the stethoscope tubing down the endotracheal tube. Then listen for breath sounds in the usual manner. The length of the stethoscope tubing allows the operator a much more comfortable distance from the victim's face during the procedure (Figure 3B-46).

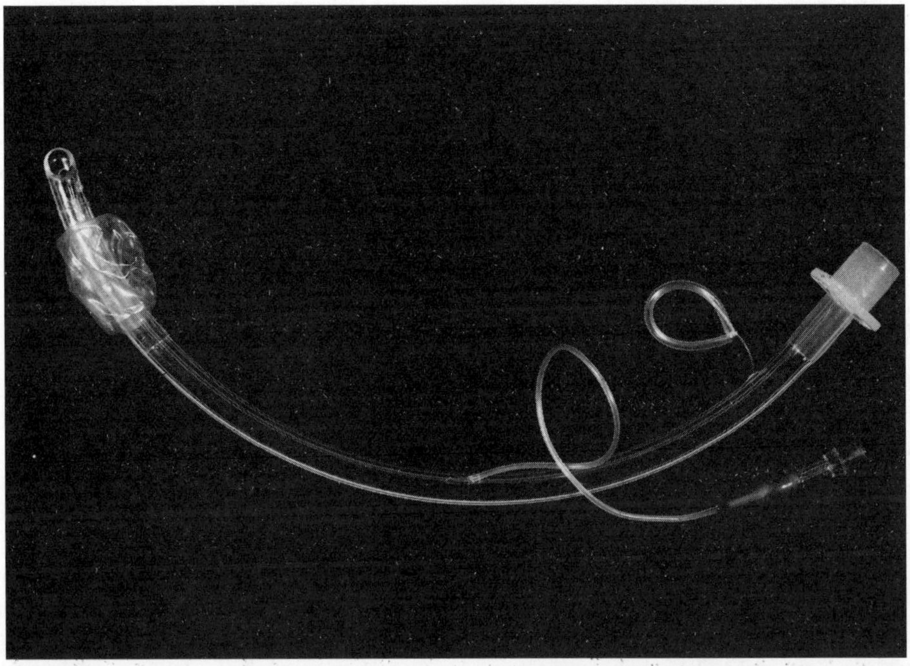

Figure 3B-45- Endotrol tube. A trigger mechanism at the proximal end of the tube allows controlled flexion of the distal end.

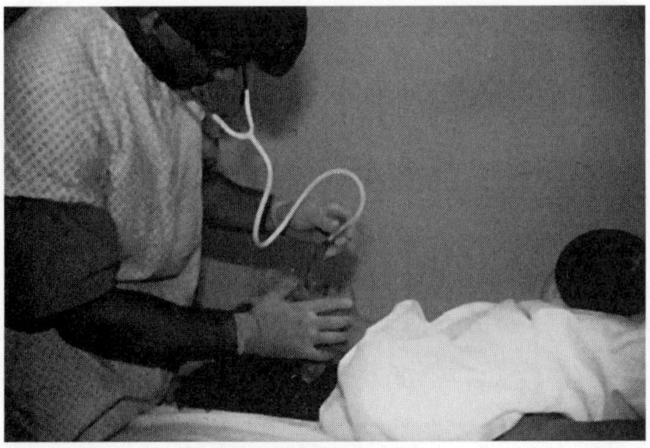

Figure 3B-46

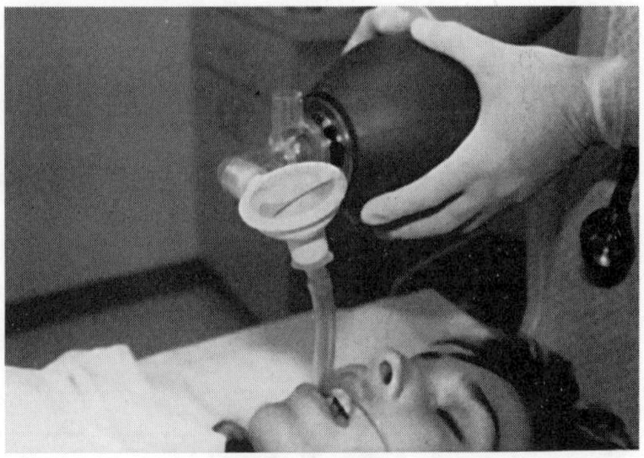

Figure 3B-47

Figure 3B-46- Use of the stethoscope for distancing oneself from the patient while listening for air movement during blind nasotracheal intubation.

Figure 3B-47- $ETCO_2$ monitor. The $ETCO_2$ monitoring device is readily attached in-line between the ET tube and the BVM.

Another way to facilitate blind nasotracheal intubation incorporates use of an endotracheal tube whistle (Beck Airflow Monitor MARK IV Endotracheal Tube Whistle, Great Plains Ballistics, Inc., Donaldsville, Louisiana). This small plastic device conveniently attaches to the 15-mm endotracheal tube adapter. Air flow through the tube produces sound that varies in intensity (becoming louder as the larynx is approached) and pitch (producing a higher-pitched sound on inspiration than expiration). This not only alerts the operator to the anatomic position of the ET tube relative to the cords, but also facilitates anticipation of the next inspiratory phase (which is a decided advantage in the noisy environment that is so common in emergency care settings).

Is the ET tube truly placed correctly?

Throughout this chapter we have emphasized the importance of verifying proper endotracheal tube placement after intubation. Verification begins at the bedside (or in the field in the prehospital setting) with auscultation of the lungs for equal bilateral breath sounds and visualization of good bilateral chest excursion. It continues with the use of modalities that assess the adequacy of oxygenation, such as oximetry and/or $ETCO_2$ determinations. Final confirmation of proper ET tube placement requires a chest x-ray.

The point we wish to emphasize is the potential fallibility of the physical exam *by itself* as a means of confirming proper tube placement. Even when highly experienced providers judge their intubations to be successful- suboptimal tube placement (right mainstem intubation or final tube placement too close to the carina) is still possible. Physical examination is simply not as reliable a method as one would like for confirming proper endotracheal tube placement! Obtaining a chest x-ray is therefore *essential* for confirmation- especially in emergency situations. Unfortunately, while ordering a chest x-ray is easy to do in a hospital setting- it is obviously impossible in the field. As a result, $ETCO_2$ monitoring (as discussed earlier) is becoming increasingly used for assessing proper tube placement (Figure 3B-47).

An additional clinical finding to be aware of that suggests correct tube placement is *condensation* of moisture on the *inside* of the endotracheal tube during ventilation.

Algorithm for Management of the Adult Airway

To help conceptualize the material covered in this chapter, we have developed an Algorithm for Management of the Adult Airway (Figure 3B-48). The management sequence begins with the rescuer simultaneously assessing ventilation and the level of consciousness (**1**).

Note- Many definitions exist for the terms conscious, semiconscious, and unconscious. For the purpose of determining optimal management of the airway, we have defined these terms in the following manner:

- **Conscious** - a patient who is alert, awake, and responding appropriately.
- **Semiconscious** - a less alert patient who may not be awake and only responds to verbal or painful stimuli. The gag reflex may still be intact.
- **Unconscious** - a patient who cannot be aroused and does not respond to either verbal or painful stimuli. The gag reflex is absent.

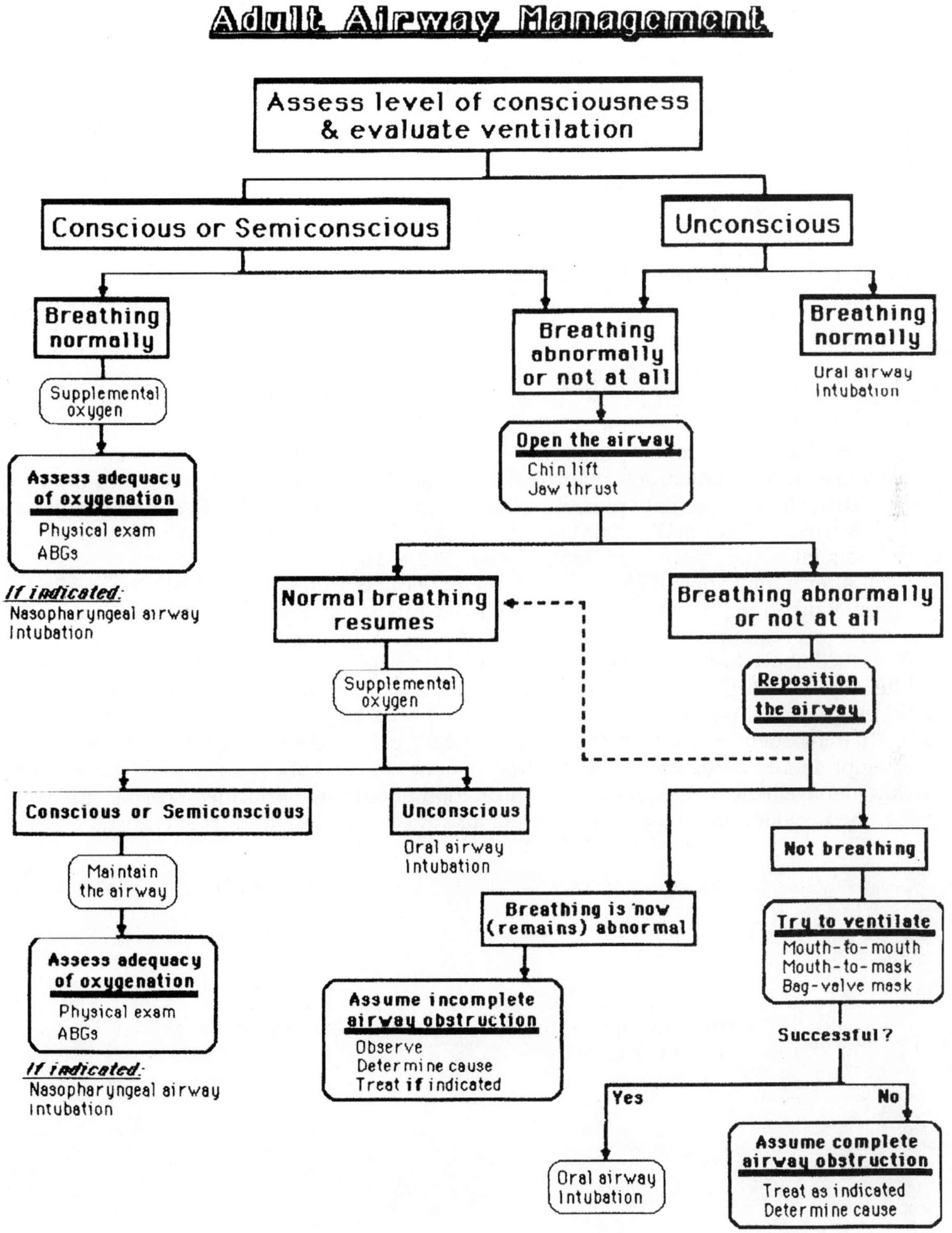

Fig. 3B-48- Algorithm of adult airway management.

If a patient is conscious or semiconscious and spontaneously breathing in a normal manner- all that may be needed is supplemental oxygen (**1-2-4**). The rescuer should then evaluate the adequacy of oxygenation (**5**). This may be done by physical examination (as described earlier in this section), oximetry, and/or by arterial blood gas sampling (if indicated). If this evaluation suggests that oxygenation is inadequate- more definitive management of the airway (either by insertion of a nasopharyngeal airway or endotracheal intubation) is needed.

> **Note**- Unconscious patients- even if they are breathing normally, require definitive airway management with endotracheal intubation (**1-3-7**).

For patients who are breathing abnormally (and for those who are not breathing at all)- appropriate management of the airway is the same regardless of the state of consciousness (**1-2-6**) or (**1-3-6**). In either case, the airway should be manually opened by either the chin-lift or jaw-thrust maneuver (**8**). If this results in resumption of normal breathing (**9**)- supplemental oxygen should be administered. For the unconscious patient, definitive airway management with endotracheal intubation is again the treatment of choice (**6-8-9-11**). On the other hand, if the patient is conscious or semiconscious (**10**)- less definitive therapy may be needed. Manually maintain the airway. Further management will then hinge on assessment of the adequacy of oxygenation (**6-8-9-10-12**).

If after initially opening the airway, the patient continues to breathe abnormally (or is still not breathing at all)- the rescuer should reposition the airway (**6-8-13-14**). If this results in resumption of normal breathing, management should follow the course described above (**8-9-10-12**) or (**8-9-11**). On the other hand, if breathing is still abnormal after repositioning the airway (**15**)- the rescuer should assume incomplete airway obstruction is present, and treat accordingly (**6-8-13-14-15-16**).

If the patient remains in respiratory arrest even after repositioning the airway- an attempt should be made to ventilate the patient (**14-17-18**). If successful, definitive airway management with endotracheal intubation should be performed (**19**). If unsuccessful, the rescuer should assume complete airway obstruction, and treat accordingly (**20**).

CHAPTER 4

Putting It All Together: *Practice for MEGA Code*

The essentials of running a code are contained within the algorithms presented in Chapter 1. The problem is that memorization of material presented in "algorithmic" form is often difficult unless one is able to practice applying it. Unfortunately being able to recite the exact sequence of an algorithm in the peace and quiet of one's own study facility does not necessarily correlate with the ability to command instant recall of the same material in an emergency situation *(or when you are being tested at the MEGA CODE station!*).

The exercises in this chapter have been selected to provide you with an opportunity to *"put it all together"* - and *apply* the information covered up to this point. Five basic scenarios of cardiac arrest are presented (in Sections 4A through 4E). The rationale for the treatment given in each of these scenarios closely follows the protocols laid out in the algorithms and commentary presented in Chapter 1. *The material is probably very similar to what will be presented in the Clinical Stations and in MEGA CODE.* It also comprises the *KEY* core content of what you need to know to successfully manage most real code situations.

To obtain maximum benefit from these exercises, *mentally transport YOURSELF to the bedside for each case.* Imagine the events transpiring before you as they might actually occur. Then assume the position of the code director- *and take over the management of each case!*

CASE STUDY A

You are working in the emergency department and are called to the bedside of a patient who has suddenly become unresponsive. No pulse can be felt, and the patient is having agonal respirations.

- The patient is a middle-aged man who weighs about 70 kg.
- A ***defibrillator*** (and team of rescuers) are at the bedside.
- *Quick-look paddles* are applied and reveal the rhythm shown in Figure 4A-1.

How would you proceed?

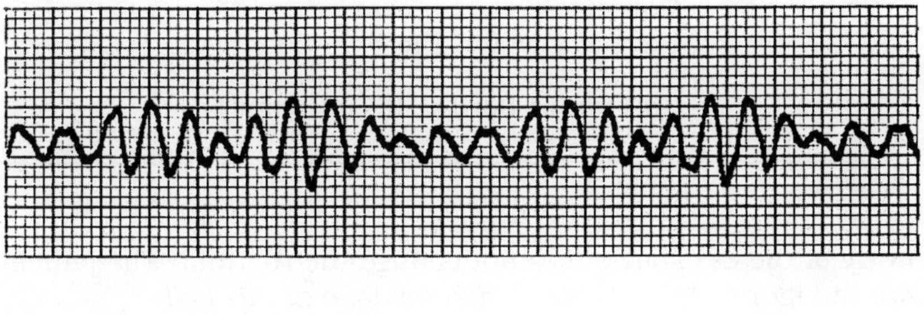

Figure 4A-1: Initial rhythm of the patient in Case Study A (as demonstrated by application of quick-look paddles).

Analysis of Figure 4A-1 and Plan:

There is a total lack of organized electrical activity. The rhythm on the monitor appears to be ***Ventricular Fibrillation* (V Fib)**.

1) *Verify* that the patient is *pulseless* and *unresponsive* (i.e., that the rhythm is *truly* V Fib- and *not* artifactual!).

2) **Defibrillate** with **200 joules**.

The *sooner* a patient in V Fib is defibrillated- the *better* the chance for long-term survival. In this particular case, quick-look paddles facilitated early recognition of V Fib. Given the presence of a defibrillator- *immediate* defibrillation takes precedence over all other actions (including performance of CPR)!

The patient is defibrillated with 200 joules. The rhythm initially seen on the monitor (Figure 4A-1) has *not* changed. *What should be done now?*

Plan:

3) **Defibrillate** again. Increase the energy for this 2nd defibrillation attempt to **300 joules**.

Pulse checks are no longer recommended between shocks that are given in stacked sequence ! AHA Guidelines advise that "as long as a properly connected monitor clearly displays persistent V Fib (and there is no unavoidable delay)- that rescuers should *not* pause for a pulse check between defibrillation attempts" (AHA Text- Pg 1-15). The appropriate action in the scenario presented here is therefore to *immediately* defibrillate the patient with 300 joules (as suggested above).

Delivery of the 2nd shock does *not* result in a change in the rhythm. *What next?*

Plan:

4) **Defibrillate** the patient a 3rd time- increasing the energy for this 3rd attempt to **360 joules**.

The recommended approach for treatment of V Fib (as well as for *pulseless* VT) is to shock *up to* **3 times** in ***stacked* sequence**. The following energy levels are recommended:

- **200 joules** (for the **1st** attempt)
- **200-300 joules** (for the **2nd** attempt)
- **360 joules** (for the **3rd** attempt)

Delivery of the 3rd shock does not change the rhythm. The patient remains in V Fib (as shown in Figure 4A-1). *What should be done at this point?*

Plan:

Failure to respond to the initial defibrillation series (of countershock with 200, 300, and 360 joules) is an indication to attempt other treatment measures. In preparation for this you accomplish the following:

5) Initiate CPR (if not already started).

6) Ventilate the patient. Use supplemental ***O**xygen.* Intubate if possible.

7) Try to establish ***I**V access.*

8) Hook the patient up to a ***M**onitor* (and/or to a 12-lead ECG machine).

AHA Guidelines suggest thinking of ***O**xygen-**I**V-**M**onitor* as a *single* "word"- to facilitate easy recall and rapid implementation of this series of actions that should be accomplished at the earliest opportunity in the managment of cardiopulmonary emergencies.

The patient remains pulseless and unresponsive. You have intubated and established IV access with a large-bore catheter in the antecubital fossa. Monitoring leads have been attached- and a slightly different rhythm is now seen (Figure 4A-2). *How does this rhythm differ from the rhythm that was seen in Figure 4A-1?*

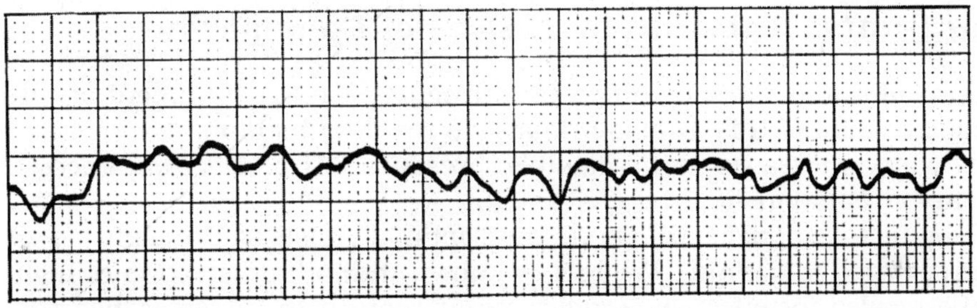

Figure 4A-2: Rhythm displayed on the monitor after completion of the initial defibrillation series. The patient is still pulseless and unresponsive.

Analysis of Figure 4A-2:

The rhythm is still V Fib- albeit with a somewhat decreased amplitude of deflection than was seen in Figure 4A-1. Assuming that the monitor gain has *not* been turned down- this is now *"fine"* V Fib.

> **Note-** Distinction between *"fine"* and *"coarse"* V Fib is made on the basis of the *relative* size of fibrillatory activity. In general, larger amplitude (i.e., ***"coarse"***) **V Fib** is more likely to be of recent onset, and is generally more readily corrected by prompt defibrillation. In contrast, smaller amplitude (i.e., ***"fine"***) **V Fib** is more likely of longer duration, and tends to be less responsive to treatment (AHA Text- Pg 3-3). Caution is needed in making this distinction to be sure that technical factors are not operative (such as alteration of the amplitude gain on the monitor or a change in leads).

The patient is in *fine* V Fib. *What should be done at this point?*

Plan:

9) *Verify* that intubation has been correctly performed and that the patient is being adequately oxygenated. Check for:

- presence of good bilateral breath sounds?
- adequate chest excursion with ventilation?
- assessment of patient color and ABGs/O_2 saturation (as/if available).

10) Give ***Epinephrine***- either **IV** or by the **ET** route (depending on *whichever* access route is established first):

- ***Initial* IV Dose**- **1.0 mg** by **IV** bolus (= 10 ml of a 1:10,000 soln).

- *OR* -

- **ET Dosing** = 2-2.5 times the IV dose (= **2-2.5 mg** of a 1:10,000 soln.)- instilled down the ET tube- and followed with several insufflations of the Ambu bag (before resuming chest compressions).

Teaching Points : The "Optimal" Dose of Epinephrine

Epinephrine is the most important drug used in the treatment of cardiac arrest. The beneficial action of this drug is primarily a result of its alpha-adrenergic (vasoconstrictor) effect- which increases aortic diastolic pressure. This effect enhances blood flow to the coronary circulation.

Despite this beneficial action, the "optimal" dose of Epinephrine to use in cardiac arrest remains uncertain. While it is known that administration of higher doses of drug may be needed for effective coronary circulation in the arrested heart (and higher doses may increase the chance of restoring a spontaneous pulse)- it has *never* been shown that increasing the dose will lead to improved survival.

AHA Guidelines acknowledge the uncertainty surrounding the dosing of Epinephrine during cardiac arrest. As a result, they allow for *flexibility* in the amount administered. The following regimens are suggested (AHA Text- Pg 1-16):

- ***Initial* Epinephrine Dose**- Give **1.0 mg** by **IV bolus** (= 10 ml of a 1:10,000 soln). This amount of drug is referred to as ***SDE*** (= *Standard-Dose Epinephrine*).

- ***Subsequent* IV Dosing**- Epinephrine should be repeated *at least* every 3-5 minutes in cardiac arrest. After the initial 1 mg IV dose- one may *either* continue with ***SDE*** amounts of drug (i.e., giving 1 mg IV Epineprhine every 3-5 minutes)-

- *OR*- chose between several ***HDE***
(= *High-Dose Epinephrine*) ***alternatives*** :

- Administration of **2-5 mg** IV boluses- *OR* -
- *escalating* **1- 3- 5 mg** IV boluses- *OR* -
- dosing at **0.1 mg/kg** as an IV bolus.

To emphasize their allowance of *flexibility* in Epinephrine dosing, AHA Guidelines explicitly state that ***"Use of HDE can neither be recommended nor discouraged"*** (AHA Text- Pg 7-4). SDE dosing should *always* be used first. Thereafter, dosing is left to the discretion of the treating clinician (*See pages 123-127 in Section 2B for further discussion*).

An initial SDE dose (i.e., 1 mg) of ***Epinephrine*** has been given IV- but the rhythm on the monitor (seen in Figure 4A-2) has not changed. *What now?*

Plan:

11) *Verify* that the patient is still *pulseless* and *unresponsive.*

12) **Defibrillate** a 4th time- using **360 joules** for this 4th countershock attempt.

Regarding initial treatment of the patient in V Fib- actions completed in this Case Study up to this point include:

- Shock X 3 (@ 200, 300, and 360j)
- *Epinephrine* (giving 1 mg as the initial IV dose)
- Repeat *shock* (@ 360j).

> **Note-** Instead of administering a 4th shock @ 360j (as was done in this case)- AHA Guidelines allow for alternative administration of another ***stacked* sequence** of shocks (i.e., another series of 3 successive shocks at 200-360j). Delivery of stacked shocks would be especially appropriate at this point- *IF* for any reason administration of medication was to be delayed.

Teaching Points : General Considerations Regarding Defibrillation

The patient in this Case Study has persistent V Fib requiring repeat defibrillation. Points to consider regarding the implementation of defibrillation include the following:

- Always *verify* that the rhythm is truly V Fib *before* defibrillating (i.e., that all monitoring leads are on- and that the patient is truly pulseless and unresponsive). If the patient responds when shaken- *then the rhythm is not V Fib.*
- Minimize time between successive countershock attempts. This reduces transthoracic resistance (TTR) of the chest wall- and therefore helps optimize the amount of *current* that will flow *through* the chest at any given energy level.
- Apply firm pressure to the paddles when defibrillating (i.e., pressing down with ≈25 lbs of force)- as this also reduces TTR.
- Be sure to coat the paddle surface with conductive gel (or use defibrillator pads).

- Take pains to ensure that everyone on the scene is *CLEAR* from the patient's bed *before* discharging the paddles (i.e., regular use of a ***"Clearing Chant"***).
- If medications are used (i.e., Epinephrine, Lidocaine, Bretylium, etc.)- be sure to *circulate* the drug for 30-60 seconds after administration *before* the next defibrillation attempt.
- If a *Nitroglycerin patch* is on the victim's chest- *remove* it prior to defibrillation.
- If the victim has *either* an implanted pacemaker or ICD (implanted cardioverter-defibrillator)- *avoid* placement of the defibrillator paddles or pads over (or close to) the generator unit.

Teaching Points : Regarding the Use of Sodium Bicarbonate

Remarkable for its absence up to this point in the code is any mention of Sodium Bicarbonate. This is because the acidosis that occurs during the *initial* minutes of cardiac arrest is primarily respiratory in nature (due to hypoventilation). Recommended treatment for this respiratory acidosis is to improve ventilation- *not* to give Sodium Bicarbonate.

Problems associated with the use of Sodium Bicarbonate during cardiac arrest are that:

i) It has *never* been shown to improve prognosis from cardiac arrest.

ii) It does *nothing* to correct the principal cause of acidosis during the *early* minutes of arrest (i.e., giving Bicarb does *not* correct *respiratory* acidosis that results from *HYPOventilation*).

iii) *Despite* improving ABG pH values- treatment with Bicarb is likely to paradoxically *exacerbate* the degree of acidosis at the *cellular* level. This may further depress myocardial function.

Bottom Line- The acidosis of cardiac arrest is best treated by *HYPERventilation*- especially during the *early* minutes of a code. Indications for use of Bicarb in the setting of cardiac arrest are extremely limited (perhaps to severe metabolic acidosis that persists *beyond* the first 5-15 minutes of the code- and/or to cardiac arrest in a patient *known* to have a severe *preexisting* metabolic acidosis *prior* to the arrest)- ***IF* Bicarb is ever indicated at all . . . .**

Special resuscitation situations in which Sodium Bicarbonate may be useful include treatment of *hyperkalemia* and *Tricyclic overdose.*

Sequential countershock (X 3), Epinephrine, and repeat countershock have been ineffective up to this point. The patient remains pulseless and unresponsive.

How would you interpret this clinical situation (Figure 4A-3)? *What should be done next?*

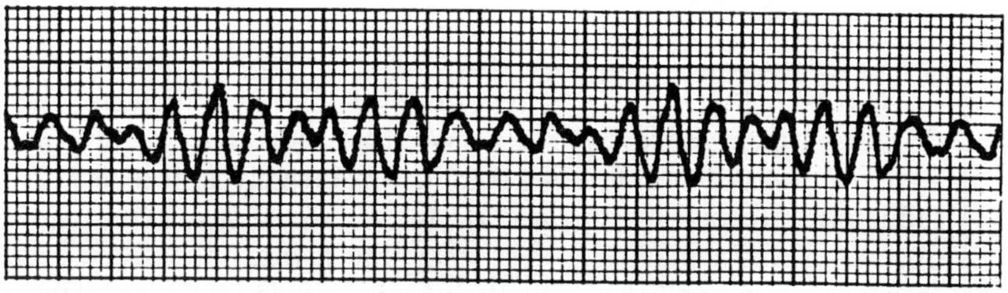

Figure 4A-3: Despite countershock and Epinephrine, the patient remains in persistent V Fib.

Analysis of Figure 4A-3 and Plan:

V Fib persists. Failure to respond to the initial series of countershocks, intubation (and ventilation), Epinephrine, and repeat countershock- is referred to as ***"refractory V Fib"***, and is indication to consider ***antifibrillatory therapy***. AHA Guidelines list Lidocaine as the *first* agent to use in this situation.

13) Give ***Lidocaine***- in an *initial dose of* **1.0- 1.5 mg/kg** (≈50-150 mg) by IV push.

14) Circulate the drug for 30-60 seconds with CPR; then defibrillate again with 360 joules.

> **Note**- Drug delivery of *any* medication to the central circulation may be enhanced by *following* IV drug administration with a ***20-30 ml IV bolus*** of fluid- and by *elevating* the arm.

15) *If V Fib persisted beyond this point*- one might then consider any (or all) of the following actions (*See also Figure 1B-2 on page 38*):

- giving a second dose of Lidocaine
- administration of one (or more) doses of ***Bretylium***
- administration of one (or more) doses of ***Magnesium***.

Teaching Points : Lidocaine Dosing for V Fib

Lidocaine is generally accepted as the *antifibrillatory* agent of choice for *initial* medical treatment of *refractory* V Fib. Reasons for this recommendation are that emergency personnel are generally more familiar (and comfortable) with the use of this drug- and that it is *faster-acting* and probably *safer* than Bretylium (and other agents) in the setting of cardiac arrest (AHA Text- Pg 1-19).

- In the *spontaneously beating heart*- the half-life of Lidocaine is short (i.e., ≈10 minutes). As a result, an IV infusion of the drug *must* be started *within* 5-10 minutes of giving an IV bolus (or the effect of the bolus will be dissipated).

- Lidocaine pharmacokinetics differ in the ***arrested heart.*** This is because clearance of the drug is *markedly reduced* in this situation. It is therefore *not* essential to start an IV infusion right after a bolus is given to a patient in cardiac arrest. In acknowledgement of these altered pharmacokinetics- AHA Guidelines now allow for use of a *single* (**1.5 mg/kg**) **IV bolus** dose of Lidocaine as treatment for V Fib.

> **Note**- AHA Guidelines recommend giving Lidocaine *only* by IV bolus during cardiac arrest. We differ with this recommendation because of our feeling that the relatively small amount of Lidocaine infused during a code (at a rate of 2 mg/minute) will probably *not* be harmful- and because *it may be all too easy to forget* to start the Lidocaine IV infusion once the patient is converted out of V Fib.
>
> **Bottom Line**- If you chose not to begin a Lidocaine maintenance infusion at the time of IV loading- it is *essential* to remember to do so *as soon as* the patient is converted out of V Fib !

A single IV bolus of 100 mg of ***Lidocaine*** has been given (to this ≈70 kg patient) and circulated with CPR. Repeat countershock (with 360j) produces the rhythm shown below (Figure 4A-4).

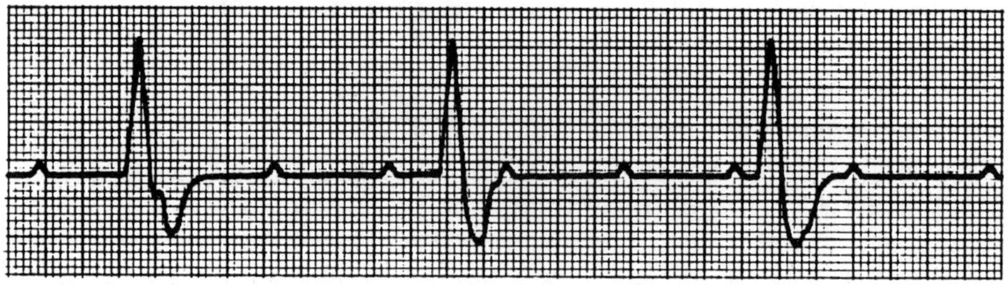

Figure 4A-4: Rhythm seen on the monitor after Lidocaine and repeat countershock.

The rhythm in Figure 4A-4 is associated with a weak pulse and blood pressure reading of 60 palpable. The patient is still unresponsive. ***What has happened?*** *What should be done?*

Analysis of Figure 4A-4 and Plan:

Antifibrillatory therapy (with Lidocaine) and repeat defibrillation have succeeded in restoring a spontaneous pulse. The rhythm appears to be **complete (3°) AV Block**- as suggested by the presence of a regular ventricular rhythm and regular atrial rhythm- *but NO relation between the two.* P waves "march through the QRS complex"- failing to conduct anywhere (despite having *more than adequate opportunity* to do so). The ventricular rate is *slow* (i.e., *less* than 40 beats/minute- since the R-R interval is more than 8 large boxes).

In view of the slow heart rate, low blood pressure (of 60 palpable), and the patient's persistent unresponsive state- one must interpret this bradyarrhythmia as being ***hemodynamically* significant**. *The patient is clearly in need of treatment.* Either of two therapeutic options might be tried:

16a) Give ***Atropine***- in an *initial* dose of **0.5- 1.0 mg IV**.

- and/or -

16b) Institute ***TCP*** **(*TransCutaneous Pacing*)**.

> **Note**- While treatment is begun (with either Atropine and/or TCP)- attention should *also* be directed to accomplishing the ***Supportive Actions*** that are listed in Figure 1D-4 on page 105. In addition to control of airway/ventilation and *Oxygen-IV-Monitor* (that have already been attended to)- other actions include brief review of the patient's history and medical chart, performance of a *targeted* physical exam, and obtaining appropriate laboratory tests as feasible and indicated (i.e., chext X-ray, 12-lead ECG, serum electrolytes, ABGs, etc.).
>
> An important point to emphasize is that *other* potentially correctable factors (i.e., hypoxemia- hypovolemia- electrolyte disturbance- etc.) may also be responsible (at least in part) for either causing or perpetuating the bradyarrhythmia.

Teaching Points : Atropine and/or TCP?

It is sometimes difficult to decide between Atropine and pacing in treatment of the patient with bradycardia. Because both therapeutic options have advantages and disadvantages- *judgement is needed in clinical decision making.*

- Decided advantages of ***Atropine*** are ready availability and rapid onset of action. AHA Guidelines still recommend this drug as "the *initial* pharmacologic agent of choice for treatment of symptomatic bradycardia"- especially when signs/symptoms from bradycardia are only "mild" (AHA Text- Pg 1-30). Atropine is most likely to be effective in the treatment of bradycardia when used during the first few hours of acute *inferior* infarction in patients who develop Mobitz type I 2° AV block, or 3° AV block with a narrow QRS complex escape rhythm.

  The drawback of Atropine is that the drug is not benign. Because it blocks parasympathetic output, Atropine may unmask previously undetected (and underlying) *sympathetic* activity- and thus precipitate ventricular tachyarrhythmias! Administration of Atropine has become especially controversial when the rhythm being treated is *advanced* AV block with ventricular escape- in which case use of the drug could (at least theoretically) result in paradoxical *slowing* of the ventricular response (AHA Text- Pg 1-30).

- Advantages of ***TCP*** (*TransCutaneous Pacing*) are that the device is entirely *non-invasive*- is easily and *rapidly* applied- and provides *effective* pacing in most cases. As a result, AHA Guidelines now state that use of TCP is appropriate (if not preferred) as the *initial* intervention in the treatment sequence- *IF* the device is available- and *IF* the bradycardia is severe and/or the patient is unstable (AHA Text- Pg 1-31). Pacing is clearly preferable to Atropine for treatment of advanced AV block with QRS widening (for the reasons we state above).

Potential drawbacks of TCP are that the device will *not* always produce mechanical contraction (i.e., the pacer may occasionally fail to capture)- and that pacing stimuli may be uncomfortable for the conscious patient.

> **Note**- Practically speaking, implementation of pacing and administration of Atropine are often attempted *simultaneously*. Thus, an initial IV dose of Atropine may be given while the pacer is being sent for. Alternatively, TCP may be applied while attempts are made to achieve IV access. The point to emphasize is that when the patient is symptomatic, treatment should *not* be delayed (AHA Text- Pg 1-29).

In the case at hand- the bradycardia shown in Figure 4A-4 on page 320 is clearly *advanced* AV block (it is 3° AV block), the QRS complex of the escape rhythm is widened, and the escape rate is slow. In addition, the patient is markedly symptomatic (BP is 60 palpable). As a result, application of TCP is the intervention of choice *as soon as* the device becomes available.

The external pacemaker has been ordered and sent for. You are told that its arrival "may take a few minutes". In the meantime, 0.5 mg of ***Atropine*** is given, but this fails to produce a response (i.e., the patient *remains* unresponsive- with a *weak* pulse- and a BP = 60 palpable).

What should you do now?

Plan:

17) Be ready to apply the transcutaneous pacer *as soon as* it arrives.

18) While awaiting TCP- *consider* repeating the **Atropine**:

- May give **1 mg** at a time for severe bradycardia (up to a total dose of **0.4 mg/kg**- or ≈ **3 mg**).
- May give Atropine *more frequently* (i.e., as often as every 1-3 minutes) when there is marked hemodynamic compromise.

> **Note**- As discussed above, use of Atropine is controversial for treatment of 3° AV block with QRS widening. Given the marked hypotension and *unavailability* of TCP (for at least "a few minutes") in this case scenario- *cautious* administration of one or more doses of Atropine would clearly be appropriate. Alternatively, use of a *pressor agent* could be considered instead of Atropine at this point in the code.

Teaching Points **: What if the patient had no pulse and no blood pressure in association with the rhythm shown in Figure 4A-4?**

If no pulse and no blood pressure were obtainable in association with the electrical rhythm that appears in Figure 4A-4- then the patient would be in PEA. AHA Guidelines now classify the diverse group of cardiac rhythms that manifest *electrical* activity (i.e., an ECG rhythm on the monitor)- but *NO pulse-* as ***PEA*** (*Pulseless Electrical Activity*) **rhythms**. Although some meaningful ventricular contraction may occur in association with many (if not most) of these rhythms- it is clinically *insufficient* "to produce a BP detectable by the usual methods of palpation or sphygmomanometer" (AHA Text- Pg 1-21).

Practically speaking- ***PEA rhythms*** are diagnosed by the finding of an ECG rhythm on the monitor in a patient who is pulseless. These rhythms are clinically unified by the fact that they are most often the result of *some other* underlying disorder- and that by definition they are *non-perfusing* (or at most no more than *minimially* perfusing) rhythms.

As discussed in detail in Section 1D (and in Figure 1D-2 on page 93)- recommendations for management of PEA reflect application of the above concepts:

- *Continue CPR-* since by definition PEA is a *non-perfusing* (or at most *poorly* perfusing) rhythm.
- *Search for a cause of the PEA rhythm-* and try to *correct* this if at all possible (*See Table 1D-1 on page 96*). Practically speaking, realistic chances for saving a patient with PEA depend on identifying and correcting the underlying cause of the disorder.
- *Give* ***Epinephrine***- in an attempt to optimize coronary perfusion. Atropine may help- but should *only* be given if the rhythm is slow. The rhythm is still the same as was shown in figure 4A-4.

A total of 2 mg of Atropine have been given to this patient without any effect. You learn that the only external pacemaker in the hospital is "broken". Clinically, the patient remains *unresponsive-* with a *weak* pulse and BP = 60 palpable.

Plan:

19) Consult for emergent ***transvenous*** **pacemaker** insertion.

20) In the meantime (awaiting your *STAT* consult)- administer the ***pressor agent*** *"of your choice"* (i.e., ***Dopamine*** or ***Epinephrine***).

Use of a pressor agent should *only* be tried as a *temporizing* (= *stopgap*) measure for severe bradycardia *until* pacemaker therapy becomes available.

Note- The patient in this case scenario received a total of 2 mg of Atropine. Although AHA Guidelines allow for a total dose of 0.4 mg/kg (or *up to* ≈3 mg) to be given- practically speaking it is *unlikely* that additional Atropine will produce the desired response if 2 mg have failed to do so. Thus, although one *could* give another 1 mg of Atropine to this patient (for a total dose of 3 mg)- a *change* in treatment (i.e., trial of a pressor agent) would be completely appropriate at this time (until the arrival of pacemaker therapy).

Teaching Points : Regarding the Use of Pressor Agents

The need for a pressor agent is a common problem in emergency cardiac care. In the setting of cardiac arrest (or impending arrest)- the two pressor agents that are most commonly used are Dopamine and Epinephrine. Which agent to select is determined by consideration of clinical needs and personal preference of the treating clinician.

- AHA Guidelines currently favor beginning with ***Dopamine*** for treatment of bradycardia that is Atropine-resistant and hemodynamically significant. IV infusion of ***Epinephrine*** is usually used when clinical symptoms are more severe (AHA Text- Pg 1-31).
- When used as a *pressor agent* (i.e., to treat *symptomatic* bradycardia)- ***Epinephrine*** should *not* be given by IV bolus. Moment-to-moment *titratability* (as afforded by IV infusion) is clearly preferable in this situation. The problem with IV bolus dosing of Epinephrine is that if too much is given- *"you can't take a bolus back"*. IV bolus dosing of Epinephrine is best reserved for treatment of the patient in true cardiac arrest (i.e., V Fib, asystole, PEA).
- Although in the past, *Isoproterenol* had been commonly used as a pressor agent- use of this drug has been strongly discouraged in recent years. The pure beta-adrenegic effect of Isoproterenol produces potentially deleterious vasodilatation, and may excessively increase myocardial oxygen consumption. Administration of Isoproterenol is therefore best reserved for treatment of the patient in need of *pure* chronotropic support- *IF* the drug is to be used at all (AHA Text- Pg 8-6).
- Regarding use of the pressor agents- application of the ***"Rule of 250 ml"*** (that we introduced in Section 2C on page 157) greatly facilitates calculation of an appropriate *initial* IV infusion rate for the most commonly used drugs. The rate of infusion can then be increased as needed to obtain the desired clinical effect. For example:
    - ***Dopamine***- Mix 1 amp (= **200 mg**) in **250 ml** of D5W, and *begin* the infusion @ **15-30 drops/minute** (=2-5 µg/kg/minute).
    - ***Epinephrine (SDE dose)***- Mix **1 mg** of a 1:10,000 soln. of Epi in **250 ml** of D5W, and *begin* the infusion @ **15-30 drops/minute** (=1-2 µg/minute).
    - ***Isoproterenol***- Mix 1 vial (= **1 mg**) in **250 ml** of D5W, and *begin* the infusion @ **30 drops/minute** (=2 µg/minute).

The cardiologist on call agrees with the need for pacemaker insertion and is "on his way". In the meantime, IV infusion of ***Dopamine*** is begun.

Shortly after beginning Dopamine, the rhythm shown at the top of the next page is seen on the monitor (Figure 4A-5). *What has happened? What would you do now?*

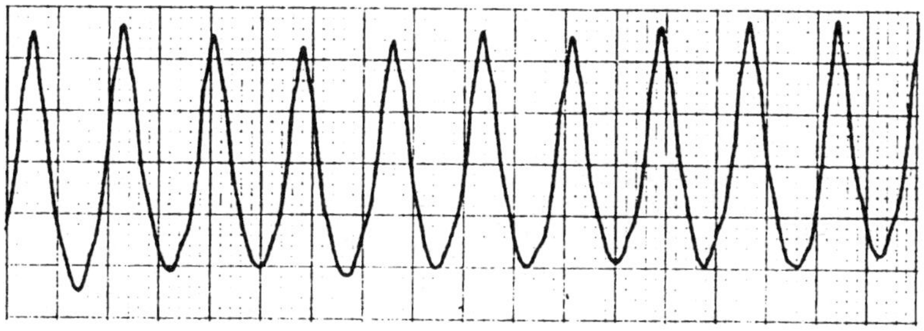

Figure 4A-5: Rhythm seen shortly after beginning the infusion of Dopamine. *What has happened?*

Analysis of Figure 4A-5 and Plan:

The monitor now displays a regular, *wide-complex* tachycardia. This must be **VT** !

21) *Stop* the Dopamine! (Arrhythmogenic effects of this pressor agent may have precipitated development of VT.)

22) Determine the patient's hemodynamic status.

> **Note-** As emphasized in Figure 1C-12- on page 80- the *KEY* to evaluation and management of VT is to determine the patient's hemodynamic status.

The patient whose rhythm is shown above (in Figure 4A-5) is still unresponsive- but a weak carotid pulse is palpable. BP is unobtainable.

Plan:

As noted, the rhythm in Figure 4A-5 is VT. The ventricular rate is ≈170 beats/minute. Although a pulse *is* present- *the patient is clearly unstable.*

23) Immediately ***cardiovert*** the patient !!! There is clearly *no time* for a trial of medical therapy (i.e., with Lidocaine) when the patient is acutely *unstable* as is the case here.

- Use **100 joules** for the *initial* attempt at emergency cardioversion of *monomorphic* VT (AHA Text- Pg 1-35).

> **Note-** AHA Guidelines distinguish between *monomorphic* VT (usually referred to simply as "**VT**")- and ***polymorphic* VT** (in which QRS morphology and heart rate are variable). Although the QRS complex of the tachycardia in Figure 4A-5 is exceedingly wide and bizarre- the *morphology* of the QRS is constant! In contrast, polymorphic VT is a much *less organized* rhythm that tends to be more resistent to treatment. As a result, AHA Guidelines recommend *beginning* with a higher energy level (of **200 joules**) for the *initial* attempt at cardioversion of *polymorphic* VT (AHA Text- Pg 1-35).

Synchronized ***Cardioversion*** with 100 joules results in conversion of VT to the rhythm shown below.

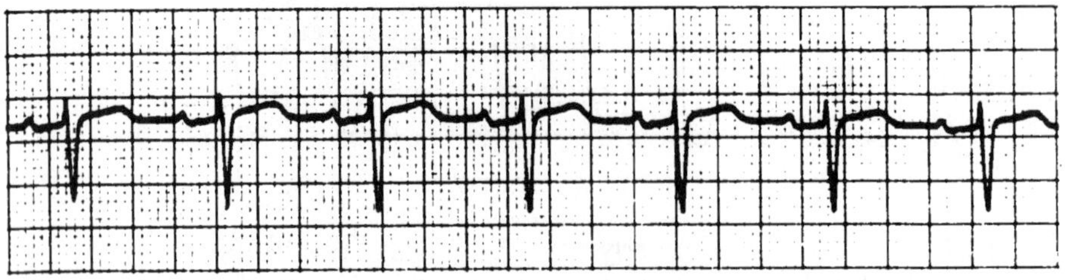

Figure 4A-6: Rhythm seen on the monitor after cardioversion of VT.

Analysis of Figure 4A-6 and Plan:

The electrical rhythm on the monitor now appears to be sinus.

Did you forget to check for something ???

Plan:

24) Check the patient for:

- presence of a pulse
- blood pressure determination
- responsiveness

> **Note-** It is *essential* to ***always*** check for a pulse after ***every*** intervention- and/or ***whenever*** the rhythm changes on the monitor! The presence of an ECG rhythm on the monitor in no way guarantees that the patient is perfusing adequately. Other parameters must be assessed (i.e., skin color, blood pressure, ABGs or pulse oximetry, etc.). The approach to management of the rhythm shown in Figure 4A-6 will clearly depend on whether or not a pulse is present in association with this rhythm.

There *IS* a good pulse in association with the rhythm that appears in Figure 4A-6. BP = 120/80 mm Hg. The patient is beginning to open his eyes! *What next?*

Plan:

This is ***normal sinus rhythm***. The QRS complex is narrow, and the PR interval is at the upper limit of normal (i.e., at 0.20 second). The patient is hemodynamically *stable.*

25) *Take a deep breath* !!!!

26) Be sure the patient is on an ***IV infusion** of **Lidocaine*** (as a *prophylactic* measure to help *prevent recurrence* of V Fib). If this has not already been started:

- ***Rebolus*** the patient now (with ≈**50-75 mg** IV Lidocaine)
- Begin ***IV infusion*** at an initial rate of **2 mg/min**.

> By the **Rule of 250 ml:** *(See pages 157-160.)*
>
> - Mix **1g** of *Lidocaine* in **250 ml** of D5W, and *begin* drip @ **30 drops/min** (=2 mg/min).

27) Verify that *NO other* IV infusions are running.

28) Recheck placement of your ET tube (by listening for symmetric breath sounds)- and reassess the adequacy of ventilation/oxygenation.

29) Transfer the patient to your critical care facility.

> - *YOU have SAVED the patient* !!!!!

Discussion :

This case illustrates the steps in the initial approach to resuscitation of the patient in V Fib (*Figures 1B-1 and 1B-2- on pages 34 and 38).* Several points are deserving of special mention:

- The likelihood of successfully resuscitating a patient in cardiac arrest is *inversely* proportional to the interval between the onset of V Fib- and the application of countershock. For this reason, defibrillation should always be implemented *as soon as* the diagnosis of V Fib is established. Delay for the purpose of intubation and/or starting an IV line (i.e.. to administer Epinephrine) is unwarranted- and may *adversely* effect the patient's chance for survival.

- Use of *quick-look* paddles facilitates rapid diagnosis V Fib. As a result, they should be applied to the unmonitored patient the moment the defibrillator arrives. This pertains *both* to arrests that occur in the hospital- as well as to those that occur outside of the hospital. *Application of quick-look paddles should only take a few seconds.* If the patient is in V Fib- *immediately* countershock *before* you do anything else.

- Initial treatment of V Fib consists of ***sequential* countershock** (with **200j**- **300j**- and then **360 joules**)- establishment of IV access/intubation- administration of ***Epinephrine***- and then repeat countershock (with *either* a single **360j** shock- *or* a 2nd series of 3 *stacked* shocks).

- Failure to respond to the above measures defines the condition as ***refractory* V Fib**- and is indication for a trial of ***antifibrillatory* therapy**. The medical treatment of choice for *refractory* V Fib is ***Lidocaine*** (which may be supplemented by Bretylium or Magnesium if V Fib persists).

- Antifibrillatory therapy with ***Lidocaine*** can be given in the form of a ***single* IV bolus** (of **1.5 mg/kg**) to patients in cardiac arrest. IV infusion need *not* necessarily be started during the code. However, once the patient is converted *out of* V Fib- it will then be *essential* to rebolus with Lidocaine and begin IV infusion (as a *prophylactic* measure aimed at preventing V Fib recurrence).

- Practically speaking, there is really no limit to the number of times that a patient may be defibrillated. As long as the rhythm in V Fib- the rhythm is *potentially* treatable.

- Persistence of V Fib should also prompt search for underlying/precipitating causes of the arrest. This point is incorporated within the **"D-D"** (= *Differential Diagnosis*) of the ***Secondary Survey*** *(see pages 14-15).*

The final point we emphasize from this Case Study is the need to ***always* check for a pulse after *every* intervention-** and/or **whenever there is a *change* in the rhythm on the monitor!** Treatment of *any* clinical situation depends on the patient's hemodynamic status. Assessing for the presence of a *pulse* is critical for this determination. If a pulse *is* present- treatment decisions will then be based in large part on the clinical significance of the arrhythmia (i.e., BP reading, mental status, patient symptoms, etc.). If a pulse is absent then the rhythm in question reflects PEA- and an entirely different set of treatment priorities will need to be implemented.

Case Study B

You are taking care of a woman admitted to the Intensive Care Unit for ***new-onset* chest pain**. The patient is alert and complaining of a "funny sensation" she feels in her chest. She has no other symptoms.

- The patient is about 60 years old and weighs about **80 kg.**
- An IV line is already in place. The patient is receiving supplemental oxygen. Sublingual NTG and morphine are the only medications that have been given.
- The patient's bedside monitor indicates the rhythm shown in Figure 4B-1.

What is the rhythm? *What would you do next?*

Lead MCL_1

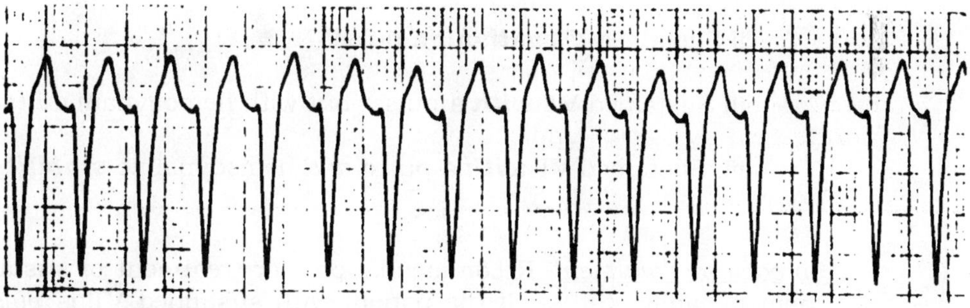

Figure 4B-1: Initial rhythm seen on the monitor for the patient in Case Study B. *What should you do next?*

Analysis of Figure 4B-1 and Plan:

The rhythm is regular and rapid (at a rate of ≈190 beats/minute). The QRS complex is *wide* (i.e., clearly *more* than half a large box in duration). Atrial activity is *not* apparent. Thus, the rhythm represents a *regular* ***WCT*** (= *Wide-Complex Tachycardia*) of *uncertain* etiology. For practical purposes-***Ventricular Tachycardia*** *must* be assumed until *proven* otherwise.

1) Determine the patient's ***hemodynamic status.***

> ***KEY***- Recommendations for evaluation and management of presumed ***sustained* VT** depend primarily on the *stability* (or lack thereof) of the patient's hemodynamic condition. As a result, the *most* important action to accomplish on encountering a patient in a rhythm such as that shown in Figure 4B-1 is to determine the *hemodynamic* status.

Teaching Points : Assessing and Treating *Sustained* VT

- *Definition*- The term ***"repetitive"* ventricular ectopy** refers to the occurrence of two or more PVCs in a row. Specifically, the occurrence of two PVCs in a row is termed a ventricular ***couplet***- and three PVCs in a row is a ***salvo*** (which is *also* the definition of ***ventricular tachycardia***). Longer runs of ventricular beats are described as ***"non-sustained"* VT**- which by definition, will *spontaneously* resolve (usually *within* a period of seconds). Ventricular tachycardia becomes ***"sustained"*** when runs are "longer" (i.e., usually 30-60 seconds- *or more* !) As might be imagined, VT of shorter duration is much *less* likely to produce symptoms of hemodynamic significance.

- *Clinical Presentation*- For practical purposes, ***sustained* VT** may present in one of three ways, as determined by the patient's hemodynamic condition. These are:

  i) Sustained VT ***without*** a pulse.

  ii) Sustained VT ***with*** a pulse- but with hemodynamic ***instability***.

  iii) Sustained VT ***with*** a pulse *and* hemodynamic ***stability***.

- *Approach to Treatment*- Recommendations for treatment of sustained VT depend on hemodynamic status. If the patient with sustained VT is *pulseless*- the rhythm should be treated the same as V Fib (i.e., with *unsynchronized* countershock using 200-360 joules). If the patient has a pulse- hemodynamic stability should be rapidly assessed *before* deciding on specific treatment. If serious signs or symptoms are produced by the rhythm as a *direct* result of the increase in heart rate- then *immediate* synchronized cardioversion is in order (beginning at 100 joules). On the other hand, if the patient is hemodynamically stable- cardioversion need *not* be immediately performed. Instead, a trial of medical therapy (i.e., with Lidocaine, Procainamide) is appropriate- as long as the patient *remains* hemodynamically stable. Synchronized cardioversion would *become* immediately indicated if the patient's condition deteriorated at *any* time during the treatment process (*See Figure 1C-12 on page 80*).

The patient whose rhythm is shown in Figure 4B-1 is awake and alert. There is a good pulse. BP = 90 systolic. Other than the "funny sensation", there are no symptoms. *How should you proceed?*

Clinical Assessment and Plan:

Despite the tachycardia- the patient is ***hemodynamically* stable**. This judgement is made on the basis of the fact that the patient is alert, has a somewhat low but acceptable blood pressure, and is relatively asymptomatic.

2) Your first action: *Take a deep breath* !!!!

KEY - As noted above, this patient *is* hemodynamically stable. By definition, you therefore have at least *some time* to formulate an appropriate therapeutic plan.

3) *Verify* the diagnosis of VT- IF this is possible given clinical constraints (*See Teaching Points below*).

Note- AHA Guidelines recommend accomplishing the ***Supportive Actions*** that are listed at the beginning of the *Tachycardia Algorithm* (Figure 1C-1 on page 51)- *as this is possible*- during the course of evaluation and treatment.

4) Consider a trial of medical therapy.

5) Be *ready* to cardiovert *immediately* (with ≈100 joules)- IF the patient shows signs of hemodynamic decompensation at *any* time during the treatment process.

Teaching Points : Can you be *sure* that the rhythm in Figure 4B-1 is really VT? *or could it be SVT?*

- **If the rhythm is SVT- how would you explain the QRS widening?**
- **Does the fact that the patient is alert with a BP = 90 systolic make the diagnosis of VT less likely?**
- **For *how long* can a patient remain in sustained VT?**

One cannot be certain from inspection of the single monitoring lead shown in Figure 4B-1 that this rhythm is truly VT. All one can say is that a regular WCT is present- and that the diagnosis of VT should be assumed until *proven* otherwise.

- Three clinical entities should be considered in the differential diagnosis of a regular WCT. They are:

  i) Ventricular tachycardia
  ii) SVT with *preexisting* bundle branch block
  iii) SVT with *aberrant* conduction.

Because VT is the most serious of these three entities, as well as being the most common (*by far!*)- one should ***always* assume** that the rhythm is **VT until *proven* otherwise**. The patient should be treated accordingly (i.e., *as if* the rhythm is VT).

- Even if the etiology of a WCT turns out to be VT- this does *not* mean that the patient will immediately decompensate. Some patients may remain in *sustained* VT for surprisingly *long* periods of time (i.e, for minutes- hours- *and even days!*). If the patient is hemodynamically stable, you have at least *some time* to formulate an appropriate therapeutic plan.
- Sustained VT is clearly more likely to persist when the ventricular rate is *not* excessively fast (usually *less than* ≈150 beats/minute) and the patient has relatively good left ventricular function. However, even *elderly* patients with *impaired* LV function and *rapid* ventricular rates may sometimes remain conscious and relatively asymptomatic for long periods of time- *despite persistence of sustained VT.*
- ***Blood pressure*** determination is *not* reliable as a diagnostic discriminator for distinguishing between sustained VT and SVT (with either aberration or preexisting bundle branch block). BP may even be *increased* in some patients with sustained VT.
- ***Level of consciousness*** is equally *unreliable* as a discriminating factor. Some patients with sustained VT are mentally alert. *Others are not.* Whether a patient is conscious or not is of *no assistance* in the differential process.
- ***Duration of the tachycardia*** is also *not helpful.* As noted above, selected patients may remain in sustained VT for hours (or more!)- *without any change in hemodynamic status.*

> **Bottom Line**- Assessment of clinical parameters (i.e., *heart rate- BP- level of consciousness-* etc.) is *not* at all helpful in the diagnostic process of determining whether a *WCT* (*Wide-Complex Tachycardia*) is supraventricular or ventricular in origin.

Teaching Points : How to proceed if *uncertain* about the etiology of a WCT?

As emphasized, it will sometimes *not* be possible in emergency situations to determine *with certainty* the true etiology of a *WCT* (*Wide-Complex Tachycardia*). For example, if the *only* information available in the Case Scenario presented here was the rhythm strip shown in Figure 4B-1 and knowledge that the patient is hemodynamically stable- *definitive diagnosis of this WCT would simply not be possible.* In this case, the following points should be strongly considered in formulating your approach:

i) Be aware that the differential diagnosis of a regular WCT includes SVT with either preexisting bundle branch block or aberrant conduction. Having said this- ***always* assume** that the rhythm is **VT** *until* ***proven*** *otherwise.* ***Treat the patient accordingly*** (i.e., *as if* the rhythm is VT).

ii) Optimal management of sustained VT depends *most* on the patient's clinical condition. Since the patient in this case is *hemodynamically stable-* a trial of medical therapy is perfectly appropriate. AHA Guidelines still recommend ***Lidocaine*** as the antiarrhythmic agent of choice for this purpose (Figure 1C-12 on page 80).

iii) <u>Alternatively</u>- AHA Guidelines also allow for *empiric* use of ***Adenosine*** in the treatment protocol of WCT when the etiology of the rhythm is *uncertain*- and the patient has *not* responded to Lidocaine (Figure 1C-13 on page 85). Use of Adenosine is especially appropriate when a strong possibility exists that the WCT is supraventricular.

iv) AHA Guidelines caution *against* reliance on ECG criteria to determine the etiology of a WCT (AHA Text- Pg 1-38). While *fully agreeing* with this reservation- *we also maintain* that attention to three simple actions *may* provide insight that helps to *verify* the etiology of the arrhythmia:

- Brief review of the patient's medical history (i.e., *older patients* with a history of *underlying heart disease* are much *more* likely to develop VT).
- Comparison with prior tracings in the medical chart.
- Obtaining a 12-lead ECG *during* the tachycardia.

If all clinical indicators suggest that the rhythm is VT, but Lidocaine fails to convert the tachycardia- consider the use of ***Procainamide*** (Figure 1C-12).

v) If the patient decompensates at *any* time duirng the process of evaluating/treating the tachycardia- *STOP and immediately cardiovert!*

vi) If in doubt about the etiology of the rhythm- *go back to **Point #i)** on the previous page* !!!!

The patient remains in the rhythm shown in <u>Figure 4B-2</u>. Assume that the diagnosis of VT has been confirmed. The patient is still alert- with a good pulse- and a BP = 90 systolic.

What might you do now?

Lead MCL$_1$

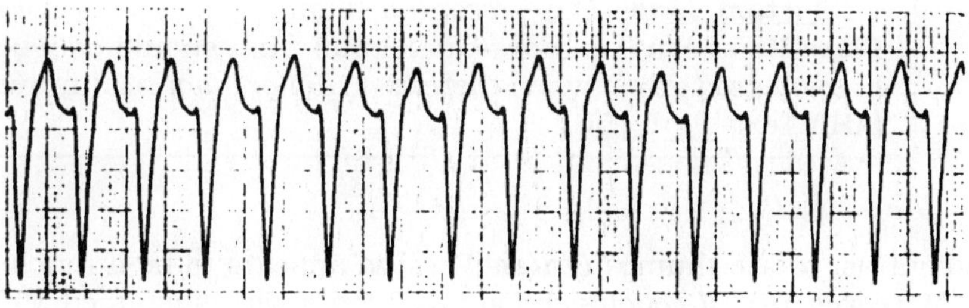

<u>Figure 4B-2</u>: The patient remains in *sustained* VT.

Analysis of Figure 4B-2 and Plan:

Sustained VT persists in this patient who remains hemodynamically stable.

6) Administer ***Lidocaine*** :

- Give an *initial* **IV bolus** (of **≈75-100 mg**).
- After giving the bolus, begin a *continuous* **IV infusion**- starting at a rate of **2 mg/minute**. By the *Rule of 250 ml* :

▪ Mix **1g** of *Lidocaine* in **250 ml** of D5W- and *begin* the infusion @ **30 drops/minute** (=2 mg/minute).

7) Remain *ready* to cardiovert *immediately* (with ≈100 joules)- IF the patient shows signs of hemodynamic decompensation at *any* time during the treatment process.

> **Note-** Lidocaine is recommended as the treatment of choice for the patient with *sustained* VT who is hemodynamically stable. AHA Guidelines advise beginning with **1.0-1.5 mg/kg** for the ***initial* IV dose**. Since we were told that the patient in this Case Scenario weighs "about 80 kg"- an appropriate amount for this initial IV bolus is ≈75-100 mg (as suggested above). Smaller IV loading boluses (i.e., of ≈50-75 mg) are recommended for lighter patients. In general, *no more* than 100 mg of Lidocaine is given at any one time in an IV bolus.

Teaching Points : Use of Cough Version/Precordial Thump

- Should either of these modalities be used for the patient in this scenario?

The ***Precordial Thump*** is *not* benign procedure. The problem with this modality is the complete lack of control over when in the cardiac cycle the energy will be delivered. Thus, although the thump *may* convert VT to sinus rhythm- it may also precipitate deterioration of VT to V Fib (or even asystole)- IF the thump is inadvertently delivered during the *vulnerable period.*

> **Bottom Line-** The *precordial thump* is now classified as a **Class IIb** action (i.e., *possibly* helpful)- that should *only* be used in *witnessed* arrest when there is *no defibrillator* readily available (AHA Text- Pg 1-15).

In contrast to the thump- ***Cough Version*** appears to be a much more benign procedure. Moreover, use of *cough version* in patients with sustained VT may convert a surprising number of these individuals to sinus rhythm. As a result, there appears to be "little to lose" by a trial of ***forceful coughing*** in a *conscious* patient who presents in sustained VT- as is the case in this scenario.

> **Note-** AHA Guidelines do *not* specifically comment on the use of *cough version.* (We discuss use of the precordial thump and cough version in more detail in Section 2D on pages 169-171).

An *initial* IV bolus of ***Lidocaine*** has been given, and a *continuous* IV infusion of this drug has been started at a rate of 2 mg/minute. The patient remains hemodynamically stable- but the rhythm shown in Figure 4B-2 has *not* changed.

What would you do now?

Plan:

8) Repeat the ***Lidocaine*** :

- Give ≈**50-75 mg** for the **2nd IV bolus**.
- May thereafter administer additional IV boluses (of ≈50-75 mg) every 5-10 minutes- *up to* a total of 3 mg/kg (or *up to* ≈**225 mg**).
- *Continue* the IV infusion at 2 mg/minute.

> **Note-** One need *not* necessarily increase the infusion rate of Lidocaine each time that a bolus is given! This is especially true during the initial period of IV loading with Lidocaine (when steady state levels of drug have *not* yet been reached!). Higher infusion rates (i.e., 4 mg/minute) will usually *not* be needed in most patients- and may predispose to development of toxicity.

9) *If VT persists*- Consider ***Procainamide*** :

- Give Procainamide in increments of **100 mg IV**- infusing each increment *slowly* over a 5 minute period (or at ≈20 mg/minute).
- Continue IV loading *until* a total dose of **17 mg/kg** (≈1,000 mg) has been given- and/or the arrhythmia is suppressed. Stop infusion sooner if hypotension occurs and/or the QRS widens by ≥50%.

- *If VT is suppressed by IV loading*- may begin a *maintenance* IV infusion of Procainamide at ≈**2 mg/minute**. By the *Rule of 250 ml* :

> - Mix **1g** of *Procainamide* in **250 ml** of D5W- and *begin* the infusion @ **30 drops/minute** (=2 mg/minute).

A second bolus of Lidocaine is given *without* effect (i.e., the sustained tachycardia shown in Figure 4B-2 continues). Slow IV loading of Procainamide is begun. The patient suddenly begins to lose consciousness- the pulse becomes faint- and the BP is now *only* 60 palpable.

What should you do now?

Clinical Assessment and Plan:

The patient has become ***hemodynamically* unstable**! She is losing consciousness and BP is now only 60 palpable.

10) *Stop* the IV loading Procainamide infusion.

- In this acutely unstable situation there is *no longer time* for a trial of medical therapy. Moreover, the IV Procainamide infusion may well be contributing (or the cause) of the hypotension.

11) Prepare to *immediately* ***cardiovert*** *the patient* !!!

- Use **100 joules** for this 1st attempt.

> **Note**- When *synchronized cardioversion* is used to treat sustained VT on a less emergent basis (i.e., in a patient who *remains* alert and perfusing)- there *ideally* will be time to *sedate* the patient and call anesthesia to the bedside for assistance.
>
> Because the patient in this case scenario is losing consciousness, sedation would not appear to be needed. Moreover, because of the abrupt nature with which this patient decompensated, there probably would *not* be time to sedate the patient anyway.

Teaching Points : On Implementing *Synchronized* Cardioversion

Be *sure* that the amplitude of the QRS complex is of sufficient size on the monitor to be detected. If it isn't- *adjust* R wave amplitude accordingly. Having said this- *IF* for *any* reason you are *unable* to activate the synchronization mode of the defibrillator (or otherwise get the machine to work)- *and* the patient you are treating is acutely unstable- *forget about cardioversion*! Instead, *immediately defibrillate* the patient (i.e., with *unsynchronized* countershock).

> **Note**- In most cases, delivery of *unsynchronized* countershock will successfully convert sustained VT to sinus rhythm. In an acutely *unstable* situation- *delivery of unsynchronized energy is far superior to delivery of no energy at all.*

Preparation for *synchronized* cardioversion- should include the following steps (AHA Text- Pg 1-35):

- Turn the defibrillator on- and attach monitoring leads.
- Be sure to keep an *ongoing* ECG recording of the entire procedure. (This may be of *invaluable* assistance later for definitive interpretation of the patient's rhythm.)
- ***Sedate*** the patient- *IF time allows.* It may also be helpful to *call anesthesia* to the bedside (so that someone *other than YOU* can take care of the Airway- and allow *YOU* to attend solely to the cardioversion).
- Press the control switch to *activate* the ***"SYNCH"*** *Mode.*
- Look for ***markers*** on the QRS (that ensure the machine is *sensing* each complex of the tachycardia- and indicate the point in the cardiac cycle at which the electrical discharge will be delivered). *The "SYNCH" Mode switch should be flashing when the machine is sensing.*

- Select **100 joules** for the 1st cardioversion attempt.

- Apply conductive gel to the paddles (or use defibrillator pads).

- Shout **"Clear"** (or other appropriate ***Clearing Chant***)- and then *verify* that *all* health care providers have indeed heeded your warning. *Don't* discharge the paddles- *until YOU are sure that no one is touching the patient or the bed.*

- Apply firm pressure (i.e., ≈25 lbs of force) to each paddle. Then press both "discharge" buttons *simultaneously*, being sure to *maintain* both buttons depressed- until the electrical discharge occurs!

- Be ready to immediately defibrillate the patient- *IF* cardioversion inadvertently precipitates deterioration to V Fib. (Most defibrillators *automatically* default back to the *unsynchronized* mode after cardioversion- a feature that facilitates immediate defibrillation in the event it is needed).

Teaching Points **: In view of the fact that this patient has become hypotensive with the tachycardia- would it be helpful to administer a pressor agent *prior* to cardioversion?**

NO !!!! The treatment of choice for sustained VT in a patient who is hemodynamically unstable consists of *immediate* cardioversion. Use of a *pressor* agent (such as Dopamine or Epinephrine infusion) is *contraindicated* in this situation. If anything, the arrhythmogenic effect of these catecholamines is likely to precipitate V Fib.

> ***KEY***- *Pressor agents* may be helpful in the treatment of hypotension that occurs in association with a hemodynamically significant bradyarrhythmia. They have *NO place* in the treatment of hypotension that results from VT !

Application of *synchronized* **cardioversion** (with 100 joules) to the rhythm seen in Figure 4B-2 on page 333 results in the tracing below (Figure 4B-3). *What to do now?*

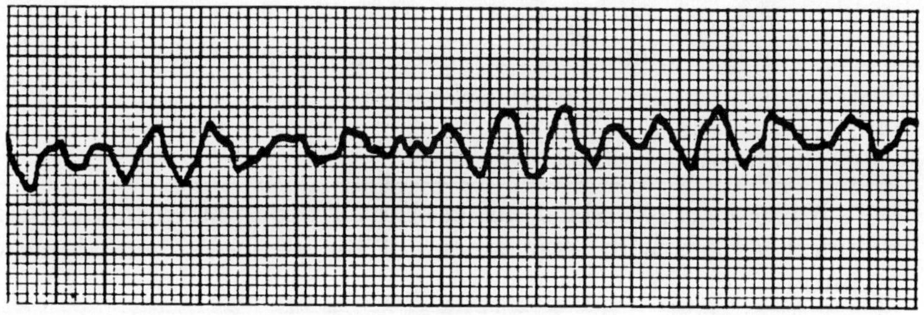

Figure 4B-3: Rhythm seen on the monitor immediately following synchronized cardioversion of VT. *What to do now?*

Analysis of Figure 4B-3 and Plan:

Synchronized cardioversion has precipitated deterioration of VT to V Fib.

12) *Verify* that the patient is pulseless and unresponsive (i.e., that the rhythm is *truly* V Fib!).

13) **Defibrillate** with **200 joules**.

It will often be helpful to try to *anticipate* potential adverse effects that *might* occur as the result of any intervention. For example, *awareness* that synchronized cardioversion can occasionally precipitate V Fib should enhance your *readiness* to respond appropriately (i.e., with *immediate* defibrillation).

If cardioversion does precipitate V Fib, comfort can at least be taken in the fact that your chance for converting such a patient *out of* V Fib should be excellent (since you have anticipated this possibility- and are therefore ready to *immediately* defibrillate the patient).

Defibrillation (with 200 joules) of the rhythm seen in Figure 4B-3 results in the tracing below (Figure 4B-4). *What should you do now?*

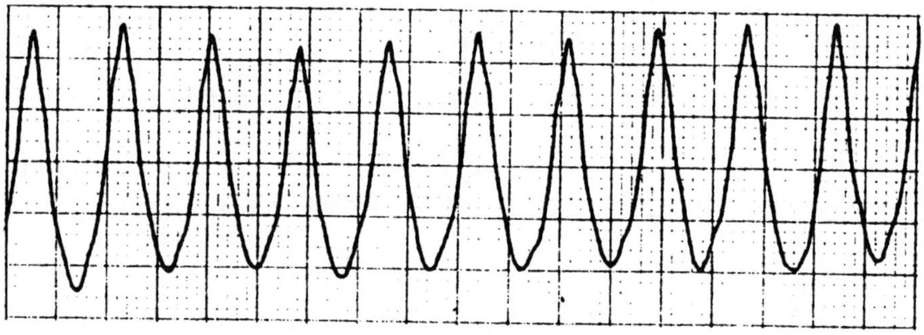

Figure 4B-4: Rhythm seen on the monitor following defibrillation.

Analysis of Figure 4B-4 and Plan:

There is now a regular, *wide-complex* tachycardia (*WCT*)- *without* any evidence of atrial activity. *The rhythm is VT.*

14) Check the patient for:

- presence of a pulse
- blood pressure determination
- responsiveness.

> **Note-** As emphasized earlier- the *KEY* to the treatment of *sustained* VT lies with assessment of the patient's hemodynamic status.

The patient whose rhythm is shown in Figure 4B-4 remains unresponsive. There is *no pulse* felt in association with this rhythm. *What next?*

Plan:

The patient is in sustained VT. *No pulse is palpable.*

15) **Defibrillate** the patient (with **200-360 joules**).

AHA Guidelines emphasize that ***pulseless VT*** should be treated the *same* as **V Fib** (i.e., with immediate *unsynchronized* countershock).

> **Note**- In addition to the fact that the patient in this Case Scenario has become pulseless- the ECG rhythm in Figure 4B-4 is *not* one conducive to an optimal response from synchronized cardioversion. This is because it is virtually impossible to distinguish between the QRS complex and the T wave in this tracing. It may therefore *not* be possible to avoid the "vulnerable period"- and deliver the electrical discharge on the "upstroke" of the R wave. (**Hint**- If *YOU* have trouble distinguishing between the QRS complex and the T wave- chances are that the machine will have similar difficulty.)

Defibrillation (with 200 joules) of the rhythm seen in Figure 4B-4 results in the tracing below (Figure 4B-5). *How would you respond?*

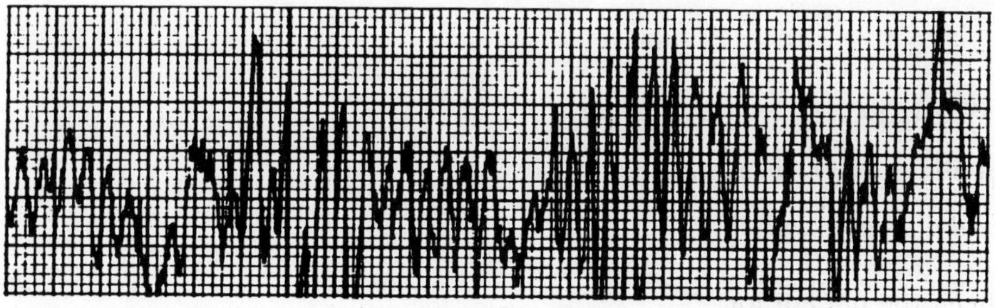

Figure 4B-5: Rhythm seen on the monitor following defibrillation of Figure 4B-4.

Despite the rhythm that is seen above- *there IS a good pulse* !

How can this be ???

Analysis of Figure 4B-5 and Plan:

The presence of a good pulse in association with the rhythm seen in Figure 4B-5 suggests that the tracing must reflect ***artifact*** !!!!

16) Check the patient to see that *all* leads are on !!!!!

> **Note**- *Artifact* should be suspected when exceedingly rapid (i.e., >300/minute) geometric-appearing spikes are seen (as in the case here)- *especially in the presence of a good pulse* !

A monitoring lead had fallen off. *After* it is put back on, the ECG monitor shows the rhythm below (Figure 4B-6).

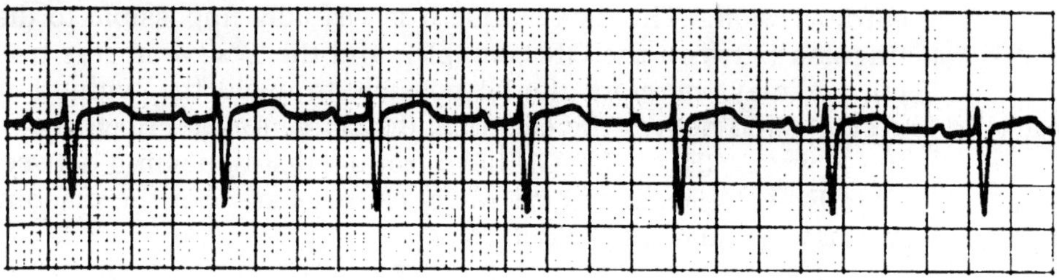

Figure 4B-6: Rhythm seen on the monitor after reattachment of the fallen monitoring lead.

A strong pulse is felt in association with the rhythm seen in Figure 4B-6. *What now?*

Analysis of Figure 4B-6 and Plan:

The patient is now in normal sinus rhythm.

17) *Take a deep breath* !!!!

18) Assess the patient further (i.e., for responsiveness, blood pressure determination, spontaneous respiration, etc.).

> **Note**- Use of the steps and actions encompassed in the ***Primary*** and ***Secondary Surveys*** (and/or in the ***Universal Algorithm***) may greatly facilitate your reassessment of the patient.

The patient begins to breathe spontaneously and is opening her eyes. There is still a good pulse. BP = 120/80 mm Hg. *What next?*

19) *Verify* that **Lidocaine** is still infusing at a *continuous* rate of ≈2 mg/minute.

> **Note-** A continuous IV infusion of ***Lidocaine*** is indicated for this patient- both as a *treatment* measure (for the sustained VT that was present at the beginning of this case)- as well as for *prophylaxis* (i.e., to *prevent* VT/V Fib recurrence). A continuous IV infusion rate of **2 mg/minute** will usually result in adequate serum antiarrhythmic drug levels for most patients.

20) Ask the patient if that "funny sensation" in her chest has gone (now that she is back in normal sinus rhythm).

21) *Take another deep breath* !!!!

> - *YOU have SAVED the patient* !!!!!
>
> \- at least *for the moment . . .*

22) Complete your reassessment of the patient. Specifically- you'll want to determine if the ***new-onset* chest pain** experienced by this patient was the result of *acute myocardial infarction* !

A 12-lead ECG is obtained on this patient- and reveals *marked* ST segment elevation in the anterior leads. Q waves have not yet formed. The patient is now alert and breathing spontaneously. She is still having chest pain. BP = 120/80 mm Hg. The overall clinical picture suggests ***Acute MI*** (*Myocardial Infarction*) in this 60 year old woman.

How would you proceed? Specifically, what are the actions/interventions that should be considered for this patient with Acute MI? What drugs should you order? *Is the patient a candidate for thrombolytic therapy?*

Teaching Points : Considerations in Treatment of Acute MI

Although this patient's chest pain may be solely the result of her acute evolving MI- it could also be due (at least in part) to the defibrillation/cardioversion attempts that she underwent during resuscitation. A sustained tachycardia (such as her sustained VT) could also produce chest pain- although *tachycardia-related* chest discomfort will most often dissipate soon after the arrhythmia resolves.

Actions/interventions/drugs to consider in management of this patient with *evolving* **Acute MI** include the following:

- ***Oxygen***- AHA Guidelines advocate use of "*Oxygen-IV-Monitor*" as a *single* word- to be routinely implemented in virtually all emergency cardiopulmonary situations.

- ***Aspirin (ASA)***- Assuming no contraindications- *all* patients with acute ischemic chest pain should receive ***ASA*** (in a dose of **160-325 mg**). The order should be written for *"ASA- given ASAP!"* - since the beneficial effect of this drug begins to work *within* 30 minutes.

- ***Nitroglycerin (NTG)***- is generally accepted as the drug of choice for acute ischemic chest pain. Although the drug may be administered by many routes- use of ***IV NTG*** is clearly preferable in the emergency situation when chest pain is severe and persistent.

- ***Morphine Sulfate***- remains an effective drug for relieving the chest pain of Acute MI- especially as an *adjunctive* measure when chest pain persists despite use of NTG.

- ***Thrombolytic Therapy/IV Heparin***- Assuming no contraindications, the patient in this Case Scenario (i.e., a 60 year old woman with large anterior infarction)- is an *excellent* candidate for these interventions.

- ***IV ß-Blockers***- are especially helpful when given *early* in the course of acute *anterior* infarction- especially when the patient is hypertensive and tachycardic.

- ***IV Magnesium***- may be considered in the treatment of Acute MI- especially when serum magnesium levels are known (or likely) to be low.

- ***ACE Inhibitors***- constitute the newest treatment for Acute MI. Although clearly effective in the treatment of patients with associated hypertension or heart failure, ACE inhibitors also appear to favorably affect the ventricular remodeling process (that begins within hours of acute infarction). Most authorities recommend waiting at least 12-24 hours before beginning an ACE-inhibitor, and *not* using this drug if the patient is hypotensive.

- ***Calcium Channel Blockers***- have *not* been shown to reduce mortality with Acute MI. These drugs (i.e., Verapamil, Diltiazem, Nifedipine, others) should therefore *not* be used routinely in this setting- unless another indication for the drug exists (such as SVT).

Discussion :

This case illustrates the steps in the initial approach to resuscitation of the patient in ventricular tachycardia. Several points are deserving of special mention:

- *Always* assume that a regular ***W****ide-****C****omplex* ***T****achycardia* (***WCT***) is VT- *until proven otherwise* !!! ***Treat the patient accordingly*** (i.e., *as if* the rhythm is VT).

- Remember that the *KEY* to management of any ***sustained* tachycardia** depends *most* on assessment of the patient's hemodynamic status. When the rhythm is rapid (i.e., *more than* 150 beats/minute) and the patient is ***acutely unstable*** as a *direct* result of the rapid rate- determination of the specific etiology of the rhythm becomes much less important than the need for *immediate* treatment. The intervention of choice in this situation is *immediate* ***synchronized cardioversion*** (*regardless* of whether the rhythm turns out to be sustained VT- or an SVT with either aberrant conduction or preexisting bundle branch block).

- If no pulse is felt- ***pulseless VT*** should be treated the same as V Fib (i.e., with *unsynchronized* countershock).

- If the patient is in ***sustained VT***- but a pulse is felt and the patient is ***hemodynamically stable***- there is clearly more time to decide on a therapeutic approach. A trial of medical therapy is perfectly reasonable in this situation (i.e., with *Lidocaine- Procainamide-* or other appropriate agents). *Adenosine* might also be given as a diagnostic/therapeutic trial if the WCT was of *uncertain* etiology and the patient was stable- especially if a supraventricular etiology was felt to be more likely (*Figure 1C-13 on page 85*). Other actions might be considered in an attempt to help clarify the diagnosis (i.e., review of the medical history, comparison with prior tracings, obtaining a 12-lead ECG, etc.). Ultimately, cardioversion may still be needed- but usually under less urgent circumstances.

- If doubt remains about what to do- return to the initial point that we list above. That is- *always* assume that the rhythm is VT until proven otherwise. Then, treat the patient accordingly.

The final point we emphasize relates to the importance of ***thinking ahead*** as you manage the patient. ***Anticipate*** the *worst* thing that could happen- *and what you would do if this were to occur.*

> **Note-** Anticipating "the worst possible case scenario" can be helpful in two ways. First, it allows you to prepare the next line of medications and/or therapeutic modalities that you are likely to turn to if your present therapy does not work. Second (and equally important)- is that *thinking ahead* (and being able to formulate your next plan of attack) often has a *calming* effect- and increases your confidence in being able to successfully manage *whatever* future problems you might encounter.

In this particular case, the "worst case scenarios" that could develop include *sudden decompensation* of the patient (i.e., loss of the pulse and/or blood pressure)- and/or development of V Fib. The former is treated by emergency cardioversion- and the latter by immediate defibrillation.

Case Study C

A 65 year old woman is transported in full arrest to the ED where you are working. Active resuscitation is in progress.

- The arrest was unwitnessed.
- The patient "has been defibrillated". She is intubated and an IV line is in place- *but no mediations have been given yet.*
- She looks to weigh *only* about **50 kg**.
- The monitor reveals the rhythm shown in Figure 4C-1.

What would you do next?

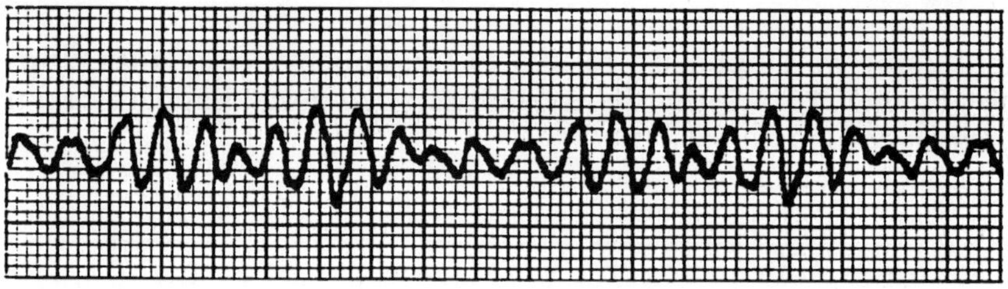

Figure 4C-1: Initial rhythm seen on the monitor for the patient in Case Study C. *What would you do next?*

Analysis of Figure 4C-1 and Plan:

The rhythm on the monitor appears to be ***Ventricular Fibrillation* (V Fib)**.

1) *Verify* that the patient is *pulseless* and *unresponsive* (i.e., that the rhythm is *truly* V Fib- and *not* artifactual!).

2) **Defibrillate** with **200 joules**.

> **Note**- Although told that the code is "in progress" and that the patient "has been defibrillated"- specific information on what has occurred is lacking. In the absence of this information, it is reasonable to begin this defibrillation series at the generally recommended energy level for "initial" defibrillation (i.e., with **200 joules**).

Defibrillation (with 200j) of the rhythm in Figure 4C-1 results in the tracing shown below (Figure 4C-2).

What should you do now?

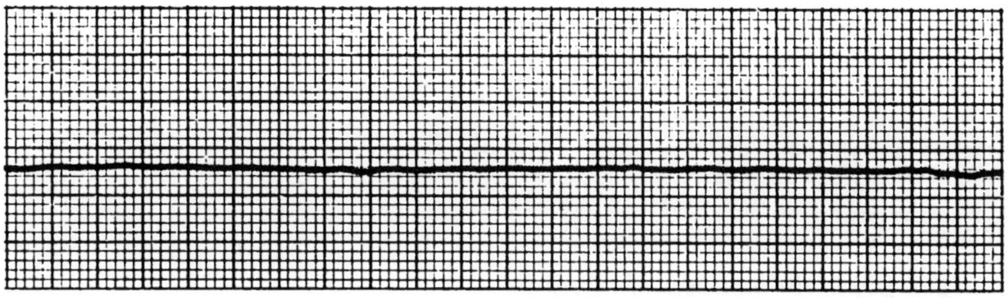

Figure 4C-2: Rhythm resulting from defibrillation of V Fib. *What should you do now?*

Analysis of Figure 4C-2 and Plan:

There is now a *flat line* recording. It therefore appears that the rhythm is now **asystole.**

3) Check the patient for:

- presence of a pulse
- responsiveness
- ET tube position
- adequacy of ventilation/oxygenation.

4) *Verify* that the rhythm seen in the above tracing is *truly* a ***FLAT line*** recording. That is- *rule out* the possibility that fine V Fib may be *masquerading* as asystole:

- Make sure the gain of the monitor has not been mistakenly turned down.
- Make sure all lead attachments are properly connected.
- Hook the patient up to a 12-lead machine (if not already done)- and check the rhythm in *other* leads !

> **Note**- It should take *no more* than a moment to accomplish the verifying actions described above (and to record electrical activity in several other leads). If the rhythm is *truly* asystole- then a flat line recording should also be seen in other leads. The importance of ensuring that this rhythm is *not* fine V Fib- is that if present, treatment would be different (i.e., repeat defibrillation would be indicated).

The *same* flat line recording that is shown in Figure 4C-2 is seen in *all* of the limb leads !!!

- The patient is unresponsive. There is *no* pulse.
- The patient is intubated, and good bilateral breath sounds are present. An IV line is in place and appears to be functioning well.

What should you do now?

Plan:

5) Resume CPR.

6) Consider *possible* ***causes*** of asystole.

- Attention to the "**D**" component (= ***D**ifferential **D**iagnosis*) of the *Secondary Survey* may sometimes suggest a potentially *reversible* etiology (*See Tables 1A-2 and 1D-1 on pages 15 and 96*).

7a) Consider *immediate* use of ***T**rans**C**utaneous **P**acing* (***TCP***)

- and/or -

7b) Administer drugs:

- Begin with ***Epinephrine*** (recommended first by AHA Guidelines in the protocol for treatment of asystole).
- Follow with ***Atropine*** .

  - See Teaching Points below for dosing of Epinephrine and Atropine.

> **Note-** To be effective- TCP *must* be started *EARLY* ! *If available*- TCP should therefore be applied *immediately* in the treatment of asystole (i.e., either *before*- and/or *simultaneously* with the use of drugs!)

In this particular Case Scenario, the duration of time that the patient has been in asystole is relatively short (since you were right here on the scene at the onset of this rhythm). It is therefore less likely that irreversible pathophysiologic changes have already set in. Prompt treatment (i.e., with TCP, Epinephrine, and/or Atropine) would therefore seem to have a much better chance for success than would be the case if asystole was prolonged.

Teaching Points : Dosing Epinephrine and Atropine in the treatment of Asystole

- *Dosing* ***Epinephrine***- The "optimal dose" of **Epinephrine** for use in cardiac arrest remains unknown. Survival rates of patients in V Fib who have not responded to defibrillation are generally low- *regardless of the dose of Epinephrine that is used* ! Nevertheless, it is possible that *some* patients in cardiac arrest *may* respond only to *higher* doses of the drug (i.e., to HDE).

  Practically speaking, it is *impossible* to overdose on Epinephrine when treating asystole. Moreover, administration of HDE to patients in asystole will *not* be harmful (i.e., *"You can't be deader than dead . . . "*). AHA Guidelines therefore recommend the following approach:

  - Begin with an **SDE** dose (i.e., **1.0 mg** by IV bolus).
  - Thereafter one may *either* continue with 1 mg IV doses- *OR chose between several* ***HDE alternatives*** (AHA Text- Pg 7-4):
    - Administration of **2-5 mg** IV boluses- OR -
    - *escalating* **1 - 3 - 5 mg** IV boluses- OR -
    - dosing at **0.1 mg/kg** as an IV bolus.

  Epinephrine should be repeated every 3-5 minutes for as long as the patient remains in asystole. Whether to continue with 1 mg (SDE) dosing- or to increase the dose to HDE is left to the discretion of the treating clinician.

- *Dosing* ***Atropine***- A higher dose of ***Atropine*** may be needed for treatment of bradyasystolic arrest than for treatment of other bradyarrhythmias. AHA Guidelines therefore recommend the following approach:

  - Begin with a dose of **1.0 mg** IV when treating asystole.
  - May repeat this 1 mg dose every 3-5 minutes- *if/as needed* (up to a *total* dose of 0.04 mg/kg- or up to ≈**3 mg** for an *average-sized* adult).

Teaching Points : What if IV access was *not* available for this patient?

- How would you treat asystole *without* IV access?

Initial actions in the management of *asystole* when IV access is *not* available are generally quite similar to those performed in this Case Study- except for the *route* of drug administration.

- Resume CPR.
- Consider potential *causes* of asystole- *and treat these if at all possible.*
- *Institute* **Pacing** (***TCP***)- *immediately* if the device is available, and/or *as soon as* it arrives!

- and/or -

- Administer drugs by the ***ET route*** until IV access *becomes* available:
    - ***Epinephrine***- Instill **2-2.5 mg** down the ET tube. May repeat in 5 minutes.
    - ***Atropine***- Instill **1.0-2.0 mg** down the ET tube.

> **Note**- Although less than ideal, certain drugs *will be* absorbed by the ET route (albeit higher doses are needed than for IV administration of these same drugs). Absorption is facilitated if ET drug administration is followed by several forceful insufflations of the Ambu bag.
>
> The mnemonic ***A - L - E*** recalls the 3 *KEY* drugs that can be given by the ***ET route*** (= *Atropine- Lidocaine- Epinephrine*).

The flat line recording shown in Figure 4C-2 has been treated with ***Epinephrine*** and ***Atropine***. Shortly thereafter the tracing below is noted (Figure 4C-3). *What has happened?*

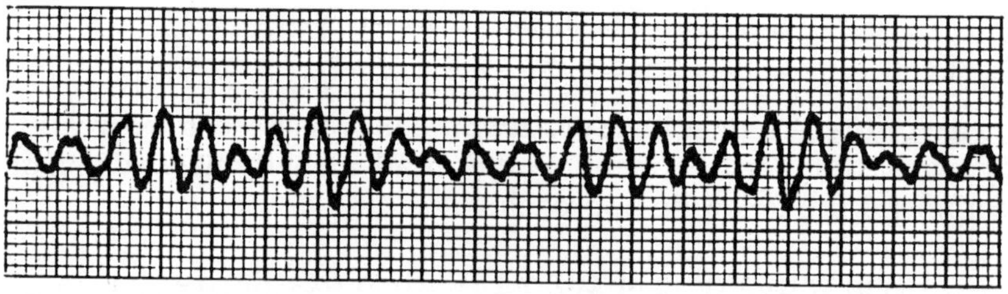

Figure 4C-3: Rhythm seen on the monitor after treatment of asystole with Epinephrine and Atropine.

The external pacer that was sent for earlier (when the patient was in asystole) has just arrived. *Do you still want to apply TCP? What should be done instead?*

Analysis of Figure 4C-3 and Plan:

The rhythm is once again V Fib.

8) *Verify* that the patient is still pulseless and unresponsive.

9) **Defibrillate** (with **200-360 joules**).

Considering that this patient was just in asystole, development of V Fib reflects a *beneficial* therapeutic response (since V Fib is potentially more treatable than asystole).

- There is *no longer* a need for TCP (since this patient is *no longer* in asystole).
- Regarding defibrillation, one might choose to shock this patient *either* with 200 joules (i.e., to restart the defibrillation series)- or with a *higher* energy (i.e., 300 or 360 joules).

Defibrillation (with 200 joules) of the rhythm seen in Figure 4C-3 results in the tracing below (Figure 4C-4). *What has happened? What should you do now?*

Lead II

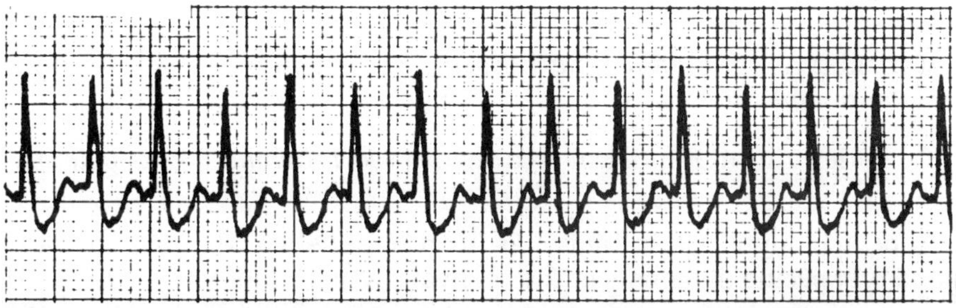

Figure 4C-4: Rhythm seen on the monitor after treatment defibrillation of V Fib.

Analysis of Figure 4C-3 and Plan:

Defibrillation has converted the rhythm seen in Figure 4C-3 to a regular *SUPRAventricular* tachycardia (*SVT*)- at a rate of ≈220/minute.

10) Check the patient for:

- presence of a pulse
- responsiveness
- blood pressure determination
- adequacy of ventilation/oxygenation.

KEY- Always recheck the above parameters *whenever* there is change in the patient's clinical status and/or cardiac rhythm.

It is admittedly difficult to determine the precise diagnosis of the rhythm shown in Figure 4C-4. This is because atrial activity is *not* clearly seen (i.e., it is impossible to be sure if the upright deflection between QRS complexes is a P wave, T Wave- or both). Moreover, the width of the QRS complex can *not* be assessed with certainty from this single monitoring lead- although it does *not* appear to be widened. Having acknowledged these uncertainties- the point to emphasize is that *specific* diagnosis of the rhythm seen in Figure 4C-4 is really is of no more than *secondary* importance- *until* the patient's hemodynamic condition has been assessed!

The patient whose rhythm is shown in Figure 4C-4 is unresponsive. Ventilation and oxygenation appear to be adequate. There is a *good* pulse. BP = 130/80 mm Hg.

How would you assess the overall clinical situation? *How should you proceed?*

Clinical Assessment and Plan:

As noted, the rhythm *appears* to be supraventricular at a regular rate of ≈220/minute. The patient is hemodynamically stable.

> **Note**- AHA Guidelines recommend accomplishing the ***Supportive Actions*** that are listed at the beginning of the *Tachycardia Algorithm* (Figure 1C-1 on page 51)- *as this is possible*- during the course of evaluation and treatment.

11) Consider use of a ***vagal maneuver*** (i.e., carotid massage)- for both *diagnostic* and/or *therapeutic* purposes.

12) Consider a trial of medical treatment (*See Teaching Points below*).

Once hemodynamic stability has been established- the *KEY* to management of SVT will depend on specific diagnosis of the tachyarrhythmia (*Figure 1C-1*). In this particular case, *regularity* of the rhythm and *rapidity* of the rate (≈220/min) suggest ***PSVT*** as the probable diagnosis (*See pages 56-58 and 63 in Section 1C*).

Teaching Points : Which drug is *preferable* for treatment of the rhythm shown in Figure 4C-4?

- Verapamil? Diltiazem? - *and/or* - Adenosine?

The choice of which drug(s) to select for treatment of the rhythm shown in Figure 4C-4 will depend on a number of factors. These include (among others)- *personal preference* of the treating clinician- and the degree of certainty *YOU* have regarding *specific diagnosis* of the type of SVT. Consider the following points:

- ***Adenosine*** :
  - Recommended by AHA Guidelines as the drug of 1st choice for the treatment of PSVT.
  - Also recommended as the drug of choice when the *specific type* of SVT is *uncertain* (i.e., as a diagnostic/therapeutic trial). Adenosine will usually slow the ventricular rate enough to allow determination of the underlying mechanism of the rhythm (i.e., "*chemical* Valsalva").
  - Highly effective for *initial* conversion of *reentry* tachycardias such as PSVT. However, the *recurrence* rate is also high (because of the drug's short half-life)- and Adenosine is *not* effective in treatment of *other* SVTs (i.e., A Fib, A Flutter, or MAT).

- ***Verapamil/Diltiazem*** :
  - Comparable efficacy as Adenosine for treatment of PSVT- with the additional advantage of being effective in the treatment of *other* supraventricular arrhythmias (i.e., A Fib, A Flutter, MAT).
  - *Slower* onset of action than Adenosine (minutes instead of seconds)- but *longer duration* of action (lower recurrence rate). Availability of *continuous* IV infusion (for Diltiazem)- and availability of oral formulations for long-term treatment/prophylaxis.

- Should *never* be used when the QRS is wide- *unless you are 100% certain that the rhythm is SUPRAventricular* !

> **<u>Bottom Line</u>**- Any of the above three drugs would be appropriate as *initial* treatment for the rhythm shown in Figure 4C-4. Other drugs (i.e., *Digoxin*, IV *ß-Blockers*) are used less commonly as initial treatment- and are probably best thought of as 2nd-line agents.

Teaching Points : How should these drugs be dosed?

- ***Adenosine*** :
  - Begin with **6 mg** by *rapid* **IV push** (i.e., over 1-3 seconds!)- followed by a fluid flush.
  - If no response in 1-2 minutes, a 2nd dose (of **12 mg**) may be given- and repeated again in 1-2 minutes if needed (for a *total* dose of 6 + 12 + 12 = 30 mg).
  - If there is no response by this time, *another* agent (i.e., Verapamil or Diltiazem) should be tried- and/or the *diagnosis* of the arrhythmia should be reevaluated!

- and/or -

- ***Verapamil:***
  - Give **2.5- 5 mg IV** over 1-2 minutes; may follow 15-30 minutes later with a 2nd dose of 5-10 mg IV. Give the drug *slower* (over 3-4 minutes) to the elderly.

- and/or -

- ***Diltiazem*** :
  - Give an *initial* **IV bolus** (of ≈**20 mg-** or ≈0.25 mg/kg) over a 2-minute period. Lighter weight patients should receive a lower dose (i.e., 0.25 mg/kg- or ≈10-15 mg, depending on body weight).
  - If the desired response is *not* obtained within 15 minutes- may increase the dose for the 2nd IV bolus (i.e., up to **25 mg**- or up to ≈0.35 mg/kg).
  - Dosing for subsequent boluses should be individualized.
  - If needed, antiarrhythmic effect may be maintained with a *continuous* IV infusion (at a rate of between ≈5-15 mg/hr).

The rhythm shown in Figure 4C-4 is treated with ***Adenosine***. Nothing happens after the 1st dose (of 6 mg)- but there is *marked* slowing of the rhythm after the 2nd dose (of 12 mg). Shortly thereafter the rhythm below is noted (<u>Figure 4C-5</u>). *What has happened?*

What should you do first?

Lead II

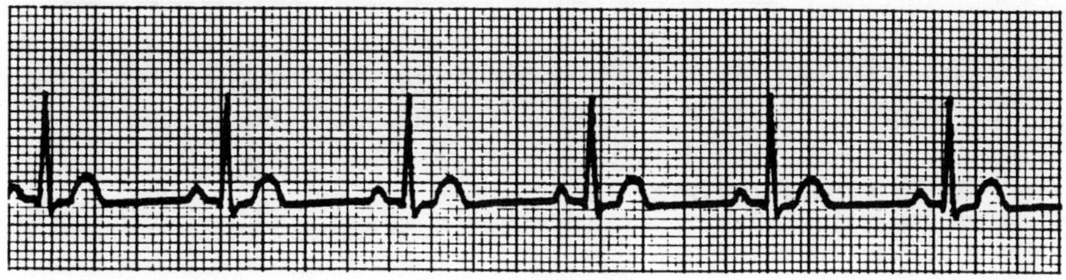

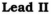

<u>Figure 4C-5</u>: Rhythm seen on the monitor after treatment of PSVT with Adenosine. *What has happened? What should you do first?*

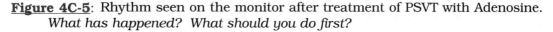

Analysis of Figure 4C-5 and Plan:

The *electrical* rhythm that is seen on the monitor is sinus.

13) Check the patient for:

- presence of a pulse
- responsiveness
- blood pressure determination.

KEY- Management decisions should *always* await assessment of hemodynamic status. Appropriate treatment depends on knowing if the patient has a pulse (and blood pressure).

The patient remains unresponsive. However, there is a *good* pulse. BP = 110/70 mm Hg.

How should you interpret the clinical situation? *What should you do next?*

Clinical Assessment and Plan:

The rhythm seen in Figure 4C-5 is sinus. Despite the fact that the patient is still unresponsive- normal sinus rhythm has been restored and the patient is *hemodynamically stable!*

14) Administer ***Lidocaine*** :

- Use of this drug is indicated as indicated a *prophylactic* measure- since the patient *had* been in V Fib at the onset of the code.
- Give an *initial* **IV bolus** (of ≈**50-75-mg**).
- After giving the bolus, initiate a *continuous* **IV infusion** to maintain antiarrhythmic effect. Begin at a rate of **2 mg/minute**. By the *Rule of 250 ml* :

■ Mix **1g** of *Lidocaine* in **250 ml** of D5W- and *begin* the infusion @ **30 drops/minute** (=2 mg/minute**).**

AHA Recommendations advise giving 1.0-1.5 mg/kg of ***Lidocaine*** for the *initial* IV bolus when the drug is used to treat patients who are *not* in cardiac arrest. Since the patient in this Case Scenario weighs about **50 kg**- an appropriate amount of Lidocaine to give for the initial IV bolus is between 50-75 mg.

The patient has received a ***Lidocaine*** bolus. She begins to open her eyes. There is a *good* pulse- and BP = 110/70. The patient remains in sinus rhythm.

What should you do now?

Plan:

15) *Take a deep breath* !!!

16) <u>*Verify*- that *ALL* is in order</u>:

- that ***Lidocaine*** is infusing @ 2 mg/minute.
- that *no other* infusions (such as Epinephrine) are still running.
- that ET tube placement is appropriate (i.e., that bilateral/symmetric breath sounds are present)- and that ventilation/oxygenation appear adequate.
- that appropriate laboratory tests (i.e, ABGs, electrolytes, chest X-ray, 12-lead ECG, etc.) have all been ordered.

17) Transfer the patient to your critical care facility.

▪ *YOU have SAVED the patient* !!!!!

<u>Teaching Points</u> **: Return for a moment to the situation presented when the patient was in the rhythm shown in Figure 4C-4 (page 349). What if the patient had been *unstable* hemodynamically?**

- Would your treatment have been different?

Yes !!! If *instead* of the situation presented in Figure 4C-4, the patient had become hemodynamically unstable- *immediate* synchronized cardioversion (with 100 joules) would have been indicated.

- AHA Guidelines emphasize that the treatment of choice for a hemodynamically significant tachyarrhythmia is *immediate* synchronized cardioversion. This holds true- *regardless of whether the rhythm is VT or SVT.*

<u>Note</u>- A tachyarrhythmia is said to be ***"hemodynamically unstable"***- <u>*IF*</u> the rhythm produces ***serious signs*** or ***symptoms*** (i.e., chest pain, hypotension, altered mental status)- as a *direct* result of the increase in heart rate. Having said this, one sometimes simply needs to *"be there"* to determine the true urgency of the situation. Thus, one might *not* necessarily cardiovert a patient with tachycardia and hypotension (i.e., a BP of 70-80 systolic)- <u>*IF*</u> the patient was also alert and clinically comfortable. In this situation, a trial of medical therapy (i.e., with *Lidocaine, Adenosine,* etc.) might be perfectly appropriate- provided one was *ready* to immediately cardiovert at the first sign of clinical deterioration.

Discussion :

This case illustrates the steps in the initial approach to resuscitation of the patient in asystole (Figure 1D-3 on page 100)- as well as for the patient in a regular SVT (Figure 1C-11 on page 74). We emphasize the following points:

- There are several *KEYS* to evaluation of a ***flat line*** rhythm. As always- *check the patient first.* If no pulse is present- *immediately* initiate CPR. Then rule out *other* potential causes of a flat line recording- including V Fib masquerading as asystole, unattached monitoring leads, or other technical problems. Asystole is confirmed by the finding of a flat line recording in multiple leads in a patient who is pulseless and unresponsive.

- The circumstances surrounding development of asystole may provide insight to the chance for successful resuscitation. In this particular Case Scenario, asystole developed immediately after the initial countershock. Although the prognosis for a patient in asystole is never good- the fact that this patient was so promptly attended to makes it at least more likely that the rhythm may respond to treatment. In contrast, the chance of successfully resuscitating a victim of out-of-hospital cardiac arrest who is found in asystole (presumably after a *long* unattended period) is virtually nil.

- Pacing is the treatment of choice for asystole- *provided that it can be implemented early.* Pacing is *unlikely* to work if it is only applied late in the process (after all other treatment has failed). In acknowledgement of this clinical reality- AHA Guidelines *no longer* recommend that pacing even be attempted in patients with prolonged asystole, for whom the chance for survival is virtually nil (AHA Text- Pg 5-2).

- Other than pacing- treatment options for asystole are unfortunately limited. They essentially consist of Epinephrine, and Atropine. Practically speaking, one can *not* overdose on ***Epinephrine*** when treating the patient with persistent asystole. Higher doses of the drug may work in some cases. Therefore, if SDE dosing fails to produce the desired response- one might consider *increasing* the dose (i.e., to **HDE**) in the hope that the patient may respond.

  A higher dose of ***Atropine*** may also be needed to treat asystole than is normally used for treatment of other bradyarrhythmias. The recommended maximum dose of this drug is now 0.04 mg/kg (or up to ≈3 mg in an *average-sized* adult) .

- Finally- don't forget the "**D**" of the ***Secondary Survey*** (= *Differential Diagnosis*) when assessing the patient with asystole. A potentially reversible cause of asystole (i.e., marked hypoxemia, tension pneumothorax, hyperkalemia, etc.) may occasionally be found.

> **Note**- If all else fails, consideration *might* be given to the use of Aminophylline- although we emphasize that this drug is *not* yet included in AHA Guidelines (*See pages 196-197 in Section 2E*).

Management of this Case Scenario took a surprising turn after delivery of the second countershock- which resulted in a regular SVT at a rate of ≈220 beats/minute (Figure 4C-4 on page 349). Points to emphasize regarding this rhythm include the following:

- The initial step in evaluation of a patient with ***SVT*** is *identical* to that for evaluation of VT- *determine the patient's hemodynamic status!* If the patient is unstable- specific diagnosis of the rhythm *no longer matters* in the acute setting (since immediate cardioversion will be needed *regardless* of what the rhythm happens to be). On the other hand, if the patient is stable- the *KEY* to management will depend on the specific diagnosis of the tachyarrhythmia (Figure 1C-1 on page 51).

- In the present Case Scenario, specific diagnosis of the rhythm shown in Figure 4C-4 is most likely PSVT. This conclusion is based on the regularity of the rhythm (which rules out A Fib), the lack of atrial activity, and the heart rate (i.e., a rate of 220/minute is too rapid for sinus tachycardia- and not consistent with what would be expected if the rhythm was A Flutter).

  The drug of 1st choice for emergency treatment of PSVT is ***Adenosine*** (so chosen because of its efficacy and rapid onset of action). Alternative agents that might also be used include *Verapamil* or *Diltiazem*. Use of a vagal maneuver may help diagnostically and therapeutically in selected patients.

Two final points should be made regarding the management of the patient in this Case Scenario:

- First- to remember to start *prophylactic* infusion of ***Lidocaine*** at the earliest appropriate moment after converting the patient *out of* V Fib. The goal of this drug is to *prevent recurrence* of V Fib now that the patient is back in a normal sinus rhythm.

- Second- to keep in mind the importance of body weight in the dosing of certain *KEY* cardioactive medications. The patient in this Case Scenario is lighter (she weighs **50 kg**) than the *"average-sized"* 70-80 kg adult. As a result- correspondingly *lower* doses of drugs should be used. Specifically:

  - ***Atropine***- is given in a dose of up to of 0.04 mg/kg. This comes out to a total of about 2 mg in this 50 kg patient. In contrast, the maximum dose of Atropine for an *average-sized* (i.e., ≈70-80 kg) adult would be closer to 3 mg.

  - ***Diltiazem***- is given in an initial IV dose of 0.25 mg/kg- which comes out to an IV bolus of 12.5 mg. This is considerably less than the 20 mg dose that is usually cited as the "typical" initial dose.

  - ***Lidocaine***- is given in an initial IV dose of 1-1.5 mg/kg- which comes out to an initial IV bolus of 50-75 mg.

  Other adjustments may also need to be made to account for this patient's smaller body size.

Case Study D

You arrive at the scene of a cardiopulmonary arrest that is occurring on a general ward in the hospital. It appears that the code has been in progress for no more than a short period of time.

- The patient is an elderly gentleman of modest body build.
- He has been shocked once (with 200j) for *presumed* ***V Fib***.
- Intubation has been difficult, but is finally accomplished.
- An IV line is in place- *but no medications have yet been given.*
- Monitor leads reveal the rhythm shown below (Figure 4D-1).

What is the rhythm? *What would you do next?*

Lead II

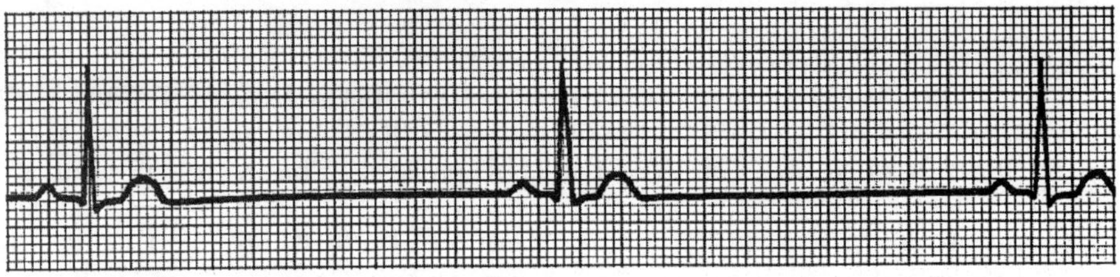

Figure 4D-1: Initial rhythm of the patient in Case Study D. *What would you do next?*

Analysis of Figure 4D-1 and Plan:

The mechanism of the rhythm is *sinus-* since upright P waves that are clearly conducting are seen in lead II. However, the rate is extremely *slow* (with an R-R interval between QRS complexes of *more* than 10 large boxes!). Thus, the rhythm is ***sinus bradycardia***- albeit with *marked* heart rate slowing. The QRS complex appears to be narrow.

1) Check the patient for:

- responsiveness
- presence of a pulse
- adequacy of ET tube placement
- blood pressure determination.

Despite restoration of a sinus mechanism, the rate of the rhythm in Figure 4D-1 is exceedingly *slow* (i.e., *less* than 30 beats/minute!). Profound bradycardia to this degree that occurs in the setting of cardiopulmonary arrest is in general a poor prognostic sign. Of even more *immediate* concern in your assessment of the situation should be the fact that this patient's clinical condition is as yet *unspecified* (i.e., there has been *no mention* at all of the presence of a pulse, the level of responsiveness, BP determination, etc.). *Clinical assessment of the patient is KEY for knowing what needs to be done next.*

The ET tube appears to be properly positioned (i.e., there is ample air movement and equal bilateral breath sounds are heard with each ventilation). The patient is unresponsive. A pulse is present, but is not very strong. BP = 60 palpable. The rhythm on the monitor remains unchanged (Figure 4D-1).

How do you assess the overall clinical situation? *What would you do next?*

Clinical Assessment and Plan:

The patient remains in an exceedingly slow *sinus bradycardia.* The rhythm is clearly of ***hemodynamic significance***- since the patient is markedly hypotensive.

2) Be sure you have *optimized* ***ventilation*** :

> ***KEY***- Inadequate oxygenation may be contributing to (or the *sole* cause of!) the bradycardia. In addition to ensuring proper ET tube placement and the presence of equal bilateral breath sounds (as you have already done)- other parameters of the adequacy of *oxygenation* should be assessed (i.e., patient skin color, ABG determination- or at least oxygen saturation, chest X-ray, etc.). Be sure that the patient is receiving supplemental oxygen at 100%.

If despite optimal ventilation- the hemodynamically significant bradycardia persists:

3a) Give ***Atropine*** :

- Administer **0.5- 1.0 mg** IV for the *initial* dose.
- May repeat Atropine (0.5- 1.0 mg IV) in 3-5 minutes- *if/as needed* (up to a *total* dose of ≈3 mg).

- and/or -

3b) Institute ***Pacing*** (*IF available*):

- Use of *TransCutanous Pacing* ***(TCP)*** is appropriate as the *initial* intervention in the treatment of bradycardia- *IF* the bradycardia is severe and/or the clinical condition unstable (AHA Text- Pg 1-31). In such situations- *one need not wait for Atropine to take effect before instituting pacing* !

It is important to emphasize that the reason for treating the patient in this Case Scenario with Atropine and/or pacing is not just that the heart rate is slow- but that *serious signs/symptoms* (in this case hypotension) are occurring in association with the bradycardia.

Teaching Points : **Would you treat this patient if BP was normal?**

- Would Atropine or pacing be indicated if the rhythm shown in Figure 4D-1 was associated with a BP = 120/80?

Despite the slow rate, immediate treatment (with *either* Atropine or pacing) would *not* necessarily be indicated for the rhythm in Figure 4D-1- IF the patient was normotensive.

- ***"Anticipatory Pacing Readiness"*** (i.e., use of TCP in the *Standby Mode*)- might be the most appropriate intervention for this clinical situation (*See page 185 in Section 2D*).
- Similar *anticipatory readiness* to use Atropine (or other drugs) is also appropriate. Because Atropine is *not* a benign medication- AHA Guidelines generally recommend that use of this drug be *reserved* for treatment of rhythms that are *truly* of hemodynamic significance. As emphasized by AHA Guidelines (AHA Text- Pg 1-30):

- "*Always* ***treat the patient***- NOT *the* ***monitor*** !" -

Bradycardia- even when *marked*- need *not* necessarily be treated if it is not producing adverse *hemodynamic* signs or symptoms.

The situation presented in Figure 4D-1 has *not* changed. The patient remains markedly bradycardic, hypotensive and unresponsive. Two doses of ***Atropine*** have been given- but without effect. You are told that the external pacer is "momentarily" unavailable. The heart rate is still less than 30 beats/minute, and BP is 60 palpable.

- *What would you do at this point?*

Plan:

4) Continue awaiting the availability of pacing:

- **TCP** is clearly the intervention of choice for this patient who has *not* responded to two doses of Atropine. TCP should be applied- *as soon as* it becomes available.

5) While awaiting TCP- Consider *other* options:

- IV infusion of ***Dopamine*** (beginning at a rate of ≈5 μg/kg/minute- and titrating the rate of infusion upward as needed)-

- and/or -

- IV infusion of ***Epinephrine*** (beginning at ≈1-2 μg/minute- and increasing as needed)-

- and/or -

- *More* Atropine (up to a *total* dose of 0.04 mg/kg- or about 3 mg).

> **Note**- Use of a ***pressor agent*** (i.e., *Dopamine, Epinephrine*) is generally reserved as a *stopgap* measure (i.e., as *temporizing* therapy)- that is best only used until TCP becomes available.
> In this particular case, given the severe degree of hemodynamic compromise and the lack of response to Atropine- use of a pressor agent would certainly seem indicated while awaiting arrival of the pacemaker.

You are told that the external pacer is "on its way". In the meantime, IV infusion of ***Dopamine*** is begun. Shortly thereafter, the rhythm below is noted. *What has happened?*

Lead II

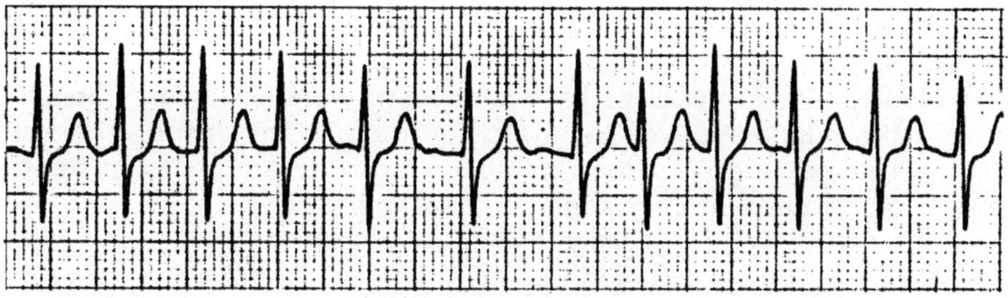

Figure 4D-2: Rhythm seen on the monitor shortly after beginning IV infusion of Dopamine. *What has happened?*

Analysis of Figure 4D-2 and Plan:

The rate of the rhythm has suddenly increased. In addition to being rapid, it is now *irregularly* irregular- and P waves are *no longer* evident. Thus, the patient has gone into ***atrial fibrillation (A Fib)***- here with a *rapid* ventricular response.

6) Check the patient for:

- presence of a pulse
- responsiveness
- blood pressure determination.

> ***KEY***- As is the case for *any* tachycardia- management decisions will depend on the patient's hemodynamic stability (or lack thereof)! Therefore, before proceeding further- it will be essential to determine the patient's clinical status.

The patient remains *unresponsive*. A weak carotid pulse is felt- but *no blood pressure* reading can be obtained.

How would you describe this patient's clinical status? *What should you do?*

Clinical Assessment and Plan:

The rhythm in Figure 4D-2 is ***rapid* A Fib**. The patient is *hemodynamically unstable* !

7) *Immediately* ***cardiovert*** *the patient* !!!

Several points should be emphasized about this case so far:

- The ***Dopamine*** that was started earlier should now be stopped. Catecholamine infusion (i.e., with *Dopamine, Epinephrine*) is *not* beneficial for treatment of hypotension when it occurs in association with a tachyarrhythmia. On the contrary, catecholamine infusion may *exacerbate* the arrhythmia.

- Rapid A Fib should *not* be treated with Adenosine. Although highly effective for management of *reentry* SVTs (such as PSVT)- Adenosine does *not* convert A Fib, and its duration of action is far too short to produce a clinically beneficial rate-slowing effect.

- Medical treatment with *longer-lasting* rate-slowing drugs (i.e., *Digoxin, Verapamil/Diltiazem*) is also *not* recommended for the situation presented here. This patient is far too unstable to tolerate any delay in treatment. Instead- *immediate cardioversion is urgently needed.*

- AHA Guidelines recommend use of a standard sequence of energy levels for emergency ***synchronized cardioversion***- in which selection of **100 joules** is suggested as the *initial* energy level for most tachycardias (AHA Text- Pg 1-35). However, because the disorganized rhythm of ***A Fib*** often requires a *higher* energy level for successful conversion- we favor beginning with ***200 joules*** for cardioversion of this arrhythmia *(See pages 180-181).*

Synchronized cardioversion of the rhythm in Figure 4D-2 results in the tracing shown below (Figure 4D-3). How would you interpret this rhythm? *What would you do next?*

Lead II

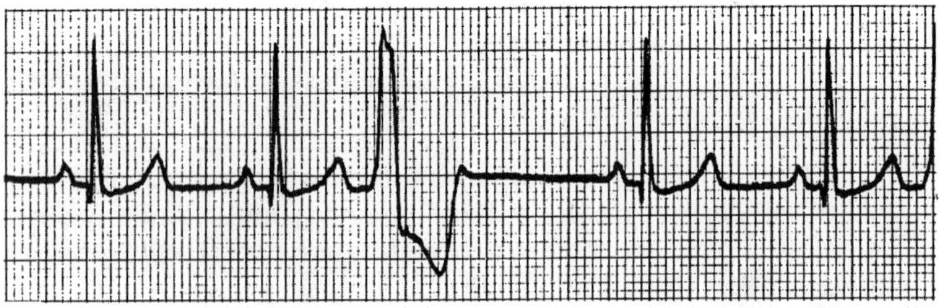

Figure 4D-3: Rhythm seen on the monitor after synchronized cardioversion of rapid A Fib. *What has happened?*

Analysis of Figure 4D-3 and Plan:

The rhythm is now ***sinus***- with ***PVCs***. Synchronized cardioversion has therefore succeeded in converting the patient *out of* A Fib- so that *electrically speaking* the rhythm is now sinus with PVCs.

8) Check the patient for:

- responsiveness
- presence of a pulse
- adequacy of ventilation/oxygenation
- blood pressure determination.

> **Note**- ACLS Instructors may become quite *devious* when assigned to the *MEGA Code* Station. Unless *YOU* develop the habit of *routinely* assessing for clinical parameters (i.e., presence of a pulse/responsiveness/BP determination)- after *each* and *every* intervention you make- *you are likely to be told that your patient has become "pulseless and unresponsive"* (i.e., that the *electrical* rhythm on the monitor is really a PEA rhythm . . .).
>
> **Bottom Line**- when taking an ACLS Course (as in any *real-life* code stuation)- *ALWAYS* remember to check the above parameters after *every* intervention- as well as *whenever* there is a *change* in the rhythm on the monitor!

The patient is unresponsive. Ventilation and oxygenation appear to be adequate. A strong (albeit somewhat *irregular*) pulse is present. The rhythm seen in Figure 4D-3 has *not* changed. BP is stable at 110/80 mm Hg. *What now?*

Clinical Assessment and Plan:

The rhythm is still sinus with PVCs. Despite the fact that the patient remains unresponsive- and despite the presence of PVCs- the patient is now *hemodynamically stable.*

9) Administer ***Lidocaine*** :

- Give an *initial* **IV bolus** (of ≈50-**75 mg**).
- After giving the bolus, initiate a *continuous* **IV infusion** (to *maintain* antiarrhythmic effect). Begin at a rate of **2 mg/minute**. By the *Rule of 250 ml* :

> ▪ Mix **1g** of *Lidocaine* in **250 ml** of D5W- and *begin* the infusion @ **30 drops/minute** (=2 mg/minute).

Administration of ***Lidocaine*** at this point in the code is especially important as a *prophylactic* measure (i.e., in the hope of *preventing* V Fib recurrence- as this patient had been in V Fib at the onset of the code).

Regarding the *dosing* of Lidocaine- AHA Recommendations advise giving **1.0-1.5 mg/kg** for the *initial* IV bolus when the drug is used to treat patients who are *not* in cardiac arrest. Since we are told that the patient in this Case Scenario is of "modest body build"- an appropriate amount of Lidocaine to administer for the initial IV bolus would be *between* 50-75 mg (and probably closer to the higher figure).

The patient is loaded with a 75 mg IV bolus of ***Lidocaine***- and started on *continuous* IV infusion of this drug (at a rate of 2 mg/minute). Shortly thereafter, the rhythm below is seen on the monitor (Figure 4D-4).

How would you interpret this rhythm? *What would you do now?*

Lead II

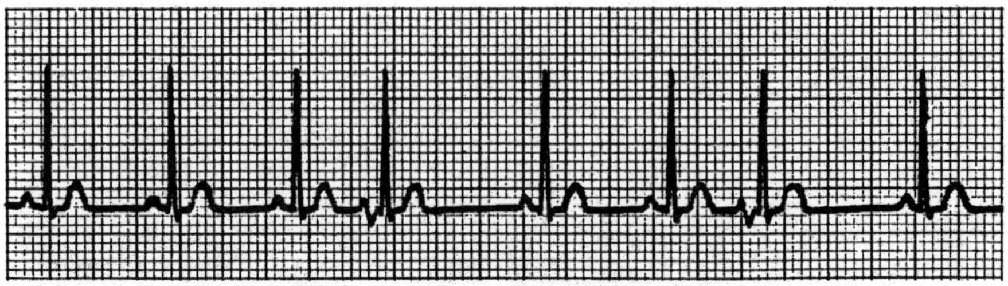

Figure 4D-4: Rhythm seen on the monitor shortly after beginning Lidocaine. *How would you interpret this rhythm?*

Analysis of Figure 4D-4 and Plan:

The *electrical* rhythm on the monitor is still sinus- but now there are ***PACs***.

10) Check the patient for:

- responsiveness
- presence of a pulse
- blood pressure determination.

Since the rhythm on the monitor has again changed (i.e., from that which was seen in Figure 4D-3)- *clinical parameters should probably again be checked* (Action #10 above).

The patient remains unresponsive. The pulse is strong (albeit slightly irregular). BP = 110/80. *What now?*

Plan:

11) *Take a deep breath!* (It appears that the patient's condition is stabilizing).

12) Verify- that *all* is in order:

- that after giving the IV bolus of ***Lidocaine***- continuous IV infusion of this drug has been started (at an appropriate rate of ≈2 mg/minute).
- that *no other* IV infusions are still running (such as the Dopamine that had been started earlier).
- that the patient is being properly ventilated- and that the ET tube is positioned correctly (i.e., that patient color is good, and that bilateral/symmetric breath sounds are present).
- that appropriate laboratory tests (i.e, ABGs, electrolytes, chest X-ray, 12-lead ECG, etc.) have all been ordered.

> **Note-** We again emphasize that the *primary* purpose of continuing IV infusion of ***Lidocaine*** is *prophylaxis* (i.e., to prevent *recurrence* of V Fib)- and *not* simply as treatment of the isolated PVCs that were seen in Figure 4D-3.

The patient begins to wake up! He is now making efforts to breathe on his own. A strong pulse is present and associated with a BP = 120/80 mm Hg. Telemetry monitoring reveals the rhythm below (Figure 4D-5). *What should you do at this point?*

Lead II

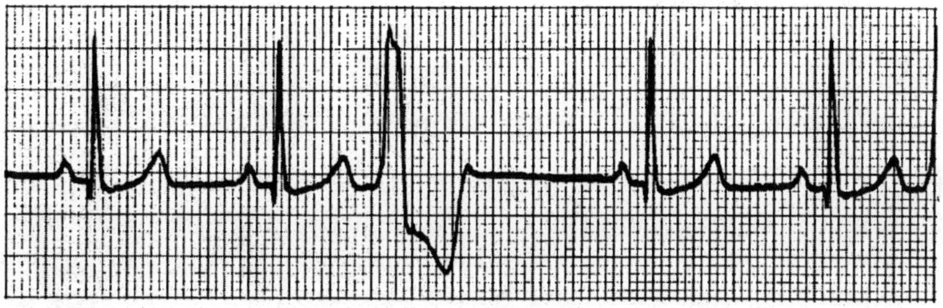

Figure 4D-5: Rhythm now seen on the monitor.

Analysis of Figure 4D-5 and Plan:

The rhythm is sinus with PVCs. This is similar to the rhythm that was seen earlier in Figure 4D-3 on page 328.

13) *Continue present therapy* (i.e., as specified above).

Despite the persistence of PVCs, one need *not* alter therapy. Specifically- one need *not* necessarily administer more Lidocaine. **Abolishment of each and every PVC is clearly *not* essential for Lidocaine to exert its protective effect against V Fib recurrence.** In general, if adequate IV loading with Lidocaine has been accomplished- *and* IV infusion is running at an appropriate rate- then the patient will *usually* be protected against the development of malignant ventricular arrhythmias (even though isolated PVCs may persist).

On the other hand- if *exceedingly frequent* PVCs (and runs of VT) persist *despite* appropriate Lidocaine loading and IV infusion- then *additional measures* may be needed:

- *More* Lidocaine may be given- ***and/or*** -
- *Other* drugs may be tried (i.e., *Procainamide- Bretylium- Magnesium-* and/or possibly an *IV ß-Blocker*).

The rhythm on the monitor suddenly changes (Figure 4D-6). The patient again loses consciousness- and *no pulse* is palpable. Monitor leads are correctly attached (and have *not* fallen off). *What has happened?*

Lead II

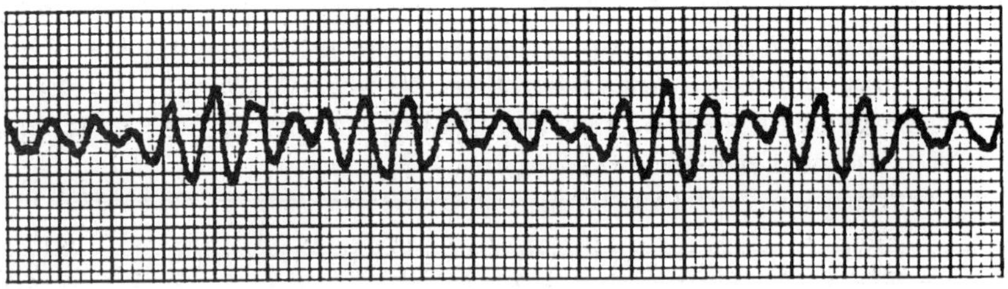

Figure 4D-6: The rhythm has suddenly changed. *What has happened?*

Analysis of Figure 4D-6 and Plan:

Despite appropriate "prophylactic" treatment with Lidocaine- the patient has gone back into ***V Fib***.

14) **Defibrillate** the patient (with **200**-360 **joules**).

- The chance for converting a patient *out of* V Fib is *inversely proportional* to the amount of time from the onset of this rhythm until defibrillation. Since *YOU* are right *on the scene* (i.e., able to defibrillate this patient *immediately* !)- the chance for successful conversion to a normal rhythm should be quite good.

> **Note**- The patient in this Case Scenario has *already* been defibrillated (i.e., with 200 joules at the *onset* of the code). One might therefore select an energy level of *between* 200-360 joules for this next countershock attempt. *Our preference* is generally to drop back to the lower value (i.e., **200 joules**)- and then to increase this amount (i.e., to 360 joules) if defibrillation at the lower level is not successful. *(See pages 172-173).*

Defibrillation (with 200 joules) of the rhythm in Figure 4D-6 results in another change on the monitor (Figure 4D-7).

What has happened? *What to do now?*

Lead II

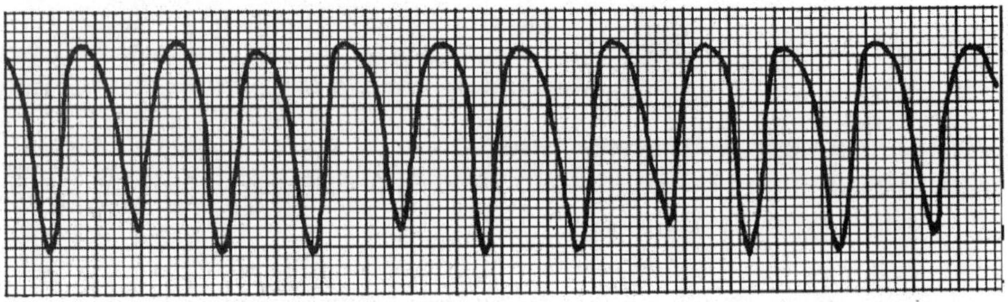

Figure 4D-7: Rhythm seen on the monitor after defibrillation of the rhythm in Figure 4D-6.

Analysis of Figure 4D-7 and Plan:

The monitor now reveals a fairly regular and definitely ***W**ide-**C**omplex* **T**achycardia (***WCT***)- *without* any sign of atrial activity. One *must* assume that the rhythm is ***VT*** (until *proven* otherwise)- *and proceed with evaluation and treatment accordingly.*

15) Check the patient for:

- responsiveness
- presence of a pulse
- blood pressure determination.

> **Note-** Even though the rhythm in Figure 4D-7 is almost certainly VT- assessment of the patient's *hemodynamic status* is still the *first* step in the mangement protocol. Recommendations for treatment of ***sustained VT*** are dramatically different depending on whether a pulse is present- and on whether the patient is hemodynamically stable.

The patient is completely unresponsive in association with the rhythm shown in Figure 4D-7. There is *no pulse* !!!

What now?

Clinical Assessment and Plan:

The rhythm is VT. The absence of a pulse in association with this rhythm defines the condition as ***pulseless VT*** .

16) **Defibrillate** the patient (with **200-360 joules**).

AHA Guidelines strongly recommend that ***pulseless VT*** be treated the *same* as V Fib- with *immediate* and *unsynchronized* countershock.

Repeat defibrillation (with 300 joules) of the rhythm in Figure 4D-7 results in the tracing below (Figure 4D-8). *What next?*

Lead II

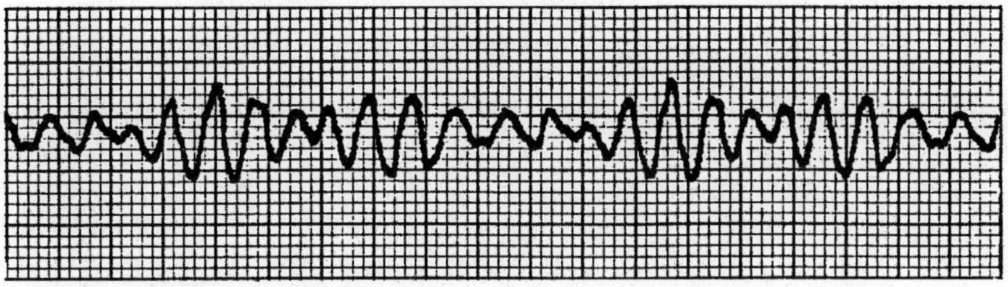

Figure 4D-8: Rhythm seen after defibrillation of pulseless VT.

Analysis of Figure 4D-8 and Plan:

The patient is once again in V Fib.

17) *Verify* that the patient is pulseless and unresponsive (i.e., that the patient is *truly* in V Fib).

18) ***Defibrillate*** the patient (with **360 joules**).

AHA Guidelines now advise that ***pulse checks*** are *no longer* necessary between defibrillation attempts *within* a particular series of "stacked" counter-shocks- IF - *"a properly connected monitor clearly displays persistent VT/V Fib"* (AHA Text- Pg 1-50). In the case presented here, however- taking a moment to verify pulselessness *is* reasonable- since the rhythm on the monitor *has* changed (i.e., from the pulseless VT of Figure 4D-7- to the V Fib shown on Figure 4D-8.

Defibrillation (with 360 joules) of the rhythm shown in Figure 4D-8 results in the tracing below (Figure 4D-9).

What has happened. *What would you do first?*

Lead II

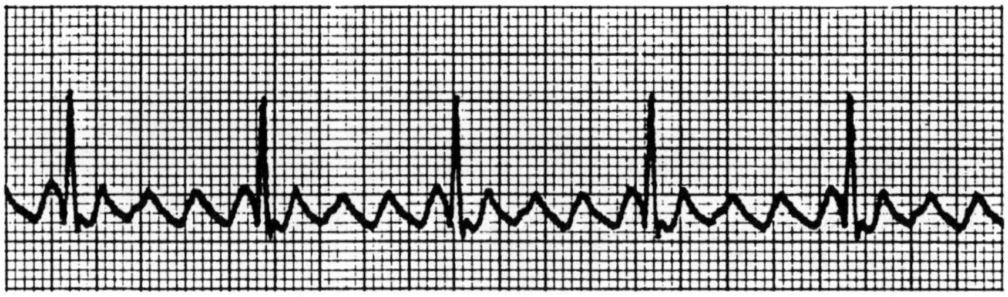

Figure 4D-9: Rhythm seen after defibrillation of V Fib. *What to do first?*

Analysis of Figure 4D-9 and Plan:

The rhythm is now ***atrial flutter (A Flutter)***- seen here with 4:1 AV conduction.

19) Check the patient for:

- presence of a pulse
- responsiveness
- blood pressure determination
- adequacy of ventilation/oxygenation.

Electrocardiographically- ***A Flutter*** is recognized by the appearance of rapid and regular atrial activity that occurs in a *sawtooth* pattern at a rate of approximately 300/minute (usual range ≈250-350/minute in adults). Because there are 4 flutter waves for every QRS in this example- the rhythm is described as *A Flutter* with ***4:1 AV conduction***.

Clinically- because the rhythm has once again changed (i.e., from the V Fib that was present in Figure 4D-8 to the rhythm in Figure 4D-9)- *patient parameters should once again be assessed* (as suggested in Action #19 above).

The patient remains unresponsive. However, there is now a strong pulse- and BP = 140/90 mm Hg. *How would you assess the patient's clinical status?*

Clinical Assessment and Plan:

20) *Take a deep breath* (since you have once again restored the patient to a hemodynamically stable rhythm)!

21) Verify- that *all* is in order:

- that ***Lidocaine*** is infusing (@ ≈2 mg/minute).
- that *no other* IV infusions are still running.
- that the patient is being adequately ventilated and oxygenated.
- that appropriate laboratory tests (i.e, ABGs, electrolytes, chest X-ray, 12-lead ECG, etc.) have all been ordered.

> **Note-** The actions/interventions suggested above comprise many of the measures routinely performed during the period of ***Post-Resuscitation Care*** (defined as the period *between* return of spontaneous circulation- and transfer to the intensive care unit). Additional concerns for consideration during this period are discussed on pages 44-45 in Section 1B.

The patient begins to open his eyes. There is now a strong pulse. BP = 140/90. Nevertheless, the rhythm shown in Figure 4D-9 persists. ***Lidocaine*** is infusing (@ 2 mg/minute).

What would you do at this point?

Plan:

22) Transfer the patient to your critical care facility.

> ▬ *YOU have SAVED the patient* !!!!!

Despite the fact that sinus rhythm has *not* been restored, the patient *IS* hemodynamically stable- and can (should) be transferred to the ICU at this point in the code. Additional treatment measures (as discussed on pages 66-72 in Section 1C) might then be implemented in an attempt to convert A Flutter (and restore sinus rhythm). However, the point to emphasize is that such measures need *not* be implemented at this time on an emergency basis !

Discussion :

This case illustrates the steps in the initial approach to resuscitation of the patient in Bradycardia (*See Figure 1D-4 on page 105*)- as well as for the patient with A Fib/Flutter. Several points are deserving of special mention:

- The *KEYs* to management of ***Bradycardia*** are to determine the *hemodynamic stability* of the patient (or the lack thereof)- and *to treat the patient accordingly.*
  - Bradycardia (even if marked)- need *not* necessarily be treated with Atropine if the patient is hemodynamically stable.
  - TCP is appropriate as the *first* intervention (*simultaneously* with- *or even before* Atropine)- *IF* the bradycardia is severe (and/or the clinical condition unstable).
  - Use of a ***pressor agent*** (i.e., *Dopamine, Epinephrine*) is generally reserved as a *stopgap* measure (i.e., as *temporizing* therapy until TCP becomes available)- to be considered for the patient who is markedly symptomatic but has not responded to Atropine.

- The need for treatment of other arrhythmias is also dependent on the patient's clinical status:
  - Rhythms such as sinus with PACs and A Flutter need *not* be treated emergently- *IF* the pt is hemodynamically stable.
  - Emergency cardioversion *is* indicated as treatment of rapid A Fib- *IF* the patient is symptomatic and/or hypotensive as a *direct* result of the rapid rate.
  - Pulseless VT should be treated as V Fib (i.e., with immediate *unsynchronized* countershock.

CASE STUDY E

You are working on an ambulance unit and are called to the scene of a cardiac arrest. Onlookers indicate that they directly observed the victim collapse "*about* 5-10 minutes" earlier. Help was summoned- and *multiple* shocks have already been delivered by an ***A**utomatic **E**xternal **D**efibrillator* (**AED**) that was brought to the scene. *Nothing else has yet been done.*

- The victim is an elderly woman who looks to weigh about **60 kg**.
- As one rescuer performs the *Primary Survey*- another applies quick look paddles- which reveal the rhythm shown in Figure 4E-1.

How would you interpret this rhythm? *What should you do first?*

Lead II

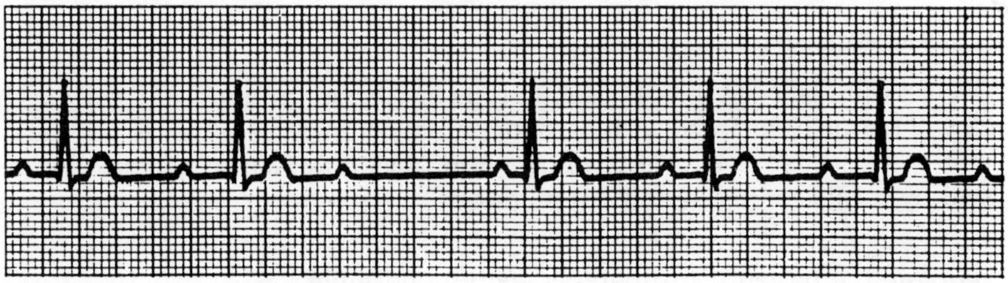

Figure 4E-1: Initial rhythm of the patient in Case Study E as seen on quick look paddles. What is the rhythm? *What should you do?*

Analysis of Figure 4E-1 and Plan:

The *electrical* rhythm on the monitor is **2° AV block- *Mobitz type I*** (i.e., ***Wenckebach***)- recognized by the presence of regular atrial activity and *progressive* lengthening of the PR interval until a beat is dropped. In this case, the P wave seen after the second QRS complex is not conducted. Following the pause the cycle resumes, with the next beat (i.e., the third QRS complex in this tracing) being conducted with a shorter PR interval- that then progressively lengthens for the last two beats on the tracing. The QRS complex is narrow (as it usually is with this conduction disturbance).

1) Check the patient for:

- responsiveness
- adequacy of ventilation/oxygenation
- presence of a pulse
- blood pressure determination.

Although the patient in this case presumably was just in V Fib (suggested by multiple shock delivery from the AED)- an *organized* rhythm has now been restored (Figure 4E-1). Clinically however, the presence of this rhythm would mean little- *unless* it was associated with a pulse. Therefore, among the *first* actions to accomplish on arrival at the scene should be assessment of the *clinical patient parameters* that are listed above.

Of special concern in this case is the amount of time that may have elapsed between collapse of the victim and the arrival of help. Witness reports are unfortunately an *unreliable* indicator of the true duration of this interval. It is also unclear as to whether the victim received layperson CPR. A final concern is that *multiple* shocks were apparently needed to convert this patient out of V Fib.

The patient is unresponsive. There is *no spontaneous respiration.* A weak carotid pulse is present in association with the rhythm shown in Figure 4E-1. The patient's BP is *only* 60 palpable.

How would you interpret the clinical situation?

Clinical Assessment and Plan:

The rhythm is 2° AV block- Mobitz type I. Although much of the time this form of AV block will not be associated with hemodynamic compromise- this is *not* the case here. The patient in this Case Scenario is *apneic* and obviously *hemodynamically unstable* (as evidenced by a BP reading of only 60 palpable).

2) *Ventilate* the patient. Intubate as soon as possible.

3) Establish IV access.

4) Attach monitoring leads.

5) *Consider* the need to perform external chest compression.

- Perfusion may or may not be adequate with a BP of only 60 palpable. Clinical clues that might suggest inadequate perfusion (and the need to perform external chest compression) include the presence of cool and blue or mottled extremities.

6a) Give ***Atropine*** :

- Administer **0.5- 1.0 mg** IV for the *initial* dose.
- May repeat Atropine (0.5- 1.0 mg IV) in 3-5 minutes- *if/as needed* (up to a *total* dose of 0.04 mg/kg- or ≈3 mg for an *average-sized* adult).

- and/or -

6b) Institute ***pacing*** (*if/when* available):

- Use of ***TransCutanous Pacing (TCP)*** is appropriate at this point in the code- and may be applied either *simultaneously* with (or *even before!*) giving Atropine because the patient is so unstable (AHA Text- Pg 1-31).

> **Note**- As mentioned above, Mobitz I 2° AV block is often a well tolerated conduction disturbance that requires little or no treatment. Unfortunately, this is *not* the case here- since the patient in this Case Scenario is markedly hypotensive. Thus, treatment is clearly indicated.

The patient is intubated and IV access is established. One dose of ***Atropine*** (0.5 mg) is given- but *without* effect (i.e., the rhythm shown in Figure 4E-1 persists). Pacemaker therapy is "not yet available". BP is still only 60 palpable. *What next?*

Plan:

7) *Consider* additional ***Atropine*** (while awaiting TCP).

- A total dose of *up to* **0.04 mg/kg** of Atropine may be given. This comes out to a dose of up to ≈**2.5 mg** in this relatively light **60 kg** woman (i.e., 0.04 X 60 = 2.4 mg).

8) Consider use of a ***pressor agent*** (*See boxed KEY on top of next page*):

- IV infusion of ***Dopamine*** (beginning at a rate of ≈5 µg/kg/minute- and titrating upward as needed)-

- and/or -

- IV infusion of ***Epinephrine*** (at ≈1-2 µg/minute).

9) Be sure you have *optimized* ventilation:

- Inadequate oxygenation may be the *cause* of (or at least a contributing factor to) the bradycardia.

10) Consider causes *other than* the rhythm disturbance for the patient's hypotension:

- Could the hypotension be due to a *volume* problem? to *decreased* vascular resistance? and/or to a *"pump"* problem (i.e., Acute MI with cardiogenic shock)?

In view of the fact that the overall heart rate for the rhythm in Figure 4E-1 is not greatly reduced- one or more of the other components in the *Cardiovascular Triad* is likely to be operative (*See page 230 in Section 3A- Clinical Issue #15*). Consideration might therefore be given to *empiric* administration of a ***fluid challenge*** (of **150-500 ml** of normal saline) if hypotension persists despite administration of Atropine and/or application of TCP. Fluid administration may be tried *instead of* (and/or in conjunction with) use of a pressor agent- depending on particulars of a given clinical situation.

> ***KEY***- Administration of a ***pressor agent*** (i.e., *Dopamine, Epinephrine*) is generally reserved as a *stopgap* measure (i.e., as *temporizing* therapy)- to *only* be used *until* TCP becomes available. Fluid infusion is more appropriate treatment than use of a pressor agent if the patient is hypovolemic.

A total of 2 mg of Atropine is given- but *without* effect. TCP is still "unavailable". In the meantime (i.e., while *awaiting* TCP)- an empiric fluid challenge is given (with rapid administration of 300 ml of normal saline). IV infusion of ***Dopamine*** is also begun. Shortly after starting the Dopamine, the rhythm below is seen (Figure 4E-2). *What has happened?*

Lead II

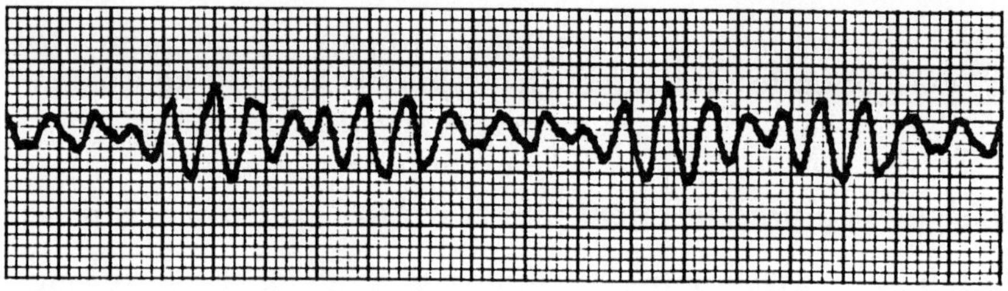

Figure 4E-2: Rhythm seen on the monitor shortly after beginning IV infusion of Dopamine. *What has happened?*

Analysis of Figure 4E-2 and Plan:

Infusion of Dopamine has precipitated development of V Fib.

11) *Verify* that the patient is pulseless and unresponsive.

12) ***Defibrillate*** the patient (with **200-360 joules**).

An ***AED*** was used on the scene at the *onset* of this code- and the patient was defibrillated multiple times (*See Figure 1A-4 on page 29*). AHA Guidelines advise that once ACLS providers arrive- they should take over care in a *coordinated* manner from AED operators who initiated the resuscitation effort. Shocks *already* delivered by AED operators count as part of the ACLS protocol (AHA Text- Pg 4-14). Selection of an energy level *between* 200-360 joules would therefore be reasonable in this case- as this defibrillation attempt may be initiating another series of "stacked" countershocks.

Defibrillation (with 200 joules) of the rhythm shown in Figure 4E-2 fails to change the rhythm. *What now?*

Plan:

13) ***Defibrillate*** the patient again (with 300-**360 joules**).

> **Note**- There is *no need* to perform a pulse check between defibrillation attempts in this case- because a "properly connected monitor clearly displays *persistent* VT/V Fib" (AHA Text- Pg 1-50). Since defibrillation at a lower energy level (i.e., 200 joules) was *not* successful- an *increase* in energy (i.e., to 300-360 joules) should be tried for this next attempt.

Defibrillation (with 360 joules) results in another change on the monitor to the rhythm shown below (Figure 4E-3). As already noted, the patient has been intubated. Ventilation and oxygenation appear to be adequate.

What has happened? What should you do now?

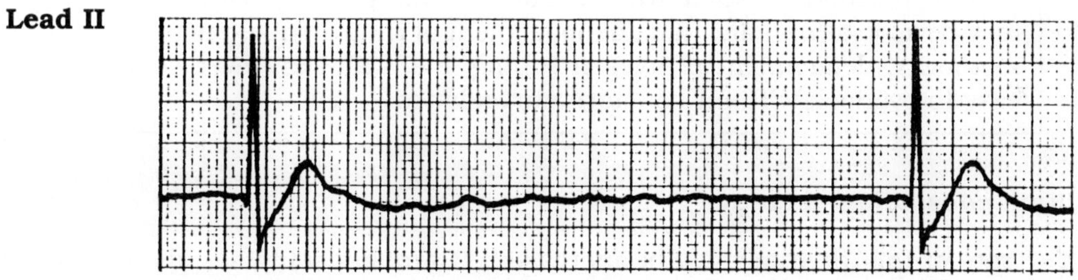

Figure 4E-3: Rhythm seen on the monitor after repeat defibrillation. *What has happened?*

Analysis of Figure 4E-3 and Plan:

There is *profound* bradycardia. The QRS complex appears to be wide and suggests a ventricular escape focus (at the exceedingly *slow* rate of *less* than 20 beats/minute). Atrial activity is absent. The rhythm is most likely to be a ***slow IVR*** (*IdioVentricular Rhythm*).

14) Check the patient for:

- responsiveness
- presence of a pulse
- blood pressure determination.

The patient is still unresponsive. A weak carotid pulse *is* palpable in association with the rhythm shown in Figure 4E-3. BP is now only 40 palpable.

How do you assess the situation? *What would you do?*

Clinical Assessment and Plan:

The rhythm is slow IVR. There is obviously marked hemodynamic compromise. The overall clinical situation *overlaps* a number of the AHA algorithms. Technically the patient has ***bradycardia***. Practically speaking, however- patients with IVR at this slow a rate are generally "quite close to the state of ***PEA***- or even ***asystole***" (AHA Text- Pg 1-31). *Alternatively*- one might interpret the problem primarily as ***hypotension*** (since there is an ECG rhythm and a pulse is present). Regardless of the classification chosen, priorities for management will be the same. They are- continuation of *CPR*- implementation of *pacing*- and administration of *Epinephrine.*

15) Continue CPR:

- With a BP of 40 palpable- perfusion for the rhythm shown in Figure 4E-3 will be clearly inadequate. Performance of CPR is therefore essential until the patient's hemodynamic condition can be improved.

> **Note-** Endotracheal tube placement and the adequacy of ventilation/oxygenation should be *continually* monitored and constantly rechecked- especially when confronted with a patient who fails to respond to standard treatment. Subtle complications may develop at *any* time (i.e., dislodgement of the ET tube, pneumothorax, detachment of oxygen tubing, etc.)- and are ever so easy to overlook without constant surveillance.

16) Institute ***pacemaker* therapy**:

- The rate of this rhythm *must* be increased. Cardiac pacing stands a reasonable chance of being effective because an organized (albeit widened) QRS complex is present in Figure 4E-3, and the patient does have a pulse. Cardiac pacing would be much less likely to work if the patient was pulseless and the rhythm asystole.

17) Give ***Epinephrine* :**

- Epinephrine is the pharmacologic agent of choice for treatment of the rhythm and clinical situation described in Figure 4E-3. In addition to the potent chronotropic and inotropic (beta-adrenergic) effects of this drug- its vasoconstrictor (alpha-adrenergic) effect increases aortic diastolic pressure, and thereby enhances coronary perfusion.

- Use of an IV infusion of Epinephrine may be preferable here to bolus therapy since the patient *does* have a pulse- as well as an *organized* rhythm. The potential problem with use of bolus therapy is that if too much of the drug is given- *"you can't take the bolus back"*. As a result- bolus therapy is probably best reserved for treatment of cardiac arrest rhythms (i.e., V Fib, asystole, PEA- *See page 125 in Section 2B*).

- Begin with ***SDE*** dosing (i.e., @ **1-2 µg/minute**)- and *rapidly* titrate the dose upward as needed until the desired clinical response is achieved.

Teaching Points : Regarding Atropine/Epinephrine/Dopamine

- **Why was Atropine *not* included among the recommended actions for the rhythm shown in Figure 4E-3?**
- **Why might Epinephrine be *preferble* to either Dopamine or Isoproterenol for treatment of this rhythm?**
- **How much Epinephrine should be given?**

- ***Atropine*** was not included among the recommended treatment actions because the *usual* "full atropinization dose" (i.e., ≈2 mg) has already been administered. Although *up to* 0.04 mg/kg of this drug *can* be given (which comes out to ≈2.5 mg for this 60 kg patient)- use of this maximal dose is usually best reserved for treatment of patients in bradyasystolic *arrest* (AHA Text- Pg 7-5). Practically speaking, it is *unlikely* that an additional dose of Atropine will produce the desired clinical response in this patient if 2 mg (that have already been given) have failed to do so.
- In general, AHA Guidelines favor beginning with ***Dopamine*** for treatment of bradycardia that is Atropine-resistant and hemodynamically significant. AHA Guidelines allow that when clinical symptoms are *more severe* (as they are in this case)- "clinicians can go *directly* to IV infusion of ***Epinephrine*** " (AHA Text- Pg 1-31).

  As already noted, AHA Recommendations for treatment of bradycardia with a pulse are to use ***IV infusion*** of Epinephrine (rather than bolus therapy)- and to begin at a *low* rate (i.e., at ≈ **1-2 µg/minute**). However, rapid titration upward to much higher doses may be needed if the patient fails to respond .
- Because of adverse hemodynamic effects (excessive tachycardia, peripheral vasodilatation)- use of ***Isoproterenol*** has been strongly *discouraged* in recent years. This drug is now only recommended for treatment of normotensive patients in need of pure chronotropic support or for the transplant patient with a denervated heart (AHA Text- Pg 8-6).

IV infusion of ***Epinephrine*** is begun for the rhythm shown in Figure 4E-3. Soon thereafter the rhythm below is noted on the monitor (Figure 4E-4). *What now?*

Lead II

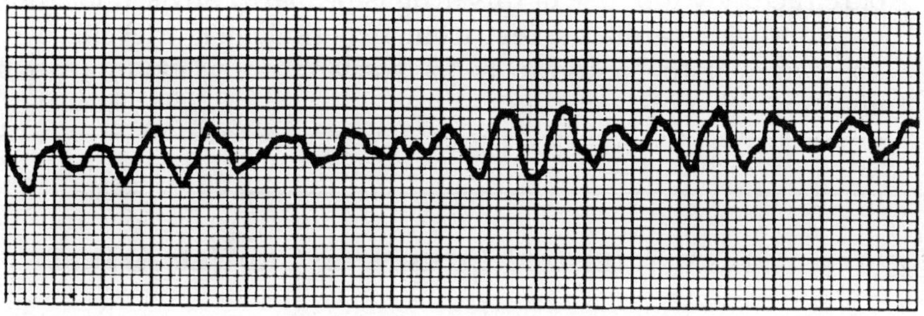

Figure 4E-4: Rhythm seen on the monitor soon after beginning IV infusion of Epinephrine.

Analysis of Figure 4E-4 and Plan:

The patient has once again gone back into V Fib.

18) *Verify* that the patient is pulseless and unresponsive.

19) ***Defibrillate*** the patient (with **200-360 joules**).

Defibrillation (with 360 joules) of the rhythm shown in Figure 4E-4 is ineffective. V Fib persists. *What else may be going on with the patient?*

What actions might you consider at this point in the code?

Clinical Assessment and Plan:

The patient in this Case Scenario has *recurrent* V Fib. She is *not* responding to standard therapy.

20) Consider *other* potential causes of *persistent/recurrent* V Fib (*See Teaching Points below*).

21) Consider a trial of ***antifibrillatory* therapy**:

- Use ***Lidocaine*** first. May give in a *single* IV bolus (of **1.5 mg/kg**) for cardiac arrest. Resume CPR for 30-60 seconds (after giving Lidocaine)- *and then shock again.*

22) *If Lidocaine is ineffective*- Consider *other* measures:

- ***Bretylium***- initially in a dose of 5 mg/kg (*or* a single **500 mg IV** bolus = **1 amp**)- with repeat dosing if needed. A second IV bolus (of 10 mg/kg- or ≈1-2 amps) may be given in 5 minutes if V Fib persists (up to a total dose of 30-35 mg/kg).
- ***Magnesium***- initially in a dose of **1-2 g IV**- which may be repeated if needed.

> **Note**- Although ***Sodium Bicarbonate*** should also be *considered* among potential therapeutic options available for treatment of refractory V Fib- use of this drug is primarily advised for those patients with cardiac arrest from hyperkalemia, tricyclic overdose, and/or those known to have severe *preexisting* metabolic acidosis.

Teaching Points : Other *Potential Causes* of Cardiac Arrest

The *"other"* causes of cardiac arrest that are most important to consider are those that are ***potentially reversible*** (or at least *potentially* treatable). Recall of these causes is facilitated by thinking of the **3** *basic* ***cause categories***- and then using the letters "**H**" and "**T**" to *prompt* recollection of specific entities:

1) *Potentially Reversible* RESPIRATORY *Causes:*

- **H**ypoxia (from *whatever* cause)- *recheck adequacy of ventilation and oxygenation!*
- **T**ension pneumothorax

2) *Potentially Reversible* CIRCULATORY *Causes:*

- **H**ypovolemia (from *whatever* cause)
- Cardiac **T**amponade
- Acute MI (i.e., **H**eart attack)

3) *Potentially Reversible* METABOLIC/MISC. *Causes:*

- Severe acidosis (i.e., $\mathbf{H}^+$ excess)
- Electrolyte disturbance (i.e., **H**yper- K^+/**H**ypo- K^+/Mg^{++})
- **H**ypothermia
- Drug overdose (i.e., **T**oxic)

> ***Remember***- "The *only* possibility of successfully resuscitating a person *may* (sometimes) lie in *searching* for- *finding*- and *treating* a *reversible* cause of the cardiac arrest" (AHA Text- Pg 1-10).

Lidocaine, ***Bretylium***, and ***Magnesium*** have *all* been given in appropriate doses. The patient has received multiple additional shocks. Despite this, she remains pulseless and unresponsive. *No potentially correctable cause of the arrest has been found.* The rhythm below is now seen on the monitor (Figure 4E-5). *What is the rhythm? What should you do?*

Lead II

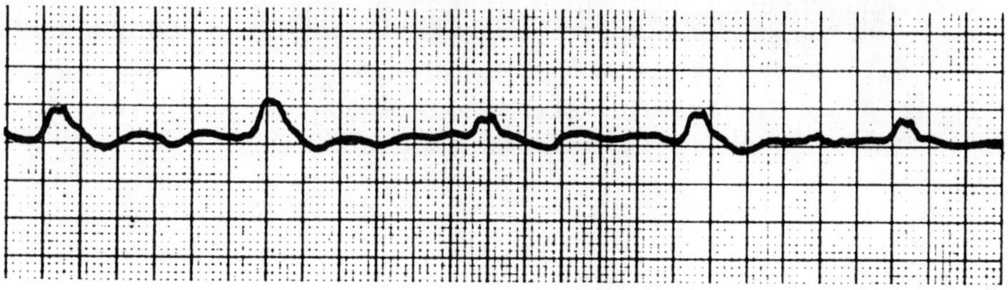

Figure 4E-5: Rhythm seen on the monitor after Lidocaine, Bretylium, Magnesium, and multiple shocks. *What is the rhythm?*

Analysis of Figure 4E-5 and Plan:

QRS complexes are bizarre in shape and markedly widened. Atrial activity is absent. This is an ***agonal rhythm***.

23) Therapeutic options at this point in the code are unfortunately limited:

- *Verify* again that the patient is truly pulseless.
- *Verify* again that the ET tube has been properly placed- and that ventilation and oxygenation are adequate.
- Continue external chest compression (since by definition *agonal* rhythm is a *nonperfusing* rhythm).

- Give *more* Epinephrine. Consider the use of HDE (if this is not being done).
- Give *more* Atropine (*up to* a total dose of 0.04 mg/kg).
- Try pacing (if/*as soon as* it becomes available).
- Continue to search for a *potentially correctible* underlying cause.

Note- Clinical implications and treatment considerations are virtually the same for ***agonal* rhythm** as they are for ***asystole***. Prognosis is likely to be grim almost *regardless* of what interventions are tried.

Epinephrine in increasing doses (i.e., ***HDE***) is ineffective. A total dose of 2.5 mg of ***Atropine*** has been given. Application of the ***external pacer*** (which finally arrives)- is unable to produce ventricular capture. *No potentially correctable cause of V Fib is found.* The rhythm below is now seen on the monitor (Figure 4E-6). *How would you assess the situation?*

What would you do now?

Lead II

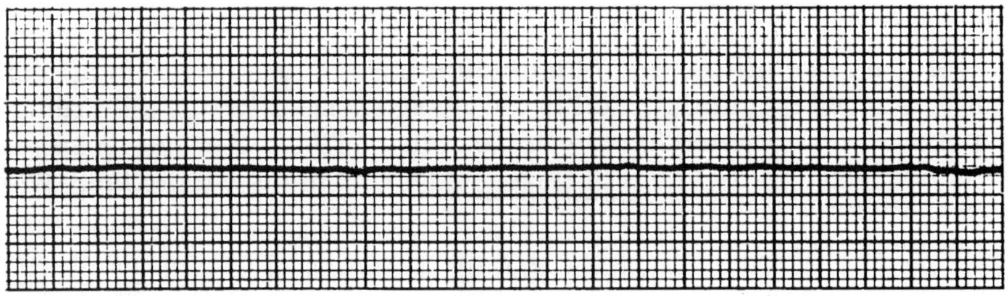

Figure 4E-6: Rhythm seen on the monitor despite Epinephrine, Atropine, and pacing. *How would you assess the situation?*

Analysis of Figure 4E-6 and Plan:

The rhythm is now *flat line* (= ***asystole***).

24) *Verify* that the rhythm is *truly* a ***FLAT line*** recording. That is- *rule out* the possibility that fine V Fib might be *masquerading* as asystole:

- Make sure the gain of the monitor has not been mistakenly turned down.
- Make sure all lead attachments are properly connected.
- Check the rhythm in *other* leads.

25) Continue with the ***Recommended Actions*** suggested above . . . .

- Add *more* Epinephrine . . . .

- Remain open to input from other members of the resuscitation team . . . .

Note- When *all* else fails (i.e., for what would otherwise be lethal bradyasystolic arrest)- you may want to consider administration of ***Aminophylline.*** Preliminary studies suggest tht use of this drug may be effective in the treatment of some cases of otherwise refractory bradyasystolic arrest (*See pages 196-197 in Section 2E*). The dose suggested for this indication is administration of **250 mg IV** over a 1-2 minute period- which may then be repeated. We emphasize that Aminophylline is *not* yet included in AHA Guidelines- and that further studies are needed to clarify the role of this drug.

Time passes. *Nothing works.* The rhythm remains *flat line* in all leads *despite* all interventions.

Resuscitative efforts are terminated. *The patient has died.*

- *What should you do at this point?* -

Plan:

26) Acknowledge the efforts of those on *your* resuscitative team.

27) *Talk* to the family.

- It is imperative to inform the family of what happened at the *earliest* possible moment. Offer appropriately explicit details of events leading up to- *and including-* the cardiac arrest. Although this information may not be needed or wanted by some family members- it is immensely important to others in helping to understand and *accept* the death of their loved one. Be sure to allow family members an opportunity to express their feelings and/or to ask questions. Remember the *special* importance of having a member of the resuscitation team be the one to inform the family.

28) Notify the attending physician (if this has not already been done).

29) *Document* the events of the code (i.e., in a progress note, on the code sheet, etc.).

30) Don't forget- to reserve a moment to ***rethink* the process** (in a *constructive* manner!)- *in an attempt to see if anything might be done different/better the next time.* If appropriate, consider *sharing* your thoughts with a trusted colleague.

KEY- Although this last step is often an exceedingly difficult one- it is *by far* the best way to learn from the events of the code (and to improve patient care in the management of future resuscitations).

Discussion :

This case highlights a number of important points in the management of cardiac arrest. Foremost among these is the fact that the patient died.

Why did the patient die? Could you have done anything different (better?) in running the code that might have prevented the patient's demise?

- The importance of asking yourself this very difficult question cannot be overstated. Only by regular retrospective review of events that transpired during the code can one hope to optimally benefit and improve on one's future performance. This process of soul-searching review is best carried out as soon as possible after the code- either by oneself, or as a collective constructive effort (with one or more trusted colleagues).
- Practically speaking- it is unlikely that *any* intervention could have saved the patient in this Case Scenario. Fate factors augured poorly from the start (since the arrest occurred *out* of the hospital- and the period of time before help arrived was probably prolonged). It is also unclear as to whether the victim received layperson CPR. If not, this would make for an additional factor that reduces the chance for meaningful long-term survival *(See pages 3-5).*
- The *initial* mechanism of arrest was presumably V Fib (since multiple shocks were delivered on the scene with an AED). Failure to respond to multiple defibrillation attempts during the early minutes of resuscitation is yet another poor prognostic indicator. And although conversion to a *supraventricular* mechanism *did* occur initially (Figure 4E-1 on page 337)- hemodynamic stability for this patient was *never* achieved.
- *All appropriate interventions were tried.* Despite multiple countershocks, *Epinephrine* in high doses, antifibrillatory therapy, *Magnesium, Atropine,* and pacing- *nothing worked.*
- In conclusion- *realistic* chances for *meaningful* long-term survival in this case were probably small from the start. The unfortunate reality is simply that many patients who unexpectedly develop cardiac arrest will die- *regardless of what interventions are tried.* Knowing this clinical reality may help with acceptance of the end result when even the best of our efforts fail.

Appendix: *Value Added Drug Table*

Epinephrine *(See also pages 123-127, 158, 162-163, 207-210, 220)*

Indications	Dose & Routes of Administration	Comments
- V Fib or pulseless VT - Asystole - EMD/PEA - Use of Epinephrine (by IV infusion) may also be considered for treatment of hemodynamically significant bradyarrhythmias that have *not* responded to Atropine.	***Initial* IV Dose**- **1.0 mg** by IV bolus = **SDE** (= 10 ml of a 1:10,000 soln). ***Subsequent* IV Dosing**- Epinephrine should be repeated every **3-5 minutes** in cardiac arrest. After the initial **SDE** (= 1 mg) IV dose- one may either *continue* with 1 mg IV doses- *or* chose *between several **HDE alternatives*** : - Administration of **2-5 mg** IV boluses- *- O R -* - *escalating* **1- 3- 5 mg** IV boluses- *- O R -* - dosing at **0.1 mg/kg** as an IV bolus. **ET Route**- *recommended for use if IV access is unavailable.* Instill 2-2.5 times the IV dose (i.e., **2-2.5 mg** of 1:10,000 soln.) down the ET tube- and follow with several forceful insufflations of the Ambu bag.	The alpha-adrenergic (= vasoconstrictor) effect of Epinephrine is the most important one in cardiac arrest (because this effect increases aortic diastolic pressure). Blood flow to the coronary arteries is favored, and there is preferential shunting of blood from the external to the internal carotid artery. The *"optimal dose"* of Epinephrine remains unknown. AHA Guidelines clearly allow for *flexibility* in Epinephrine dosing by stating that *"use of HDE can neither be recommended nor discouraged"* (AHA Text- Pg 7-4). Use of HDE for pts with refractory V Fib may increase the likelihood of ROSC (return of spontaneous circulation). Unfortunately- because of the longer time until discovery and treatment of many of these pts, there is also a greater chance of permanent neurolgic sequelae. Judgement is therefore needed in deciding whether or not to use **HDE**- and if so, under what circumstances. The effect of an IV bolus of Epinephrine peaks in 2-3 minutes (which is the reason AHA Guidelines now allow for repetition of each bolus as often as every 3 minutes for as long as the pt remains in cardiac arrest).

Epinephrine *(Continued)*

Indications	Dose & Routes of Administration	Comments
	--- **<u>IV Infusion of Epinephrine</u>**- may be administered in both standard and high dose form: - **<u>Standard Dosing (= SDE)</u>**- Mix **1 mg** of a **1:10,000** soln. of Epinephrine in **250 ml** of D5W- and *begin* the infusion @ **15-30 drops/min** (=1-2 μg/min). Titrate the rate of infusion upward as needed. - **<u>High-Dose Epinephrine (= HDE)</u>**- Mix **50 mg** of a **1:1,000** soln. of Epinephrine in **250 ml** of D5W- and *begin* the infusion @ **30-60 drops/min** (=100-200 μg/min). Titrate the rate of infusion upward as needed. --- NOTE- An IV infusion rate of **200 μg/min** will deliver 1,000 μg = **1 mg** of Epinephrine every **5 min** (= 200 X 5 = 1,000 μg)- *which is comparable to an SDE dose of Epinephrine* !	When Epinephrine is used to treat pts who are *not* in cardiac arrest (i.e., for treatment of symptomatic bradycardia with a pulse)- a *lower dose* of drug (i.e., SDE) should be used- and the Epinephrine should be administered by *continuous* **IV infusion** instead of by IV bolus. This is because if adverse effects do occur- "you *can't* take the effect of a bolus back". Use of Epinephrine by continuous IV infusion allows *moment-to-moment* titration of dose. Compared to Dopamine- Epinephrine may be preferable for use as a *pressor* agent in the treatment of bradycardia with more severe hemodynamic impairment.

Lidocaine *(See also pages 128-131, 158, 159-160, 213)*

Indications	Dose & Routes of Administration	Comments
- Drug of choice for *refractory V Fib* and acute treatment of ventricular ectopy (*PVCs, VT*)- when such treatment is indicated. - Appropriate for treatment of *wide-complex* tachycardias of unknown etiology (which statistically are most likely to be VT).	**IV Bolus** (Treatment of PVCs/VT)- Give **1.0-1.5 mg/kg** (= 50-150 mg) as an *initial* bolus. Repeat boluses of ≈50-75 mg may be given every 5-10 minutes up to a total of ≈3 mg/kg (i.e., ≈225 mg). - - - - - - - - - - - - - - - - **IV Infusion**- Mix **1g** in **250 ml** of D5W- and begin drip @ **30 drops/min (= 2 mg/min).** - The usual *range* of IV infusion = 0.5-4.0 mg/min (although most pts are adequately treated at a rate of between 1-2 mg/minute). - - - - - - - - - - - - - - - - **IV Bolus** (Treatment of V Fib)- Give **1.0-1.5 mg/kg** (= 50-150 mg) as an *initial* bolus. May repeat in 3-5 minutes- *although a single* IV dose (of **1.5 mg/kg**) is acceptable in cardiac arrest. NOTE- IV infusion is *not* necessarily needed while the pt remains in V Fib! **ET Tube**- Use 2 to 2.5 times the IV dose (=100-150 mg) to obtain equivalent blood levels as with IV administration.	Remember to start a *prophylactic* IV infusion of Lidocaine immediately after converting a pt out of V Fib (in the hope of preventing recurrence of V Fib). For pts who only received IV boluses during cardiac arrest- rebolus of the drug may be needed prior to starting the IV infusion. In the *spontaneously beating heart,* the half-life of Lidocaine is short (i.e., ≈10 minutes). As a result, an IV infusion of the drug *must* be started *within* 5-10 minutes of giving an IV bolus (or the effect of the bolus will be dissipated). However, because clearance of Lidocaine is markedly impaired during cardiac arrest- one need *not* necessarily begin the IV infusion until after the pt is converted out of V Fib. Not every PVC need be eliminated for Lidocaine to exert a protective effect. Maintenance of a therapeutic serum level of Lidocaine may be all that is needed to protect against development of VT/V Fib- even if "breakthrough" PVCs are still occurring.

Bretylium *(See also pages 132-133, 158)*

Indications	Dose & Routes of Administration	Comments
- Drug of 2nd choice for *refractory V Fib* (after Lidocaine). - 3rd-line agent for acute treatment of PVCs/VT. NOTE- The sympathomimetic effects of Bretylium may on some occasions initially aggravate ventricular arrhythmias- which is why use of the drug is now generally reserved for those pts who are truly symptomatic from their arrhythmia.	**IV Bolus** (*for Refractory V Fib*)- 5 mg/kg initially (*or* a single **500 mg** bolus = **1 amp**). Defibrillate ≈1 min later. If V Fib persists, a **2nd dose** (of 10 mg/kg *or* ≈1-2 amps) may be given 5 min later. This 10 mg/kg dose may be repeated *twice* at 5-30 min intervals (up to a total loading dose of 30-35 mg/kg). - Be sure to circulate the drug with CPR (for ≈1-2 min) after each administration- and then *defibrillate* again. **IV Infusion**- Mix **1g** in **250 ml** of D5W- and begin drip @ **15-30 drops/min (=1-2 mg/min).** **IV Loading Infusion** (*for VT*)- Dilute **500 mg** (≈1 amp) in 50 ml of D5W, and infuse over ≈10 minutes (i.e., giving a dose of ≈5-10 mg/kg). May repeat IV loading of another 5-10 mg/kg (i.e., ≈500 mg) in 10-30 minutes (again infused over ≈10 min).	Bretylium has been used less in recent years for a number of reasons: - The drug has *not* been shown to be superior to Lidocaine for treatment of V Fib. - Lidocaine appears less likely to produce adverse hemodynamic effects during CPR. - Most clinicians are more familiar (and comfortable) with the use of Lidocaine. Although the onset of action of Bretylium is usually within a few minutes when treating V Fib- its onset may sometimes be *delayed* for up to 2-20 minutes (especially when the rhythm is VT!). The duration of action of a Bretylium bolus is 2-6 hrs. Use of a **Bretylium IV infusion** (@ 1-2 mg/min) may help to maintain the effect of the drug- especially for pts with *refractory V Fib* who only responded after Bretylium was added. Hypotension is the most common (and limiting) side effect of IV maintenance infusion with Bretylium.

Procainamide *(See also pages 134-136, 158)*

Indications	Dose & Routes of Administration	Comments
- Drug of 2nd choice (after Lidocaine) for acute treatment of ventricular ectopy (PVCs, VT). - Treatment of A Fib/Flutter (similar action as Quinidine that may help in conversion of A Fib/Flutter to normal sinus rhythm). - *Possibly* for refractory V Fib (although *not* nearly as effective as Lidocaine and Bretylium for this indication). - May be invaluable in the treatment of *wide-complex tachycardia* of uncertain etiology (since this drug may effectively treat *both* VT and PSVT- *as well as* rapid A Fib with WPW).	**IV Loading**- Give in increments of 100 mg *slowly* over a 5 minute period (@ ≈20 mg/min)- *until* one or more of the following *end points* are reached: - the arrhythmia is suppressed - hypotension occurs - the QRS widens by ≥50% - a total loading dose of **17 mg/kg** has been given (which comes out to ≈1,000 mg for the *average-sized* adult). ***Alternative* IV Loading Regimen**- Mix ≈500-1,000 mg of drug in 100 ml of D5W- and infuse this over 30-60 minutes (keeping in mind the *end points* of infusion noted above). - - - - - - - - - - - - **IV Infusion**- Mix **1g** in **250 ml** of D5W- and begin drip @ **30 drops/min (=2 mg/min).** - - - - - - - - - - - - - Use of an **IV infusion** may be considered to *maintain* the drug's effect following IV loading. - Usual *range* of infusion = 1-4 mg/min.	Hypotension is exacerbated with more rapid IV infusion of Procainamide (i.e., @ >30 mg/min). Hypotension is the major limiting factor in IV use of this drug. Procainamide is available in both oral and IV forms- which is a decided advantage for pts in need of long-term maintenance therapy. Even when IV Procainamide does not convert a pt out of sustained VT- it may slow the *rate* of the VT (which may allow the pt to tolerate the arrhythmia better). Procainamide works in the treatment of rapid A Fib with WPW by slowing conduction in the *antegrade* direction down the accessory pathway. Procainamide should *not* be used for treatment of *Torsade de Pointes* (since use of this drug may further prolong the QT interval- and therefore exacerbate the arrhythmia).

Magnesium *(See also pages 136-138, 226)*

Indications	Dose & Routes of Administration	Comments
Torsade de Pointes- for which Magnesium is clearly the medical treatment of choice! **Refractory VT/V Fib**- for which the mechanism of action of the drug is unclear. However, *empiric* use of Magnesium may be helpful in some pts- *even when serum levels are normal* (especially when standard measures have failed). - **Acute MI/PVCs/SVTs** (including PSVT, MAT, and A Fib)- use is controversial, although the drug *may* be helpful. - **Suspected body depletion of Magnesium**- regardless of serum levels, *intracellular* Magnesium deficiency is likely in pts who manifest other electrolyte disturbances (i.e., hyponatremia, hypokalemia, hypocalcemia, and hypophosphatemia). Strong consideration should be given to *empiric* administration of 1-4 g over several hours in such pts.	**For V Fib**- Give **1-2 g IV** of Magnesium Sulfate (= 2-4 ml of a 50% soln.)- by **IV push**. May repeat in 1-2 minutes if no response. **For VT or Torsade de Pointes**- Give **1-2 g IV** of Magnesium Sulfate (= 2-4 ml of a 50% soln.)- over 1-2 minutes. May repeat in a few minutes if no response. Significantly higher doses (of up to 5-10 g) are sometimes needed for treatment of Torsade. **For *Less Urgent* Treatment Situations** (i.e., treatment of **PVCs** and/or **Acute MI**)- consider *more gradual* IV infusion of ≈1-2 g of Magnesium Sulfate over ≥20 minutes. Alternatively, may add the drug to the pt's IV fluids and infuse it over a period of hours (i.e., at a rate of between ≈0.5-1 g/hour for up to 24 hrs). - - Give *lower* doses of Magnesium to pts with renal failure.	Dosing of Magnesium is largely *empiric* ! The exact amount of drug required in a given clinical situation is simply *not* known! Clearly the drug needs to be given *faster* for life threatening arrhythmias (i.e., by IV push for V Fib- or over 1-2 minutes for VT). It may be given by more gradual IV infusion for less urgent clinical situations (such as for treatment of PVCs and/or Acute MI). Comfort can be taken in the fact that with rare exceptions- IV administration of Magnesium (*even in large doses!*) is surprisingly free of adverse effects. Most often nothing more is seen than transient flushing, slight hypotension or transient bradycardia- all of which usually resolve with *slowing* of the rate of IV infusion. Ready availability of **Calcium Chloride** is suggested as a "safeguard" when administering Magnesium- in the rare event that marked hypotension or asystole is produced.

Atropine *(See also pages 138-141, 211)*

Indications	Dose & Routes of Administration	Comments
- Hemodynamically significant bradyarrhythmias (including **"relative bradycardia"**)- for which Atropine remains the pharmacologic intervention of choice (AHA Text- Pg 1-30). - Asystole - PEA	<u>**IV Bolus:**</u> - ***<u>Not in Cardiac Arrest</u>***- Give **0.5-1.0 mg IV**; may repeat every 3-5 minutes- *if/as needed* (up to a total dose of 2-3 mg). - ***<u>In Bradyasystolic Arrest</u>***- Give **1.0 mg IV** at a time; may repeat every 3-5 minutes- *if/as needed* (up to a total dose of **0.04 mg/kg**- or ≈3 mg).	Although 2 mg will be the *full atropinization dose* for many pts- up to **0.04 mg/kg** (i.e, *up to* ≈**3 mg** in an *average-sized* adult) may occasionally be needed to obtain maximal effect. In general, lower doses of Atropine (i.e., **0.5 mg IV**) are preferred for *initial* treatment of pts with bradycardia who are *not* in cardiac arrest- especially if symptoms are less severe. Higher doses (i.e., **1 mg** at a time) may be tried in pts with more severe symptoms- and/or for those who fail to respond to a 0.5 mg dose. Use of a maximal dose of Atropine (i.e., ≈3 mg) is most often *reserved* for treatment of pts with bradyasystolic cardiac arrest. AHA Guidelines allow for more frequent dosing of Atropine (*as often as every 1-3 minutes!*) for pts with *marked* hemodynamic compromise from bradycardia. Use of Atropine is *not* benign! The drug may unmask previously undetected excess sympathetic tone- and thereby precipitate ventricular tachyarrhythmias. On rare occasions, the drug may also produce paradoxical slowing of the ventricular response if given to pts with more advanced AV block. For these reasons- Atropine should *only* be used to treat pts with hemodynamically significiant bradyarrhythmias.
- Atropine is most likely to work when used to treat bradycardia in the early hours of acute *inferior* infarction (when increased parasympathetic tone is most likely to be at least partially responsible for the reduction in heart rate). - Caution is advised when using Atropine in the setting of Acute MI to treat 2° or 3° AV block with QRS widening. Use of cardiac pacing may be preferable in this situation.	<u>**ET Tube**</u>- 1-2 mg at a time (diluted in 10 ml of normal saline or sterile H_2O)- and followed by several forceful insufflations of the Ambu bag.	

Dopamine *(See also pages 141-143, 159, 161, 211-212)*

Indications	Dose & Routes of Administration	Comments
- Hemodynamically significant bradyarrhythmias that have *not* responded to Atropine (when cardiac pacing is unavailable) - Cardiogenic shock NOTE- Dopamine is generally accepted as the intitial pressor agent of choice for treatment of hemodynamically significant bradycardia when symptoms are not too severe. With more profound hypotension, IV infusion of Epinephrine may be preferred.	**IV Infusion**- Mix 1 amp **(200 mg)** in **250 ml** of D5W- and begin drip @ **15-30 drops/min (=** 2-5 µg/kg/minute**)**. Titrate to clinical response. NOTE- moderate to high infusion rates of Dopamine produce an effect that resembles Epinephrine (and may be used to maintain coronary perfusion in the arrested heart). As the infusion rate is increased even further (i.e., to ≈15-20 µg/kg/min), the drug becomes progressively more like Norepinephrine (i.e., a pure vasoconstrictor).	- At ***LOW infusion rates*** **(**i.e., 1-2 µg/kg/min- and perhaps up to 5 µg/kg/min**)**- dilates renal and mesenteric blood vessels (so urine output may increase)- but heart rate and BP will usually *not* be affected (i.e., predominant *dopaminergic* effect). - At ***MODERATE infusion rates*** **(**i.e., 2-10 µg/kg/min**)**- increases cardiac output- usually with only a modest effect on peripheral vascular resistance and BP (i.e., *beta-adrenergic* effect prevails). - At ***HIGH infusion rates*** **(**i.e., >10 µg/kg/min**)**- results in intense peripheral vasoconstriction (as *alpha-adrenergic* effect takes over)- producing a significant increase in peripheral vascular resistance and BP. NOTE- Despite the above general guidelines for dose-dependent effects of Dopamine, there is still some patient-to-patient variability in dosing. Thus, some pts may manifest predominant alpha-adrenergic effects at relatively low infusion rates- whereas in others, beta-adrenergic effects may still predominate at high infusion rates. Individualization of dosing is therefore essential.

Oxygen *(See also pages 143-144, 235-280)*

Indications	Dose & Routes of Administration	Comments
- *Suspected* hypoxemia of any cause (including cardiopulmonary arrest, acute ischemic chest pain, Acute MI, etc.).	**Nasal Canula**- 24-40% oxygen can be delivered with flow rates of 6L/min. **Face Mask/Pocket Mask**- up to 50% oxygen can be delivered with flow rates of 10L/min. **Venturi Mask**- offers a decided advantage over the nasal canula and face mask in that *fixed* oxygen rates (of 24%, 28%, 35%, and 40%) may be delivered- a particularly helpful feature for pts with chronic obstructive pulmonary disease and a history of CO_2 retention. **Non-Rebreathing Oxygen Mask**- superior device for delivering high oxygen concentrations (of up to 90%).	Oxygen is one of the truly *essential* drugs. It should *never* be withheld in an emergency situation for fear of suppressing a pt's respiratory drive. This simply *won't* happen with numerous caregivers at the bedside. Use 100% F_{IO2} during resuscitation! Oxygen toxicity may become a problem with *continual* delivery of high oxygen concentration (F_{IO2} ≥50%)- when it is given for a *prolonged* period of time (i.e., *more* than 3 days). It is *not* a problem with short term delivery of 100% oxygen during the period of cardiopulmonary resuscitation.

Morphine *(See also pages 144-145)*

Indications	Dose & Routes of Administration	Comments
- Acute ischemic chest pain - Pulmonary edema ------------------------------------ **Mechanism**- Morphine markedly increases venous capacitance (and thus reduces preload), produces mild arterial vasodilatation (thus lowering afterload to a small degree), and reduces acute ischemic chest pain and the anxiety of acute air hunger.	**IV Bolus**- Give in small (i.e., **1-3 mg**) *incremental* **IV doses**. Higher doses (i.e., of 3-5 mg) may be used if the drug is tolerated and symptoms are severe. May repeat IV dosing every 5-30 minutes (as needed).	Although IV nitroglycerin is the drug of choice for acute ischemic chest pain- incremental dosing with Morphine is still an extremely useful adjunct when symptoms are severe and persistent. Morphine may cause oversedation and/or *respiratory depression* (which *is* reversible with 0.4-0.8 mg IV **Naloxone**). Morphine may also occasionally cause bradycardia or hypotension (which is usually easily treated by placing pt in Trendelenburg position, fluids- and if needed, Atropine). Morphine remains a treatment of choice for acute pulmonary edema. The drug reduces preload and afterload- as well as attenuating the anxiety and air hunger inherent with pulmonary edema.

Verapamil *(See also pages 145-149, 233)*

Indications	Dose & Routes of Administration	Comments
PSVT- >90% success rate in converting to sinus rhythm. **MAT**- treatment of choice when rate control is needed. **Atrial Fib/Flutter**- effectively slows ventricular response. - - - - - - - - - - - - - - - - - - NOTE- Use of either Verapamil or Diltiazem is more effective than Digoxin for rate control of A Fib/ Flutter in *both* the acute and chronic setting.	**IV Dosing**- Begin with a dose of **2.5-5 mg IV** (to be given over a 1-2 min period). Give the drug *slower* (i.e., over 3-4 min) in the elderly or in those with borderline BP. - May give up to 5-10 mg in a dose (and repeat several times in 15-30 min if/as needed)- up to a total dose of ≈30 mg. **Oral Dosing**- 120-480 mg daily, divided into three equal doses (or given less often if sustained release preparations are used).	Combining small doses of Verapamil/Diltiazem with IV Digoxin- may produce a *synergistic* effect when treating rapid A Fib/Flutter. Pretreatment with **Calcium Chloride** (giving 500-1,000 mg IV over a 5-10 min period) minimizes the hypotensive response of Verapamil/Diltiazem *without* affecting its antiarrhythmic efficacy. Do *not* use Verapamil/Diltiazem to treat *wide-complex* tachycardias (WCTs) of uncertain etiology! Do *not* use Verapamil/Diltiazem to treat rapid A Fib with WPW. Do *not* use Verapamil/Diltiazem within 30 minutes of using an IV ß-blocker. Should calcium channel blocker toxicity develop (i.e., significant bradycardia/asystole)- in response to administration of Verapamil or Diltiazem- the treatment of choice is with **Calcium Chloride**.

Adenosine *(See also pages 149-152, 214)*

Indications	Dose & Routes of Administration	Comments
PSVT (and other *reentry* tachyarrhythmias including PSVT associated with WPW). Adenosine is now the drug of 1st choice for emergency treatment of PSVT.	**IV Bolus**- initially give **6 mg** by **IV push**. If no response after 1-2 min, give **12 mg** by IV push- which may be repeated a final time 1-2 min later (for a ***total* dose** of 6 + 12 + 12 = **30 mg**).	Be sure to give Adenosine by **IV push** (i.e., injecting the drug *as fast as possible* over 1-3 seconds!)- and follow each dose with a ***saline flush*** (of ≈20 ml of fluid). Otherwise the drug will deteriorate *within* the IV tubing.
As a ***diagnostic maneuver*** (i.e., "*chemical Valsalva*") in pts with SVT of *uncertain* etiology. Adenosine will probably convert the rhythm if it is a reentry tachycardia. Otherwise, it will probably produce *transient slowing* (which will hopefully enable atrial activity to be seen- so as to allow the correct diagnosis to be made).	- Higher than usual doses of Adenosine may be needed for pts receiving Theophylline. - Lower than usual doses may be needed for cardiac transplant recipients and for pts on Persantine/Tegretol.	The half-life of Adenosine is exceedingly short (i.e., *less* than 10 seconds!). As a result, little time is needed to find out if the drug will work- and any adverse effects that are produced are likely to be extremely short-lived. Realize however that a longer-acting agent may need to be added to prevent recurrence of PSVT.
Caution- Adenosine is *not* a completely benign agent. We therefore feel that the drug should *not* be given if the rhythm is *known* to be VT.	- Caution is advised in the use of Adenosine in pts with sick sinus syndrome and/or a history of AV conduction defects.	Adverse effects that may be seen include facial flushing, cough/dyspnea, chest pain, and bradycardia. The drug should *not* be given to pts with frank bronchospasm or asthma. Because of its short half-life, Adenosine is in general *unlikely* to cause deterioration of a *wide-complex tachycardia*- even if the drug is inadvertently given to a pt who turns out to have VT.

Diltiazem *(See also pages 152-154, 233)*

Indications	Dose & Routes of Administration	Comments
PSVT- >90% success rate in converting to sinus rhythm. **MAT**- treatment of choice when rate control is needed. **Atrial Fib/Flutter**- effectively slows ventricular response. - - - - - - - - - - NOTE- Use of either Verapamil or Diltiazem is more effective than Digoxin for rate control of A Fib/ Flutter in *both* the acute and chronic setting.	**IV Bolus:** - For the average-sized adult, begin with an *initial* **IV bolus** of **20 mg** (or 0.25 mg/kg)- given over a 2 minute period. - If the desired response is *not* obtained within 15 minutes- may increase the dose with a **2nd IV bolus** of **25 mg** (or 0.35 mg/kg). Dosing for any subsequent boluses should be individualized. - Remember that the doses cited above are for an *average-sized* adult! *Smaller doses* (i.e., of ≈10-15 mg) should be given to pts of light body weight. - - - - - - - - - - **IV Infusion**- Mix **250 mg** of Diltiazem in **250 ml** of diluant (to make a ***concentration*** of 1,000 mg in 1,000 ml = **1 mg/ml**). - Begin infusion at **10 mg/hr** (= 10 drops/minute). - Usual rate of infusion is between **10-15 mg/hr** (although some pts only need 5 mg/hr). - - - - - - - - - - **Oral Dosing**- 90-360 mg daily, divided into three or four equal doses (or given less often if sustained release preparations are used).	Clinical effects from an IV bolus of Diltiazem usually *begin* within 3 minutes- *peak* by 7 minutes- and *last* for 1-3 hours (after which an IV infusion may be used if needed to provide continued rate control). Characteristics of Diltiazem are generally quite similar to those of Verapamil (*See Comments under Verapamil*). However, Diltiazem does appear to offer several advantages: - availability of an approved formulation for use as continuous IV infusion (which facilitates dose titration and allows *maintenance* of antiarrhythmic effect). - less hypotension/LV depression than IV Verapamil. - minimal effect on serum Digoxin levels (whereas Verapamil may increase the serum Digoxin level by up to 50%). Perhaps the clinical niche for IV Diltiazem is treatment of rapid A Fib/Flutter- in that continuous IV infusion allows for *continued* rate control (and thereby avoids the need for repeated IV bolus dosing of Digoxin and Verapamil).

Propranolol *(See also pages 155-156)*

Indications	Dose & Routes of Administration	Comments
Emergency care situations in which ***IV ß-Blockers*** are most likely to be helpful include: - Treatment of supraventricular or ventricular arrhythmias that occur in association with (and/or because of) excessive *sympathetic* tone (i.e., in pts with acute *anterior* MI and/or when hypertension or tachycardia *precede* the arrest). - Cardiac arrest from *cocaine* (or *amphetamine*) overdose. - Severe *psychogenic* stress in the prearrest period. - Antecedent *ischemia* (i.e., ST segment depression) *prior* to the arrest. - *Empiric* use in the treatment of cardiac arrest when other (more standard) measures have failed. - In the treatment of *acute MI*- for which IV ß-Blockers have been shown to reduce mortality (especially when used *within* the first 24 hrs after onset of symptoms).	**IV Dose**- Give **0.5-1.0 mg** by *slow* IV (i.e., over a 5 minute period). May repeat as needed (up to a *total* dose of ≈3-5 mg). - - - - - - - - - - - - - - - - - - - NOTE- Because of ease of administration and familiarity with its use- **Propranolol** is the IV ß-blocker most commonly selected for treatment of pts in cardiac arrest. Alternatively, other ß-blockers could be used instead: - **Atenolol**- 5 mg IV over 5 minutes; may repeat in 10 min. - **Metoprolol**- 5 mg IV over 2 to 5 minutes; may repeat X 2 every 5 min. - **Esmolol**- *dosing is listed on page 365.*	Although *not* commonly used in the setting of cardiac arrest- there clearly are times when an IV ß-blocker is the *only* medication likely to successfully resuscitate the pt. The mechanism of action of ß-blockers appears to be *multifactorial* (due to a *combination* of antiarrhythmic effect, blocking of catecholamine stimulation, reduced myocardial contractility, decreased oxygen consumption, and lowering of BP). - - - - - - - - - - - - - - - - - - - **Caution**- IV ß-blockers should *not* be given in close proximity to either IV Verapamil or IV Diltiazem (as doing so may cause marked bradycardia- or even asystole!). **Contraindications**- acute bronchospasm, heart failure, and/or intraventricular conduction disturbances.

Digoxin *(See also pages 188-193)*

Indications	Dose & Routes of Administration	Comments
Rapid A Fib/Flutter- Dig may help with *rate control* (especially if the pt is in heart failure). **PSVT**- although *other* drugs (i.e., Adenosine, Verapamil, Diltiazem) work faster and are more effective in the acute setting. - - - - - - - - - - - - - - - - - - - NOTE- Indications for Digoxin are limited in the acute care setting. While we emphasize that use of this drug *is* still appropriate for acute treatment of A Fib/ Flutter- *other* drugs (i.e., Diltiazem, Verapamil, and/or ß-blockers) may be preferable (and more effective) for this indication. If Digoxin is selected for treatment, keep in mind that the addition of a second rate-slowing agent may be needed if Digoxin alone fails to adequately control the ventricular response.	**IV Digoxin Dosing:** - If the pt has *not* previously been digitalized, consider **IV loading** with an *initial* dose of **0.25-0.5 mg.** - This may be followed with **0.125-0.25 mg IV increments** given every 2-6 hrs (until a *total* loading dose of 0.75-1.5 mg has been administered over the first 24 hrs). - The next day, the daily *maintenance* dose may be started. - - - - - - - - - - - - - - - - - - - **Oral Digoxin Dosing:** - The daily *oral* maintenance dose of Digoxin for *most* adults under 60 yrs old (who have normal renal function)- is **0.25 mg/day**. - *Lower doses* (**0.125 mg daily**- or every *other* day) are recommended for ***older pts*** (and/or in those with impaired renal function). - If there is less clinical urgency, a pt may be slowly (and *safely*) loaded with Digoxin over a period of ≈1-2 weeks- simply by starting them on their expected daily dose. The pt and serum digoxin level should be checked at the end of this time.	Digoxin slows heart rate by increasing *vagal* (= parasympathetic) tone. It is therefore likely to be *less* effective in situations in which catecholamines (and sympathetic tone) are increased (i.e., exercise, stress, acute illness)- which explains why *other* rate-slowing agents (i.e., Verapamil, Diltiazem, ß-blockers) may be more effective in such cases. Digoxin may exert a *synergistic* (1 + 1 = 5) effect when used in small doses *in conjunction* with other rate-slowing drugs. Effects of IV Digoxin begin more rapidly than is generally appreciated (i.e., onset of action is often *within* 5-10 minutes- and certainly within 30-60 minutes). The most commonly used oral form of Digoxin (= **Lanoxin**) is *only* 65-70% bioavailable (so that an oral dose of 0.325-0.35 mg is comparable to an IV dose of ≈0.25 mg). The ***half-life*** of Digoxin is between **36 hours** (in a healthy, young adult)- and **5 days** (in an elderly pt with severe renal impairment). It may therefore take a pt with renal failure who presents with a toxic serum Digoxin level of 4.0 ng/ml about 4-5 days after stopping the drug for the Digoxin level to decrease by *half* (i.e., to ≈2.0 ng/ml)- and another few days for the level to fall back into the therapeutic range.

Esmolol *(See also pages 193-195)*

Indications	Dose & Routes of Administration	Comments
- Similar to those for Propranolol (*See description for Propranolol on page 363 in this Table*).	**IV Dosing:** - Administer an *initial* **IV loading dose** (of **250-500 µg/kg**) over a 1 minute period. - Follow with a 4 minute infusion @ **25-50 µg/kg/min.** - If desired response is not obtained, titrate the rate of infusion *upward* by **25-50 µg/kg/min** at 5-10 minute intervals (up to a *maximal* dose of 300 µg/kg/min). - May then begin oral antiarrhythmic (and taper Esmolol). - It is generally best *not* to exceed 200 µg/minute (as doing so greatly increases the incidence of hypotension).	Esmolol is a *cardioselective* ß-blocking agent with a *rapid* onset and short duration of action. Pharmacologic effects usually dissipate within 15-30 minutes after stopping the drug. Contraindications are similar to those for IV Propranolol (although Esmolol's cardioselectivity may make it somewhat less likely to precipitate bronchospasm in susceptible pts). Drawbacks of IV Esmolol are the frequency of *hypotension* (which occurs in up to 50% of pts)- and *complexity* of the dosing regimen. - **Caution**- IV ß-blockers should *not* be given in close proximity to either IV Verapamil or IV Diltiazem (as doing so may cause marked bradycardia- or even asystole!).

Amiodarone *(See also pages 195-196)*

Indications	Dose & Routes of Administration	Comments
In Cardiac Arrest- refractory V Fib. **In Emergency Cardiac Care**- life-threatening ventricular arrhythmias *not* responsive to other therapy; selected pts with refractory supraventricul ararrhythmias /tachyarrhythmias associatd with WPW.	- Until results from additional studies become available, dosing recommendations for Amiodarone in the setting of cardiac arrest will be largely *empiric.* The Medical Letter recommends the following regimen (Vol 37: 114, 1995): - Consider rapid **IV loading** of **150 mg** over a 10-minute period. May repeat (one or more times) for recurrent VT/V Fib. - May follow with slow IV infusion of 1 mg/min (= 60 mg/hour) for the next 6 hours- which may then be followed by *slower* IV maintenance infusion (of **0.5 mg/min** = 30 mg/hour) over the next 1-4 days.	IV Amiodarone has recently been approved for general use in this country. However, the drug is *not* yet included in AHA ACLS Guidelines! In the future, IV Amiodarone may assume a useful role in the treatment of pts with *refractory* VT/V Fib- especially for the pt who goes in and out of these rhythms! Use of *oral* Amiodarone is associated with *numerous* side effects- and is therefore best left to a specialist in arrhythmia management.

Aminophylline *(See also pages 196-197)*

Indications	Dose & Routes of Administration	Comments
- May be considered for *brady-asystolic arrest* (or *severe* hemodynamically significant bradycardia) that is *refractory* to standard measures.	**<u>IV Dose</u>**- Give **250 mg IV** over a 1-2 minute period; may repeat.	Aminophylline is *not* yet included in AHA ACLS Guidelines ! Postulated mechanism relates to fact that endogenously released Adenosine is a naturally occurring mediator of bradyasystolic arrest and severe ischemic states- and that Aminophylline is a *competititve antagonist* of Adenosine. - Although use of Aminophylline for treatment of bradyasystolic arrest is clearly controversial- small studies suggest that this drug may restore a rhythm in *selected* pts who fail to respond to Atropine, Epinephrine and pacing. Practically speaking- there may be little to lose in such situations (i.e., *"You can't be deader than dead"*)- so that empiric trial of Aminophylline may not be unreasonable if standard measures have not been successful.

Sodium Bicarbonate *(See also pages 198-200, 215)*

Indications	Dose & Routes of Administration	Comments
- Indications are limited in the setting of cardiac arrest to *severe* metabolic acidosis that persists *beyond* the initial phase (i.e., beyond the first 5-15 minutes)- and/or cardiac arrest in a pt *known* to have a severe *pre-existing* metabolic acidosis *prior* to the arrest- - *IF any Bicarb is indicated at all . . . .*	***IF*** Sodium Bicarbonate is felt to be indicated at all- then an *initial* dose of **1 mEq/kg** (≈1-1.5 amps) has been recommended. No more than *half* this amount should be given every 10 minutes. In the postresuscitation phase, ABGs should guide therapy.	Remember that *"good CPR is the best buffer therapy"* (AHA Text- Pg 7-15). Standard ABG studies in cardiac arrest *cannot* be relied upon (because they do *not* accurately reflect the true state of *intracellular* homeostasis).
NOTE- Severe special resuscitation situations do exist in which use of Bicarb is both appropriate and *likely* to be helpful. They include: - Hyperkalemia. - Tricyclic antidepressant overdose (aiming to keep serum pH between 7.45-7.55). - Phenobarbital overdose (aiming to alkalinize the urine). - After the code is over (if severe metabolic acidosis persists).	NOTE- If you do chose to administer Bicarb empirically in cardiac arrest- it may be advisable *not* to give the drug for the initial 5-10 minutes of the arrest (since it usually takes *at least* this long to develop a metabolic acidosis in cardiac arrest). - It should be emphasized that the initial cause of acidosis in cardiac arrest is *hypoventilation* (that is best corrected by improving ventilation- and *not* by giving Bicarb).	Drawbacks of administering Sodium Bicarbonate to pts in cardiac arrest include that: - the drug has *not* been shown to improve survival. - the principal cause of acidosis during the *early* minutes of cardiac arrest (i.e., *hypoventilation*) is *not* corrected by Bicarb administration. - the degree of *intracellular* acidosis paradoxically *worsens* (despite "improvement" of ABG pH values)! - other significant *adverse effects* may occur (including *iatrogenic* alkalosis, hyperosmolality, hypokalemia, sodium overload, impaired oxygen delivery to tissues, seizures, arrhythmias- and impaired left ventricular function from the negative inotropic effect of excess CO_2).

Calcium Chloride *(See also pages 201-203)*

Indications	Dose & Routes of Administration	Comments
Limited in the acute care setting to 4 clinical situations: 1. *Hypocalcemia.* 2. *Hyperkalemia.* 3. As *pre-treatment* prior to giving Verapamil/Diltiazem. 4. Treatment of *calcium channel blocker toxicity* (i.e., if marked bradycardia or asystole occurs following use of Verapamil/Diltiazem. - - - - - - - - - - - - - - - - NOTE- Caclium is *no longer* indicated for treatment of EMD/asystole!	<u>**IV Bolus**</u>- Give **500-1,000 mg** (5-10 ml) by *slow IV* (over 5-10 minutes). May repeat every 10 minutes if needed (up to 2-4 g). - - - - - - - - - - - - - - - - NOTE- Infusion of calcium as *pre-treatment* minimizes the hypotensive response of Verapamil/Diltiazem without diminishing their efficacy in converting/controlling the ventricular response of supraventricular tachyarrhythmias. Calcium preinfusion might be considered particularly for pts with borderline hemodynamic status (i.e., systolic BP ≤100) in association with their tachyarrhythmia.	The 10% solution of Calcium Chloride contains 1,000 mg (= 13.6 mEq) of calcium per 10 ml syringe. - - - - - - - - - - - - - - - - Don't forget that the "antidote" of calcium channel blocker toxicity is *calcium.* Although **Calcium Chloride** is clearly the most commonly used IV form of this cation- *other* preparations are available (i.e., **Calcium Gluconate**). These other preparations contain *different* amounts of elemental calcium !!!

Isoproterenol *(See also pages 158-161, 204)*

Indications	Dose & Routes of Administration	Comments
The major indication for use of Isoproterenol at this time is limited to treatment of bradycardia that develops in the denervated transplanted heart- - *IF the drug should ever be used at all . . .* (AHA Text- Pg 1-32; 8-6).	<u>**IV Infusion**</u>- Mix **1mg** in **250 ml** of D5W- and begin drip @ **30 drops/min (=2 µg/min)**. Titrate infusion to clinical effect (but do *not* exceed 10 µg/min!).	Isoproterenol has become a *deemphasized* drug. It is *contraindicated* for treatment of asystole, EMD and V Fib because it increases myocardial oxygen consumption- and its pure beta-adrenergic effect results in vasodilatation (which *lowers* aortic diastolic pressure and therefore *reduces* coronary flow!). At low doses (i.e., <<10 µg/min), Isoproterenol may provide pure chronotropic support to *selected* bradycardic pts who are not hypotensive. *The drug should not be used at higher doses.* At the present time, Epinephrine and/or Dopamine are generally preferred to Isoproterenol for use as "pressor agents".

INDEX

N

O

P

Credits

Figure 3B-1, 3B-39 From Yokochi, C Rosen JW: *Photographic Anatomy of the Human Body,* Baltimore, 1978, University Park Press.

Figure 3B-9, 3B-10, 3B-12, 3B-15, 3B-16a, 3B-16b, 3B-16c, 3B-16d, 3B-20, 3B-38, 3B-41, From Ambu, Inc. from Lotz, P Ahnefeld FW, Hirlinger WD: *A Systematic Guide to Intubation,* Atelier Flad, Eckental, West Germany.

Figure 3B-31, 3B-33, 3B-40 From Applebaum EL, Bruce DL: *Tracheal Intubation,* Philadelphia, 1976, WB Saunders.

Rapid Locator Guide

KEY Algorithms

The Patient with Tachycardia: Differential Diagnosis

Modalities

Miscellaneous Topics

Value Added Drug Table